Keystone Reconstructive Solutions for Major Surgical Defects

Springer Nature More Media App

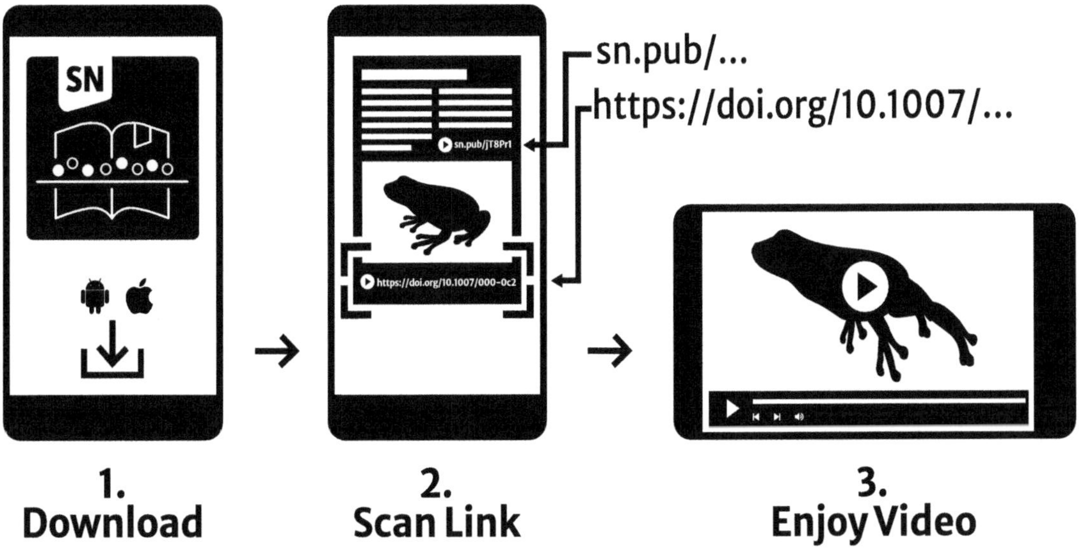

Felix Behan

Keystone Reconstructive Solutions for Major Surgical Defects

Vol. 1: Principles, Parotid, Ear, Head and Neck

Springer

Felix Behan
Department of Surgery
University of Melbourne, St. Vincent's Hospital
Parkville, Australia

Department of Plastic and Reconstructive Surgery
Peter MacCallum Cancer Centre
Melbourne, Australia

Head of Department of Plastic and Reconstructive Surgery
Western Hospital
Melbourne, Australia

This work contains media enhancements, which are displayed with a "play" icon. Material in the print book can be viewed on a mobile device by downloading the Springer Nature "More Media" app available in the major app stores. The media enhancements in the online version of the work can be accessed directly by authorized users.

ISBN 978-3-032-21715-8 ISBN 978-3-032-21716-5 (eBook)
https://doi.org/10.1007/978-3-032-21716-5

This Springer imprint is published by the registered company Springer Nature Switzerland AG
The registered company address is: Gewerbestrasse 11, 6330 Cham, Switzerland

Foreword

I worked with Professor Felix Behan for nearly 30 years. My role, and those of my colleagues in the Peter MacCallum Cancer Centre ENT/Head & Neck 'excisional team', was to excise large facial, parotid and neck tumours (usually sun-induced skin cancers) and then hand the patient with their large skin defect over to Felix and his 'reconstructive team'. The following morning's ward round was confusing: How did he close that? Where did the skin come from?

In the bad old 'good ol' days', these defects would be closed with skin grafts, multistage tubed grafts walked up from the abdomen (before my time), two-stage pedicled skin flaps like the delto-pectoral, the workhorse head and neck flap since the 1980s or the single-stage pectoralis myo-cutaneous flap.

With advances in microvascular free-tissue transfer, particularly pioneered in Melbourne, Australia, free flaps took over—those wonderful flaps can fairly reliably fill almost any defect. But free flaps are not without problems. They take a lot of surgical time, which is expensive. Not all hospitals around the world have the facilities, the time or the money for such operations. As our patient demographic has become older and developed more comorbidities, duration under anaesthetic becomes relevant. Free flaps are not without complications, and a 5% rate of return-to-theatre, often in the middle of the night, is not without consequence. Surgery comes with colour match cosmetic problems of pale flaps from distant sites to facial skin, and the excessive bulkiness of flaps from abdominal or thigh adiposity can be problematic (although, admittedly, they can undergo debulking later).

Professor Behan's innovative 'Keystone perforator island flap' (KPIF) solves many of these problems. They are quick to perform, are usually thin, have perfect colour match because they come from the face or neck and are reliable in Felix's magic hands.

These flaps defy many of the rules of surgery. Old age, infirmity, diabetes, vascular disease and even previous radiation doesn't seem to matter. Unlike most plastic surgeons, who use multiple fine interrupted sutures, Felix closes them with a hemming suture, and initially, they look like the closure of a sack of potatoes. Most surgeons are horrified when they first see these early post-operative wounds. But they heal up beautifully, and within a few months, one often can't even see the suture lines. He doesn't close the deep fascial layer, relying on the flexibility of the loose skin in these usually elderly patients to stretch into the defect—but they are equally effective in younger patients with problems such as pilonidal sinuses, leg injuries and chronic leg ulcers.

The 'red dot sign' is a true phenomenon, as part of the hyperaemic flare. The flap allows a better blood supply than the skin that it is sutured to, presumably from the surgical denervation of the skin's autonomic supply by the 'islanding' of the flap or perhaps because now the blood supply to the skin comes from deep tissue and perforators (which do not even need to be found with a Doppler) rather than from collateral skin flow.

Because these Keystone flaps break many of the accepted rules of flap surgery and are difficult to envision, understanding them and teaching them are challenging. Our reconstructive surgical teams spend a lot of time training in their microvascular skills, can understand free flaps and are keen to do many of them as a matter of pride. KPIFs are too difficult to master, and when they work (as they usually do), they seem too easy—there are no 'bragging rights' for having done them. But they should not be forgotten, and neither should Professor Behan's genius.

Stephen Kleid
Ear Nose & Throat Surgeon
Head & Neck Surgery, Nasal Cosmetic Surgery
Snoring Surgery, Masada Medical Centre
St Kilda East, VIC, Australia

Peter MacCallum Cancer Centre
Melbourne, VIC, Australia

Foreword

The outcomes of surgery for head and neck cancer are optimised by a multiteam approach, with each discipline contributing to the overall planning of the surgery and reconstruction. For over 30 years, I worked with Felix Behan treating many patients with complex cancers of the head and neck. During this time, Felix developed and refined the Keystone flap as the preferred reconstruction method for extensive soft tissue defects. I recall the initial comments by others that the technique 'could not possibly work' and 'breaks all the rules'. But advances in surgery come from those who think laterally and are not constrained by the status quo, who use existing knowledge to formulate novel ideas and who incorporate an element of artistic licence to soften the boundaries of rigid thinking. Felix epitomises this approach, and the stunning success of the Keystone technique is a testament to this. This technique has resulted in huge benefits for the patient, such as reduced surgical and anaesthetic time, reduced recovery time and hospitalisation, improved function at the reconstruction site, no donor site morbidity, a superior cosmetic result and very rare early or long-term complications. It has been successfully used even following large resections in heavily irradiated sites. The relatively short surgical time compared to other reconstructive techniques offers clear advantages to frail, cachectic, immunocompromised patients. The technique is easily taught and then executed, particularly when Felix's clear and concise descriptions, such as in this book, are followed. The Keystone technique is easy, elegant, efficient and economic and has become our reconstruction of choice in most situations.

Andrew Sizeland

Otolaryngology, Head and Neck Surgery,
University of Melbourne,
Parkville, Australia

Otolaryngology, Head and Neck Surgery,
Royal Melbourne Hospital,
Melbourne, Australia

Department of Surgical Oncology,
Peter MacCallum Cancer Centre,
Melbourne, Australia

Preface

This preface to Volume 1 can act as an introduction to Volume 2 given that both books can be viewed in the same light from adopting the same principles. The ideas about the Keystone perforator island flap (KPIF) concept leading to the angiotome are quite entrenched, and the clinical applications of the Keystone are widespread and reflections of its universal usefulness in reconstructive surgery, like tailoring, where the defects are closed with flaps governed by the dermatomal outlines and gracefully fitted into the defects thanks to the laxity of the surrounding tissue, dermatomally aligned.

If I'm allowed to diverge laterally into a musical context, I will include a quote from my colleague and eminent musician Miklos Pohl, a plastic surgeon and founder of the Australian Doctors Orchestra, that could explain why Joseph Haydn became such an eminent composer at the Esterházy Palace in Austria. He was untainted by the musical developments of the hierarchy from Mozart to Salieri and Hummel, who performed at the big concert halls of Europe. Haydn went in his own direction, creating 104 symphonies and 50 concertos and pioneering 84 string quartets (maybe I should follow this pattern and let this text be one of my final gestures). He did not have a big brother sitting over his shoulder questioning what he was doing, which I avoided at the Western Hospital in Melbourne. Haydn's compositional style, leading to his definitive work *The Creation*, whose premiere in Vienna in 1798 was a huge success in the composer's lifetime, mirrors the sequence of publications on the Keystone, from melanoma (*Atlas of Keystone Reconstructive Technique in Melanoma Management*, Springer, 2023) to orthopaedics (*Keystone Flap for Complex Orthopaedic Problems*, Springer, 2024) and now to major surgical defects. We have done this with the third book on the Keystone concept with Springer Nature. As Haydn is the father of the classical symphony, I am being presumptive in using that same terminology in my direction in reference to the Keystone; however, the similarities keep emerging. Every aspect of the Keystone's performances is illustrated in these texts, relying on the embryological background which always embraces arteries, nerves and veins as applied to the vascular and neural networks when applied to somatic and autonomic supply. These networks are supported with lymphatic input, which explains why oedema of the lower limb in cases of trauma initiate the resolution of any oedema (evident in the early postoperative phase, even overnight), which in the past would characteristically stay rigidly static, needing secondary procedures.

All cases have been included, successful or otherwise, to highlight any limitations that might surface. A separate section on complications is included for universal clinical awareness, but such episodes are rare, possibly reflecting the patient's inability to control their smoking. This book is really a duet in two volumes, featuring reconstructive elements with applications of the Keystone to cover defects, and I use that wording above, in the manner of a tailor, to create a like-for-like garment cover for the subject. Both volumes are to be reviewed in unison because they both reflect the similar principles of the Keystone but in different body locations, where sometimes different principles apply; for example, the reconstruction of the calcaneal in Volume 2 is another relevant entity. The single aim is to teach this cost-effective Keystone technique as an alternative to microsurgical reconstruction, which has dominated reconstructive thinking for a long period of time. Only when alternative methods surface does this economic and speedy execution gain its appeal in these days of severe financial constraint in the health industry. Microsurgical procedures are expensive, and tragically, we are now getting the commercial arm of management governing the likes of what procedures should be done, merely from an economic point of view. The Keystone technique, as illustrated in these volumes, helps to tackle this problem. By using this technique, surgical teams in hospital units that are disadvantaged can find another method of closure, without the need of microsurgical techniques and without the delay implications and repeat cancellations that often occur with waiting lists and emergency procedures.

Patients' willing acceptance of the good outcomes is illustrated throughout the text, with videos of patients' perspectives. In simple terms, the book shows how the technique is done, with the added advantage of operative videos explaining the technique and its refinements in detail and why such a procedure was undertaken.

I recently penned a synopsis of the Keystone principle for the uninitiated who have trouble understanding my thinking and the technique of the Keystone perforator island flap. It was titled 'The Keystone Enigma', where I tried to explain the unexplainable from wide clinical experience and a perspective on how it works, but success has been the basis for its repetition. In synoptic terms, we have tried to reduce surgical reconstruction from complexity to simplicity, which is how they describe pianist Einaudi and his portrayal of compositional presentations. We have reverted to the terminology 'bespoke' reconstruction when a pattern of repair fits the defect, as one sees in tailoring.

Umpteen surgeons around the world are doing variations of the Keystone design. Why is this so? In simplistic terms, the younger generation who have not seen me operate have tried to put into practice and writing what they perceive to be my success. But before publication, as one of the overseas authors observed, the review process for the established journals is done by those who are not aware of this technique and its applications, slowly emerging as it is. So, they converted to layperson language for the uninitiated.

I have transgressed certain principles in plastic and reconstructive surgery and removed the mindset of hunting for a perforator with its limitations, likened to a garden hose, which we know often kinks. The island flap, based on random perforators in the suprafascial and infrafascial distribution, is the lifeline governing the Keystone's success. The fascia is never repaired in closure; rather, the epidermal closure, sometimes under tension, creates the optimal aesthetic outcome and wound seal.

I have had to hark back to embryological principles to offer some basis for my scientific reasoning and use the dermatomal mark outs as aides-mémoire for design, with the laxity of the tissues facilitating any advancement, rotation or transposition of the fascial lined island flap but essentially leaving one-third of deep attachment to ensure vascular integrity, an absolute necessity. This embryological basis retains neural, autonomic, somatic, arteriovenous and lymphatic links while remaining undefined and not skeletonised. Thanks to Professor Geoffrey Hallock in the US, who synopsised my Keystone characteristics—namely pain-free, aesthetic, complication rarity, economical, and sensory recovery—with the acronym PACES, now others are communicating with me worldwide looking for an answer, as Professor Rollin Daniel in California did when he recently emailed me about my concepts, reflecting his inquisitive mind and using the word 'brilliant' to describe it in principle. Its worldwide clinical applications are being used in the present war in Ukraine because of its speed of execution and reliability of repair without reverting to multiple amputations, often a characteristic of war injuries. This statement warrants repetition: Creating an epidermal island with fascial lining produced a sympathectomy effect that explains the hypervascularity and pink flare that occurs, allowing us to close under tension.

This random overview allows the suprafascial and infrafascial circulation of Saint Cyr—which must not be undermined—but the superior epidermal cover can be closed under tension while avoiding any fascial tear, and the epidermis creates the wound seal. During this clinical series, my highlight moment came to the surface when I thought, as an overview, that I feel like a locksmith who has picked a lock. It can be universally applied because of these principles, originating from basic sciences and observational findings.

In summary, the plastic surgery literature since the times of Esser and Dieffenbach has been filled with clinical successes and repetitive eponyms for wound closure, arguably universalising flap repairs, which occurred before the microsurgical development that focuses on individual anatomical units. The word *Keystone* has gone some way towards unifying all these ideas in locoregional repair, and our new word, *bespoke*, is again something where the flaps are used to fashion the repair to cover a defect—like the habits of a tailor.

Standing on the shoulders of giants—as Newton (Fig. 1) said about his discovery of gravity in 1666 and a year earlier when a beam of light shone through a prism, creating a spectrum, when he was a student at Cambridge—was part of Newton's philosophy in his text *Philosophiæ Naturalis Principia Mathematica*, thankfully translated by Voltaire upon escaping the politics of Paris, who went to England and befriended Newton so that the translation would accurately convey Newton's ideas to the world. Let us not forget that French was the official diplomatic language in Europe at the time, so Newton could correct his translations, which no doubt would have had some questionable translations that would have been corrected by Newton.

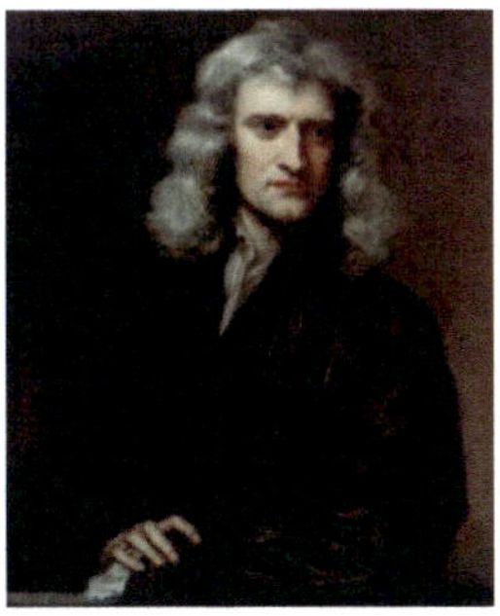

Fig. 1 Portrait of Isaac Newton (1643–1727), by Godfrey Kneller. (Public domain)

More importantly, many have contacted me from around the world about my concepts, asking for explanations and seeking my advice on how to close certain wounds (from Rwanda to Hong Kong, North Macedonia and Yemen). My clinical successes speak volumes, all published in peer-reviewed articles, as listed in this text. This leads to the wording of the Keystone 'enigma'—something unexplainable; that is, we have ventured into new fields with new designs and different theories and have finally ended up with tailoring as a metaphorical similarity. My work over 30 years has all been documented, covering over 3000 cases, leading to the publication of six textbooks and umpteen chapter inclusions. I would not be publishing if this technique was not standing up to the rigours of criticism and repeat failures. Now, microsurgery, with a boot on the other foot, has introduced a different cost factor and a different time factor into locoregional repair, for which future surgeons must have both barrels loaded; in other words, they need to be able to do both techniques.

No wonder Newton and Darwin had their problems.

The Keystone evolved from empirical development, observational findings and didactic elucidation, which summarises my concepts above.

Parkville, VIC, Australia A/Prof. Felix Behan, AM

Contents

List of Videos

1 General Embryological Principles of the Keystone Reconstructive Flap

Contents

Core Messages

Clinical observation becomes the basis of research developments, as Osler said.

In major head and neck reconstructions, particularly in the elderly population, speed, efficiency and guarantee play major roles in clinical outcomes. As we know, the quicker these patients are removed from the operating table to safely reduce operating time, the more likely surgical execution can be propitious or even prescient. The Keystone technique has this facility of being easily executed, even among inexperienced surgeons once the technique is mastered. Postoperative monitoring, a hallmark of microsurgical repair, is an expensive and time-consuming additive, hampering further by the

---

Supplementary Information The online version contains supplementary material available at https://doi.org/10.1007/978-3-032-21716-5_1. The videos can be accessed individually by clicking the DOI link in the accompanying figure caption or by scanning this link with the SN More Media App.

F. Behan, *Keystone Reconstructive Solutions for Major Surgical Defects*,
https://doi.org/10.1007/978-3-032-21716-5_1

current constraints of cost-saving healthcare management. The Keystone saves time, money and staff commitments and reduces the return-to-theatre rate accordingly. According to experiences, repeatedly using the technique substantially increases the range of reconstructive options, as evident in the table of cases.

1.1 Introduction

After an extensive career spanning 40 years in plastic and reconstructive surgery, certain tips and skills emerge to expedite wound closures and facilitate surgical reconstruction with success and minimal complications, and that is why it has been developed. Tricks of the trade are part of any emerging thinking while honouring these principles and achieving good outcomes.

Flap reconstructions are part of our toolbox because they help us to achieve objectives in wound healing. We are grateful in the reconstructive world to be the focus of referral for many surgical specialties in which problems arise with wound closures. These requests need the attention of experts in wound cover, which is really our domain, and we would be wise in principle to show others how we would close wounds simply. Teaching is part of this commitment. Thus, this publication focuses on many of the manoeuvres adopted to achieve such outcomes, including wound repairs and flap designs. This has been the basis of the Keystone [1–15] perforator island flap (KPIF) development and the emancipation of surgical thinking, which emerged to create new concepts. *Emancipation* can mean freeing a person from restraint, and we use this metaphorically in surgery to describe how new, sometimes-controversial ideas erupt, with results that speak for themselves. We must repeat Helen Keller's famous adage that yesterday's heresy becomes tomorrow's orthodoxy.

The KPIF is a surgical technique in locoregional reconstructive surgery. Its arc design goes back to the earlier format of the Moors' architectural concepts, and even every important arch in European buildings, including the Colosseum and the Arc De Triumph, has relevance in the Keystone concept in design. The Keystone is the apical stone that locks the arch into security.

The Keystone's clinical development over 40 years has led to various surgical applications, and this practice, based on experience, has led to new ideas that are being assessed only as time progresses. This has resulted in over 40 publications, all peer reviewed and then compiled into textbooks with Springer Nature, covering topics such as melanoma [14] and orthopaedics and leading to the evolution of Keystone reconstructive solutions for major surgical defects, under the domain of microsurgery and its cost restrictions and staffing implications.

The KPIF is a perforator island flap based on fascia with filamentous perforators within the dermatomal alignment. All embryology embraces neural, somatic and autonomic factors, including arterial supply, venous drainage and lymphatic support, and all the observational findings from clinical cases have been compiled such that they lead to the conclusion that the success of the Keystone concept must have an embryological basis.

The absence of experimental animal investigations may be a criticism, but it is not applicable here, because all my clinical findings have a patient focus. The best animal and documented studies have been carried out clinically if not also recorded on video, and the patient experiences are thus verifiable parts of the Keystone's success, with their own postoperative opinions recorded, thus avoiding bias.

In parallel, Carl Sagan, the astrophysicist, said years ago that 'The absence of evidence is not the evidence of absence.' Also, William Osler (1849–1919), the influential Canadian physician and professor of medicine at Oxford University, stated that 'Observation is the basis of scientific advancement in medicine.'

With over 3000 cases in Keystone clinical experiences, certain observational findings and characteristics have emerged, and thanks in part to Prof. Geoffrey Hallock's input, we now use the acronym PACES to represent the Keystone characteristics, namely pain-free, aesthetic, complications, economical, and sensory recovery. I must add that these findings derive from patient input, and patients' comments on video supplement the principle as it applies at a clinical level.

The patients find the procedure to be pain-free.

The patients find that the aesthetics match to their satisfaction, and repairing a melanoma defect of the calf with a Keystone speaks volumes about the satisfaction of wearing personal garments and avoids the cosmetic defect of a large skin graft on the leg, and the patient can now go swimming without embarrassment.

Complications occur at a vascular level, without focusing on major perforators, but the filamentous perforators in the fascial base circulation, I presume, contribute to its vascular reliability without defining perforators. Diabetic cases are problems, as are smoker cases, and they are therefore to be handled cautiously. These textbooks illustrate cases featuring such characteristics and complications in an audiovisual format with video supplements.

The economic factors are now becoming part of the surgical decision-making and govern what can be done because some of the health insurance firms are now refusing admission rights to patients because of the absurd cost of long-term microsurgical sagas, especially in the elderly 50–95 years. Unfortunately, the accountancy factors in hospital management are determining treatment variables.

Sensory recovery, particularly in facial reconstructions, is one of the keynote characteristics that patients reveal, and they feel as though they are getting back to normal [16, 17]. I must reference this researcher's innovative work, in which the somatic sensation retained in the fascia that contributes to the success of the Keystone repair is my hypothesis.

The resolution of oedema features prominently in the lower limb section in Volume 2, which sometimes disappears within 24 h of a Keystone insertion, and this again is recorded by way of clinical evidence, without scientific confirmation but rather with only the simple observation of clinical findings. All these characteristics are based on embryological science, I suspect, where somatic sensation and autonomic sensation show recovery with a good arteriovenous supply and with intact lymphatic support—an integral part of embryological development.

So, I repeat that the acronym PACES is a valid overview at a clinical level of observation findings. The flap design that is based on microperforators has led to a satisfactory solution in countries around the world without the privilege of refined microsurgical facilities.

Following my recent webinar presentation to the International Microsurgery Club, organised by Mr. Tommy Nai-Jen Chang in Taiwan and Prof. Geoffrey Hallock in Pennsylvania, the acronym PACES emerged and is gaining universal acceptance as more get attuned to the KPIF concept in wound closure. Subsequent to the webinar, I received an email from Rwanda that enabled me to help a surgeon do a reconstructive repair by using one of my own cases on file to illustrate the technique that I would have used, as requested. This has its own rewards and substantiates why we must publish, as I have done with my Springer Nature publications.

1.2 A History of Dieffenbach's V-Y Flap—A Stepping Stone Leading to the Development of the Keystone Concept [18]

The pioneering German surgeon Dieffenbach (1792–1847) in 1845 established the principle of the V-Y flap, and starting in the 1850s, this became the hallmark of his clinical expertise in locoregional repairs when doing cleft lip reconstructions. The looseness of the locoregional tissues facilitated wound closures by employing V-Y principles when necessary. The V-Y advancement locoregional flap was a consequence of repeat surgical procedures by Dieffenbach, whose experiences revealed that the patient would sit on the first floor landing without the usual theatre facilities and spill the oozing blood over the railings to the footpath below.

The history of the V-Y Flap is part of the surgical repertoire for reconstruction and is part of the toolbox we all use for closing simple defects with V-Y advancement. Those who have never been schooled in plastic surgery find this simple manoeuvre irreplaceable, but again, the incision that makes the island, leaving it attached by its stalk of the filamentous communications, is the basis of its success.

In the modern reconstructive vein, the importance of an island flap is being reassessed, and we look back to the work by Esser [19] after World War I to see what his contributions were. I must remember that Sir John Baron and his protégé Prof. Anthony Emmett carried on this concept of island flap reconstruction on the basis of random perforator supports before the purists began hunting for individual axial vessels, looking for a lifeline support. Esser's range of cases is far and wide and governed by the necessities of war, looking for quick solutions. Esser's work was subsequently adopted by the likes of Gillies, who appreciated the merits of this expeditious style of repair.

1.3 The Keystone Is a Conjoined Double V-Y Flap

Stylistically, the Keystone is designed as a conjoined double V-Y flap, but physically, fascial communication and the reliability of the V-Y have been the bases for the Keystone's success, reflecting the history of the V-Y principle. My experience since 1995, featuring 20 years of over 3000 Keystone flaps universally applied all over the body, is the basis of these publications from observational findings. Additionally, soft tissue defects are included to show the range of applications of the Keystone flap, which is really a conjoined V-Y flap based on Dieffenbach's [18] innovation in the 1850s. Once, in a tutorial, when I had just completed a Keystone reconstruction, I was looking for a simple analogy to help to explain the idea to my registrar when he asked me, 'how does the Keystone work?' I remember that afternoon drawing an arc Keystone on paper joining the points of the diagonally opposite design, and I just said simply 'really, this is only a conjoined V-Y flap; that's the basis of its success.' And I find this simplistic explanation within the mental acceptance of the emerging surgical mind.

This surgical experience, also documented photographically, is the basis of the surgical development of the KPIF for major surgical defect closure. Just as a tailor fashions the cloth to create a bespoke suit, a Keystone in a similar manner closes the surgical defect and minimises the use of grafting, which often fails from an aesthetic perspective (Figs. 1.1, 1.2, 1.3, 1.4 and 1.5).

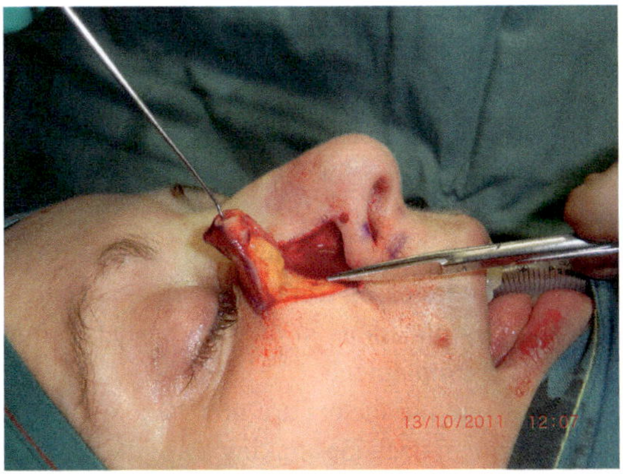

Fig. 1.1 The V-Y flap is a conjoined Keystone. Its preparation is based on filamentous attachments and has advanced into a defect. The tissues are teased and loosened to appropriately fit into the defect. Blunt dissection rather than clean incisional release preserves the integrity of the sympathetic and somatic supply, and this can be assumed only because the outcomes, as explained above, reflect an ongoing anastomotic link

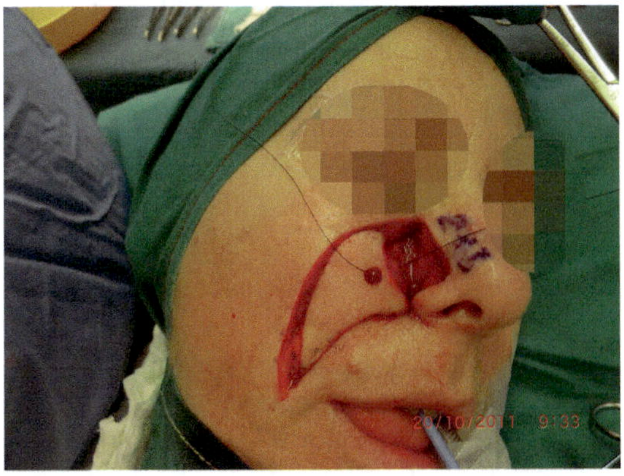

Fig. 1.2 Prior to definitive insertion, no vascular impedance is noted, and the arterialised flow is a regular observed characteristic. Close the V-Y flap with a three-point suture, and the same principles are employed for the insertion of large Keystone flaps—a conjoined V-Y unit

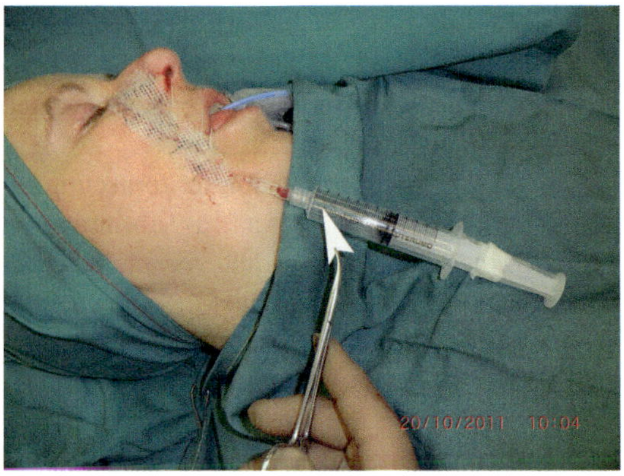

Fig. 1.3 Drainage is an appropriate surgical necessity, and one can see how this modified technique, using a syringe and tubing, is an essential requirement in reconstruction around the nose, a later development

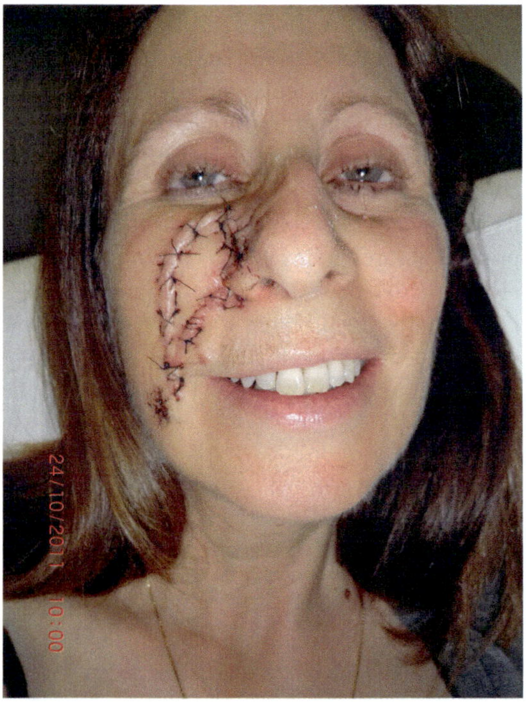

Fig. 1.4 The postoperative appearance at 24 h shows how the everted margins achieve an epidermal seal that ensures an aesthetic linear appearance in the final outcome once the cross-hatching sutures have been appropriately removed

When conjoined as a paired unit with the same reliability, the Keystone becomes the basis for larger reconstructive repairs, as used in a range of

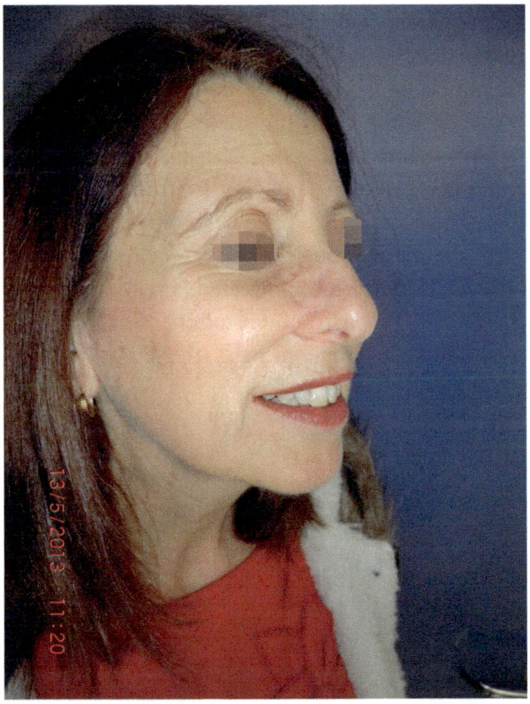

Fig. 1.5 After the final dressing has been completed and the resolution of oedema has settled, this could reflect re-anastomosis of lymphatic channels with a sympathectomy effect, which we know controls the lymphatic system

cases. This concept has been refined, and I developed the ellipsoidal V-Y variant (like a tailor), which I called the Bezier flap [20], to facilitate tight closures and soften the aesthetic line for mitotic lesions on the face in a bespoke manner. Schematically, the Keystone is a conjoined architectural shape of two V-Y flaps with V-Y points at either extreme (joining the diagonals produces the shape in a conjoined manner). My original arc flap, fascially based, totally islanded and left any communicating venous links where possible, all based on supra- and infrafascial random perforators along the dermatomal alignments. My surgical colleague, Alan Breidahl of Melbourne, suggested the word *Keystone* with its universal bespoke applications and its wider acceptance because it harks back to the architectural Moorish designs of curvatures being more reliable than straight lines aesthetically and structurally (Fig. 1.6).

The KPIF development doubles the size of the V-Y and the mark out on the calf where closure can be done correctly, even under tension, producing this aesthetic outcome (Fig. 1.7). The Keystone mark out in the calf is indicated. The looseness of the calf muscles facilitates the V-Y compression.

This Keystone name led to further observational findings which have been clinically significant regarding healing. Even closing under tension is not contraindicated, breaking one of the rules in reconstructive surgery. You might ask why. The Keystone mirrors the embryological

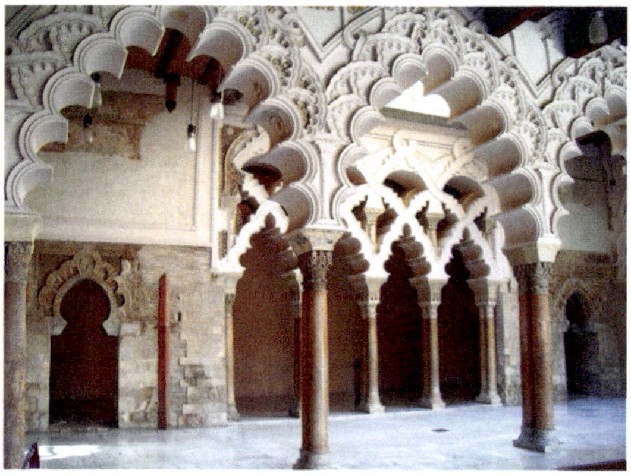

Fig. 1.6 The arched domes of the Moorish mosques have architecturally stood the test of time. In other words, arches continue to remain stable because they are self-locking, like a Keystone design, as in the Palacio de la Aljafería, Zaragoza, Spain. (Photo credit: Escarlati, figure under Public Domain, via Wikimedia Commons, https://commons.wikimedia.org/wiki/File:Testero_norte_4.jpg)

background of development. All these numerous cases have produced the acronym PACES, which represents a good summary of the Keystone applications and its characteristics.

Even *design variations* aiming to accommodate various surgical defects, as illustrated in Fig. 1.8, including squares and rectangles, have been used and have not affected the reliability of the basic V-Y design but have always been governed by the size and dimensions of the defect and have relied on the laxity of surrounding tissue planes when designed within dermatomal mark outs. But the principles of varying the design are still based on dermatomal alignment, with its intact neurovascular and lymphatic support. These embryological principles are respected in all Keystone designs as long as they are fashioned in the dermatome and leave at least one-third of deep attachment as a security and basic prerequisite in Keystone applications to preserve random vascular integrity. Specific vascular investigations of perforators through angiography have not been found necessary—another cost-saving benefit in these times of financial management under administrators—if the above principles are followed in raising Keystone reconstructive flaps. The above design precepts—i.e. fascially lined within the dermatomal mark outs and leaving one-third of deep attachment—allow one to close under tension because of the

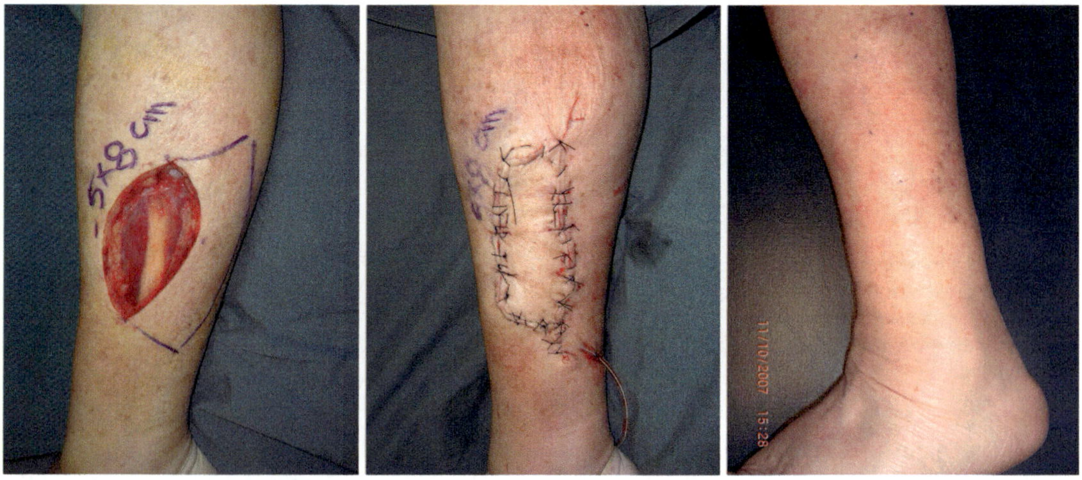

Fig. 1.7 Clearance, closure and conclusion

hypervascularity produced, which ensures safety in reconstruction.

Another architectural variant is the horseshoe *omega variant* design, facilitated by undermining and leaving fascia as the basis for security. This allows the arm of the Keystone to close variations in anatomical surgical defects. It has additional applications in closing defects of the lower limb, where the flaps can be bent in the shape of a U, as illustrated—hence the eponym the omega variant. Another clinical observation, as summarised below, is the hyperaemic phase. If these design precepts are observed, where the red dot sign is a characteristic finding of all Keystone closures in spite of wound apposition under lines of tension, this is hypothetically supposed to be a sympathectomy effect, causing vascular flare. Also, does it facilitate lymphatic drainage? The resolution of oedema of the lower limb in Keystone reconstruction is a regular finding, as illustrated in the cases included and as will be noted. Given that the perforators are not skeletonised and therefore not stripped of fine elements of autonomic and somatic nerve supply and lymphatic drainage, I assume that these are retained to support the clinical outcome of findings, as observed and shown in the postoperative results and with the patient's confirmation.

The Keystone has many bespoke design variations (Figs. 1.8 and 1.9). Some of these design variations originated from wide experience in reconstructive surgery with use of the V-Y island flap (of which the Keystone represents a duplicated version) and earlier work on the *Limberg flap* [21] and its designs on the flap integumentary surface.

The reliability of the Keystone is its main characteristic, and the main limitation of the technique is closure under tension, but should this be inappropriate, supplementary grafting can be used to minimise any areas of tension, thus avoiding necrosis. A lack of adherence to such principles, as enunciated here, may result in some necrosis from those with less experience. Presumably, undermining and disturbing support from the suprafascial and infrafascial perforators

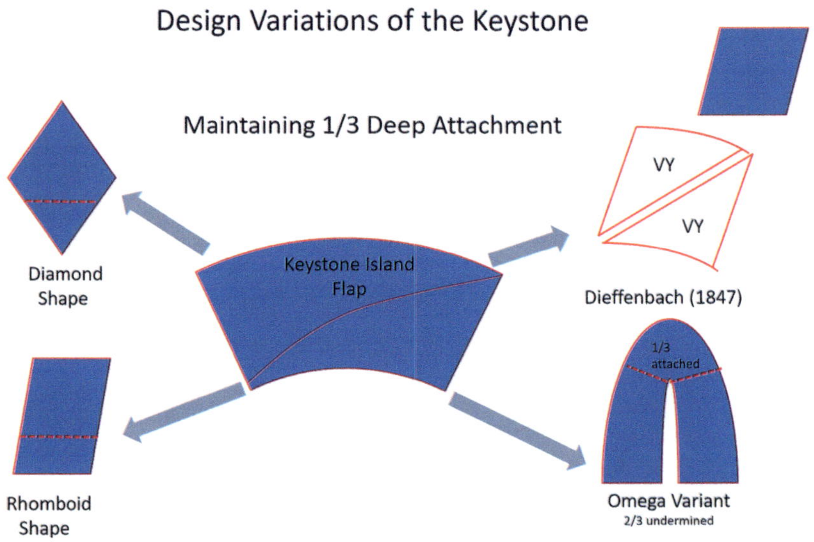

Fig. 1.8 Bespoke design variations of the Keystone flap are governed by the surgical defect needed for repair (as in tailoring) and rely on the laxity of surrounding tissues, and the angiotomes are vascular supports along the dermatomal mark outs, which are part of the embryological basis

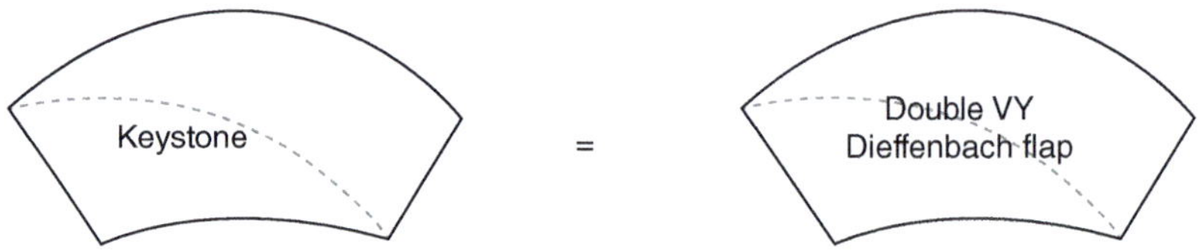

Fig. 1.9 The Keystone flap is a double V-Y Dieffenbach flap design diagonally joining opposite extremes

are the causes of any failures. In all reconstructive techniques, venous drainage must be respected, and microanastomosis and any inadvertent venous damage can thus be repaired immediately. These hairline perforator supports are thus embedded in the fascia and constitute the basis of the Keystone's success, presumably including lymphatics.

The outline of the dermatomes perforators is a guideline for vascular support. Their angiographic definition helps one with the design based on dermatomes, and this has been the pattern in this reconstructive series of Keystone applications. However, the aide-mémoire in raising the flap within the dermatomes has been clinically confirmed by the observation of the vascular flare leading to the red dot sign that is consistent with hypervascularity. If there is a dermatomal blood supply embryologically linked, there must be an accompanying blood supply with these neural mark outs, which are dragged in continuity as development continues, all expediting healing. The Keystone is really an umbrella term of tissue expanded to cover various surgical defects with V-Y points at their apices. The random pattern of the perforators is the source of vascular support that ensures the advancement, rotation and transposition (ART) of Keystone island flaps as long as one-third of the deep attachment of the cutaneous island flap is maintained as a safeguard, and the reliability of the lax surrounding tissues ensures closure. The gamut of vascular changes in the KPIF comes from observational findings, not experimental investigations, and from the usual restrictions that one observes in closing large defects, allowing wound closure. However, the Keystone principle, which is fascially based, allows one to *close under tension*—breaking one of the mandated rules of reconstructive surgery. Why is this possible? Again, observationally, this increase in vascular perfusion that we call *reactive hyperaemia* [22] has two aspects. They are the same as those of a lumbar sympathectomy effect, creating a pink foot in due course to assist in healing in elderly diabetic patients with distal perfusional restraints. This reactive hyperaemia usually emerges in 10–15 min when using the KPIF repair. However, others have observed that the island principle creates a hydrostatic barrier to perfusion, forcing the venous exit to the line of least resistance down the perforator stalks. These findings may be cyanotic from an observational point of view. Thus, if we have a combination of two hypotheses working out a combined outcome, the hyperaemia causes the *red dot sign*; the suture point site of exit through the Keystone is arterially based and red, not cyanotic bluish, which can convey any element of restricted perfusion. In summary, the repeat observations of these vascular changes might explain the sympathectomy effect surrounding the fascially based island aligned within the dermatome, similar to a lumbar sympathectomy.

As a preamble to the Bezier design of an ellipsoidal V-Y island flap—as illustrated in the dia-

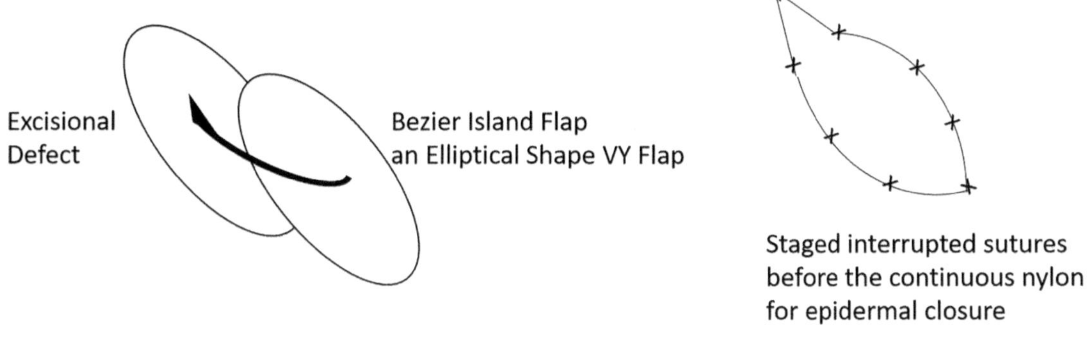

Fig. 1.10 The insertion of the Bezier flap around a curvilinear concept creates softened corners, not triangulated straight lines

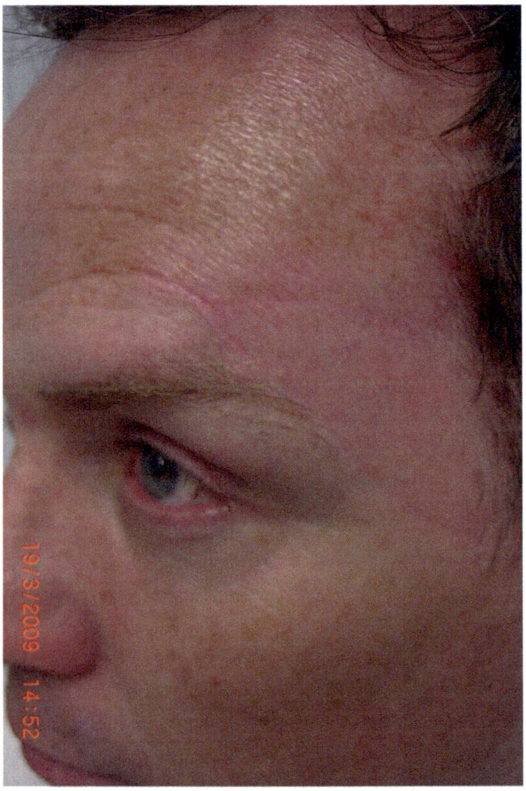

Fig. 1.11 This clinical example comes from my melanoma series using the Bezier curvilinear V-Y island flap with its subsequent applications applied in major surgical defects—a clinical outcome at 6 months

grams in Figs. 1.10 and 1.11—I add that variations in the triangular design arise by joining the opposite extremes of the rhomboidal shape. The next stage in island flap design—the Keystone—combines two conjoined V-Y island flaps. In other words, this elliptical shape allows easy apposition without lines of tension in the closure of a surgical defect, one of the limitations of the straight V-Y flap.

Any reconstruction based on a specific perforator may experience interference with their somatic, autonomic, lymphatic or humeral supply. The Keystone concept retains these neurovascular supports at the arterial, venous, somatic, autonomic and lymphatic support levels, which has clinical applications in reviewing the postoperative effect of the KPIF, leading to its acronym PACES: pain-free, aesthetic outcomes, complications are rare, economic timeframes and somatic and autonomic neural recovery and the resolution of oedema.

1.4 The Science Behind the Keystone Flap

Observed hyperaemia in the Keystone is the basis of its success, allowing it to be closed under tension as a reconstructive principle. The Keystone's success in reconstructive surgery is speculatively based on the dermatomal outlines of the body, which incorporate embryological principles in development, and each clinical illustration in this series where closure under tension has become an accepted norm realistically mimics the physiology of intrinsic expansion [23, 24] in tissue. However, if the balloon factor is necessary in tissue expansion, the Keystone under tension does this tissue closure as a single gesture, so we have tissue expansion in an immediate sense if we can apply that analogy when visualising the Keystone reconstructive applications. I repeat that closing under tension is contraindicated in sound reconstructive surgery, but because of the hypervascularity, flare and red dot signs, the circulation has been enhanced, allowing us to close under tension in this immediate sense, which is another version of tissue expansion. And what is the basis of these findings? Successful observations of these clinical principles evident throughout the series constitute the basis of these findings which implies the absolute necessity, when tissue is developing from its embryological phase, of some stimulus to make the organelle (the viscous or the limbs) develop in a way that matches the final outcomes, creating a human specimen when treated clinically or when researched in an anatomy museum. What goes where to produce the ultimate outcome? In experimental or physiological outlines, such observational findings have been the stepping stones when looking for an aetiological explanation. The history of the lumbar sympathectomy is worth recalling again as an adjunct to my findings in clinical anatomy with the Keystone.

Professor John Royle, a former Royal Australasian College of Surgeons dignitary and a former vascular surgeon, might have revealed the story of the development of a lumbar sympathectomy [25]. He was following the treatment of wounded soldiers after the Great War and thought that spasticity in muscles with still-ongoing intact motor and sensory innervation could have been a contribution from the autonomic nervous system and its sympathetic overlay. The orthopaedic surgeon who made the observation did anatomical investigations down the lumbar chain, looking for elements of the sympathetic nervous system, all of which were operational and all of which were from an anatomical point of view. Besides the sympathetic nervous system, the somatic nervous system made an important contribution to sensory protection and proprioceptive function. So, this combination of neural elements became the basis for the research before the clinical application of lumbar sympathectomy became accepted.

During the observational findings following such a procedure, the 'warm foot' observed within 24 h became the natural consequence following the operation of a lumbar sympathectomy. But as an additional finding, this hypervascularity had important implications in wound healing, with the increased blood supply providing a solution to elements of trophic ulceration in the lower limbs that were still recovering from war injuries.

Therefore, the division of the lumbar autonomic trunk had the collateral effects of vascular dilatation and increased vascular perfusion, and a corollary of these effects was expedited healing for elements of trophic ulceration, which has a diabetic or pressure origin.

Could making an island flap of the integument with a fascial base have been similar in principle to a lumbar sympathectomy and its distal foot manifestations? When creating an island flap and the division through the integument is removed, the somatic sensory response and local changes, like the swearing response, occur in an area so demarcated.

Thus, when we raise a Keystone flap, we are in fact dividing filamentous branches of somatic or autonomic nerves, allowing the remaining networks, sourced from the lumbar region, to function in accordance with their manifestations of hypervascularity. We constantly have observed with the Keystone the vascular flare, where the flap, as an island, has the apparent appearance of increased vascular flow. But more importantly, the suture point for surgical alignment bleeds more on the flap side than on the suture site.

An article by Coventry and Walsh [26] was coincidentally published in the same year and in the same journal—the *ANZ Journal of Surgery*—as my initial Keystone publication. The background to the Coventry article discusses the issue of ischaemic rest pain and notes that lumbar sympathectomy had been evident over the years, the mechanism through which improvements, achieved as both sensory and vasomotor fibres, travel along the lumbar sympathetic chain, and the effects of lumbar sympathectomy on these nerve types have been the basis of investigation. Normal and physical vapour deposition (PVD) controls had intact sensory and vasomotor nerves around dermal cutaneous blood vessels, but these were completely or almost completely lost after lumbar sympathectomy, through either chemical or surgical means. In conclusion, lumbar sympathectomy severs both vasomotor and sensory fibres, suggesting that the relief of rest pain may be explained not only by increased cutaneous and muscle blood flow but also by nociceptor sensory denervation.

Hence, through reverse thinking, when we have the vascular changes in a Keystone island flap, there must be a dominating sympathectomy effect to present the characteristics of the Keystone, which make up the acronym PACES: They are pain-free; the tissues match like for like in an aesthetic manner; the vascular complications are minimal; the procedure is economically feasible in time; and cutaneous sensory recovery occurs. But as an acknowledgement of Osler's later statement that all developments in medicine are related to observational findings, I admit that I only recently read Leonardo Da Vinci make this observation in the fifteenth century, and scientific conclusions emanate from this concept of amassed clinical findings. So, what is new in the world?

Since the publication of the Keystone concept and the reliability of a V-Y island background, as summarised above, many have attempted variations employing this principle and have developed multiple applications all over the body, from the head and neck region down. Therefore, we have unified this concept by offering a series of publications and clinical applications from my personal experiences, which have led to the Keystone series of books.

The simple fact of creating an island within the embryological outlines of the dermatomes seems to create a *sympathectomy effect*, and as illustrated with the Keystone, *hypervascularity* and *vascular flare* with its *red dot signs* at the suture points are constant observational findings. These clinical observations have become characteristic of this reconstructive technique, leading to adventurous reconstructions, which initially seem at variance with some of the established principles of plastic and reconstructive surgery (e.g. closing under tension), and it even allows one to trim dog ears in the acute phase to avoid secondary procedures for scar revision. Such success speaks volumes about the validity of these observational findings, all which, again, have been illustrated.

This led to the characteristics of the Keystone, which developed after over more than 3000 clinical cases that have been digitally documented and became the basis of publications on melanoma [4], major orthopaedic defects [5] and major surgical defects, surgeries that previously were the province of microsurgery. Their inclusion has now completed the series.

William Osler (1849–1919), the influential Canadian physician and professor of medicine at Oxford University, stated that 'Observation is the basis of scientific advancement in medicine.' My observations of the behaviour of various islanded local flaps led me to search for the physiological basis of these successes by using digital images as the background for clinical comparisons. This was inspired by other research published in the surgical literature on angiogenesis, the increased blood supply in tissue-expanded flaps, concepts in endothelial stress and facial nerve repair. These observations have not been the subject of pathology investigations to date, but according to Carl Sagan, the physicist, 'The absence of evidence is not the evidence of absence' [27]. We have repetitive observational findings with the Keystone, and all our observations are accompanied by clinical records that digitally verify the basis of our clinical success, including patient satisfaction.

The challenge was how I could come up with good *research projects* confirming the clinical findings, which have been observational. I can refer you only to the following paper: Lo [28] on the vascularity of Keystones is the only reference for these tissue findings that confirms the increased vascularity in island flaps. However, a recent verbal communication from Mr. Naveen Somia with Professor Carla Stecco, an orthopaedic surgeon from Padua University and an expert on fascial innervation and vascularity, has supported these clinical characteristics with scientific investigation, complimenting my observational findings and supporting my earlier hypothesis. As evidenced by her 2022 publications [16, 17], she affirms that there are implications for the sympathetic nervous system, as she has described in her communication. In a recent work, Stecco et al. revealed a huge innervation of the superficial fascia: The nervous structures were found above and around blood vessels and close to fatty tissue—adipocytes—but they also penetrated into the connective tissue itself and were found amid fibroadipose tissue. The diameter of the nerve fibres ranges from 2.5 to 35μm, and they include both sensitive and autonomic nerve fibres. The relative percentage of autonomic innervation was 33.82% in the superficial fascia, which was found in association with a huge vascular network that formed a plexus. Additionally, arteriovenous shunts could be detected as under the control of sympathetic innervation. In the light of these findings, the superficial fascia might play a role in thermoregulation, proprioception and pain perception. The creation of the Keystone flap can alter the sympathetic innervation of the superficial fascia, and if it does, it consequently causes the vasodilation of the vessels inside the superficial fascia. This would explain the red dot sign, and the clinical findings of the Keystone confirm this published work. In conclusion, a sympathetic, autonomic and somatic background supports my findings. I also include a synopsis of the observational findings that have been digitally recorded from clinical cases.

1.4.1 How the Red Dot Sign and Vascular Flare Illustrate the Sympathectomy Effect of the Islanding

The red dot sign and vascular flare occur at the suture point, and the flare reflects hypervascularity, as indicated in the included cases. The advantages of a noncomplicated surgical repair need no elaboration, and the KPIF has one preeminent characteristic, namely that it is neurodermatomally based within embryological mark outs. This contains the accompanying arteriovenous, autonomic and somatic supply. The Keystone has fascially lined variations for advancement, rotation and transposition (ACT) and for more-awkward locoregional repairs along the anterior tibia, and it can be undermined up to two-thirds along the peroneal L1 dermatome while preserving deep attachment to the remaining one-third over the neurovascular perforator supports. These must include lymphatic drainage. This embryological presumption has been the basis for the clinical characteristics synopsised by the acronym PACES covering pain, aesthetics, vascular complications, expeditious execution and the subsequent recovery of sensation with the resolution of oedema, presumably dilating lymphatic channels after clinical healing under sympathetic control. Again, these are all observational phenomena gleaned over the thousands of cases done to date. Conducting the delayed reconstruction after pathology evaluation (DRAPE) [29] procedure while awaiting pathology clearance is a necessary prerequisite in good clinical management with cases of mitotic malignancy of the integument (melanoma, SCC, etc.).

1.4.2 Closure Under Tension Is Now Possible

This basic dictum of general surgical principles applied universally is part of our surgical training because closure under tension produces epidermal necrosis. This sympathectomy effect precludes such setbacks, and the hypervascularity minimises this possibility of flap necrosis. However, the Keystone has reorientated the thinking of this concept because of the redirection of vascular flow—the vertical infrafascial and suprafascial perforator supports are hydrostatically superior to those of the horizontally orientated subdermal plexus, a common cause of flap necrosis, but islanding bypasses this problem. For example, dynamically, one can compare fire hydrants and garden hoses; both have their specific uses. All the cases illustrating the hyperaemic effect in the text have been closed under tension. Absolute white lines of tension are warnings to reinsert and realign the suture orientations. But in the main, the vascular flow based on fascial support ensures the dynamic effect of hyperaemia and the red dot sign of the blood at the *suture site* of the flap, which confirms its dynamic flow and is just a scientific observation, quoting Osler again. Bleeding more on the flap side than the receiving side is a characteristic on the KPIF insertion—under tensional closure, we have increased flow. Variations on the design, such as hatchet flaps, completely miss the point of this dynamic perfusion concept. They are mentioned here merely to dispel the clinical applications of such variations and to reaffirm that they reflect erroneous thinking; however on the basis of tradition from the times of Barron and Emmett [30] and their island flap designs based on Esser's work, all these historical clinical observations are relevant. From my experience of the Keystone, lax tissues in surrounding areas are important contributions to the overall repair. Again, the red dot signs are observed throughout. For example, the Keystone in the lateral peroneal compartment will cover defects closed towards the anterior tibial line, but as a precaution, Keystones should not be based centrally along the anterior tibial surface, because the muscle substance of the peroneal compartment can be closed using direct pressure. The muscle bulk facilitates this manoeuvre, and the bone of the anterior tibial margin precludes such tightness; it must be over a muscle belly. If clinical closure is necessary, skin grafting becomes a necessary adjunct to safe wound healing over the exposed bone. These elements of closing under tension happen when they have a peroneal compartment in support. Discretion must always be exercised, and when an area like the anterior tibial wall is needed as a repair site, using a locoregional Keystone to cover any bony defect based on the lateral L5 dermatome, with or without grafting over muscle, is wiser.

The repair technique employs a standard three-phase suture technique to close the wound under tension as a single layer. The locking mattress sutures combine all layers into one without using a deeper layer, and appositional alignment should this disturb the perfusion through the fascia. The rest of the wound is closed with ordinary mattress sutures as a single layer, and finally, an epidermal seal is achieved by using a continuous nylon, which is cut after 7–10 days to avoid cross marks. The tension mattress sutures can stay for up to 2–3 weeks or longer to effectuate perfect wound healing, as illustrated in the cases documented, and avoid any rupture.

Main operating clinics should observe these techniques, where the inexperience of outside units can lead to complications like rupture. Staples are avoided.

1.4.3 PACES—Clinical Outcomes from the Patient's Perspective

The Keystone management in major reconstructions employs the same principles as those in any other closure of soft tissue defects. The soft tissue defect closure in such management can be achieved either with the use of split skin grafting or by applying additional locoregional flaps and microsurgery. Cases from various regions will illustrate the adaptability of the Keystone technique, helping to establish the *clinical characteristics* of the Keystone. Patient satisfaction is the pre-eminent indicator of its usefulness, as confirmed in videotaped experiences of patients' voicing their own opinions. In many microsurgical repairs, the aesthetic outcome can be questionable, and the Keystone concept is a suitable alternative to overcome these difficulties when fulfilling clinical requirements.

The range of Keystone applications overcomes these restrictions and has led to the establishment of good clinical outcomes and options. These *clinical characteristics*, summarised by the acronym PACES, are all based on clinical observation and act as an aide-mémoire for teaching.

Pain — How are they *pain-free*? We have all experiences of surgical wounds where a nonsensate area in the healed phase along the links of the incision takes some weeks to eventually recover sensate supply. The Keystone and its island design follow the same idea that no somatic input at the integumentary level subsequently recovers, which allows the patient to say that they are totally pain-free. Could the cutaneous somatic supply divided around the arc of the Keystone create a temporary anaesthetic surface which takes some weeks to recover, as is characteristic of all linear surgical wounds? The only symptom that the patient notices is a feeling of tightness, which is one of the key features when wounds are closed under such tension; again, we have broken one of the rules in reconstructive surgery, namely to not close under tension. But such are the elements of hypervascularity with the red dot sign. Closure under tension is a clinical possibility, and it allows us to trim out dog ears, avoiding a secondary procedure, sometimes indicated for aesthetic reasons. The cases listed illustrate these observations and respond to the criticisms of the uninitiated.

Aesthetics The Gillies principle of using **like for like** is a standard reconstructive principle entrenched in history and producing outcomes which are most satisfying to the patient, particularly on exposed sites. The normal attractive appearance of the integument is lost when large defects are grafted or when microvascular free flaps are used without tissue matching to fill the soft tissue contour defects for surgical necessity.

Complications Complications and adverse outcomes are not common in vascular repair; sometimes sutures need to be realigned to eliminate any lines of tension in the flap repair, but major wound breakdown occurs when dressings are done at an outside clinic with the premature removal of sutures and when the principles of closure with the Keystone have not been respected. The surgical repair is a standard three-phase locking mattress suture technique, as illustrated throughout all the cases, and conceivably, if wound dressing is delegated to an inexperienced operator, the single layer of the locking mattress suture might lead to wound breakdown. My 3-week rule for points of tension is applied routinely, and when the locking mattress loop is cut, the suture is easily delivered without having to look for hours for the buried knot in the deep mattress suture. Vascular complications do occur, particularly in diabetic patients and patients with vascular impendence, because these flaps are based not on a singular perforator but rather on a filamentous collection, which becomes defined only with blunt dissection and the teasing apart of the tissues to achieve closure. Perforators are not precisely defined, because the reliance on the filamentous network helps to overcome the problem of blood supply. Skeletonising for perforators may strip away the filamentous autonomic, somatic and lymphatic supports along the axial channels of such vascular perforators of the suprafascial and infrafascial location. Irradiated tissue is not a contraindication in the use of Keystone applications, because of the hypervascularity principles already discussed. In a type II diabetic patient's lower limb, where the microcirculation is the centre of pathology, the elements of partial necrosis have occurred, and as a consequence, closure must be done without tension, and a generous use of skin grafting is an alternative fall-back position, particularly in elderly patients' lower limbs.

Expeditious in execution 'Time is money' is a Benjamin Franklin quote from Fisher's book of 1748. If one can operate within a reduced timeframe, this has benefits for all modalities in the treatment and care of patients, particularly elderly patients. It has also an economic factor and theatre throughput, whereas long reconstructive sagas continue to produce adverse alternatives. Microsurgical team procedures have high-cost and long-time-frame implications, particularly for staff allocation and the availability of theatre time. We all have experiences of umpteen cases being cancelled because microsurgical reconstructions are still continuing in spite of inadvertent or intermittent setbacks. The Keystone cases illustrated here will go some way to overcoming this setback, and the audiovisual account helps to facilitate the teaching process.

Somatic recovery with the resolution of oedema

These final outcome characteristics go hand in hand with surgical success, and we have tried to elaborate on certain areas to bypass any incidental complications, such as wound breakdown with any premature removal of sutures (staples are not used). As in any surgical wound, the division of the filamentous cutaneous branches creates a temporary anaesthetic field around the operative site. This may recover in the weeks that follow when the integument has healed and the scar is maturing. A final characteristic under observation is the resolution of swelling and oedema, which goes hand in hand with this recovery period of up to 8 weeks. My observational suggestion is that when the sympathectomy effect of the island fascial flap is evident with vascular flare and red dot signs, this could simply be transferred to the lymphatic network as a means to explain why swellings of the surgical site seem to resolve spontaneously.

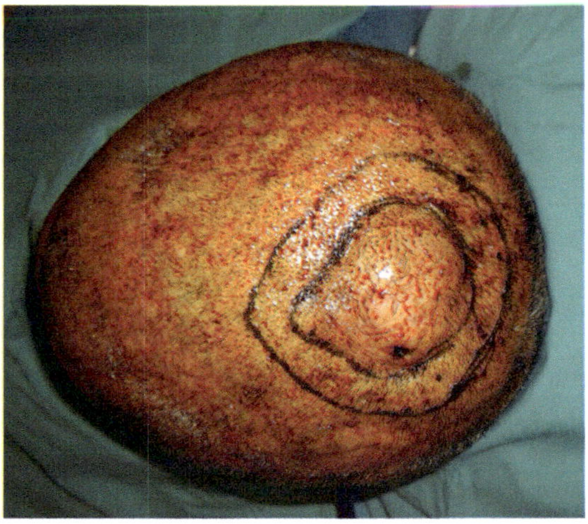

Fig. 1.12 The mark out of the macroscopic tumour and the 2 cm peripheral clearance of 1 cm into the outer table of the skull

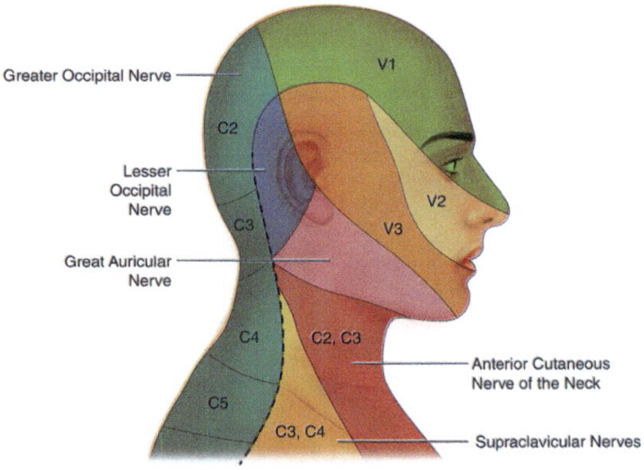

Fig. 1.13 The dermatomal mark out is the guide for the location of the random perforators coming through the fascia that support the superficial temporal artery. (Reprinted with permission from Atlas, *Reconstructive Technique in Melanoma Management* (p. 19), by Felix Behan, Springer Nature 2023)

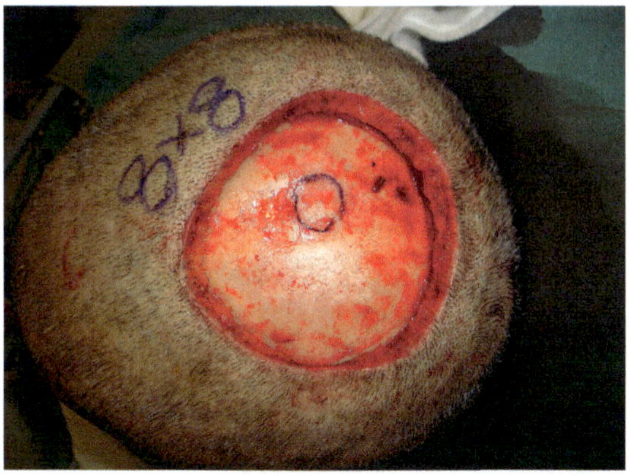

Fig. 1.14 The peripheral clearance before the additional removal of the outer table of the scalp for the clearance of the Merkel cell tumour, producing a 8 × 8 cm defect

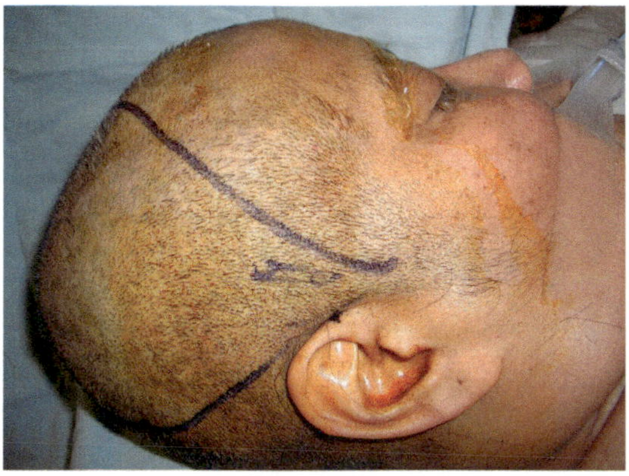

Fig. 1.15 Superficial temporal artery mark out is shown. The flap is raised while retaining and not skeletonising the axial neurovascular structures. This retains periadventitial tissue to ensure autonomic and somatic input

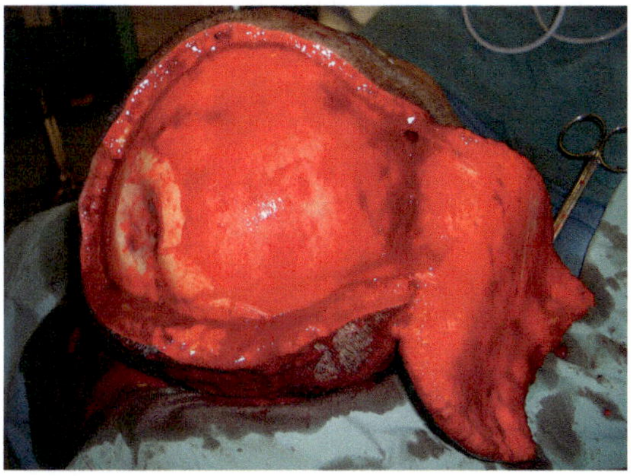

Fig. 1.16 Raising the flap using blunt dissection once the integument has been divided around the periphery

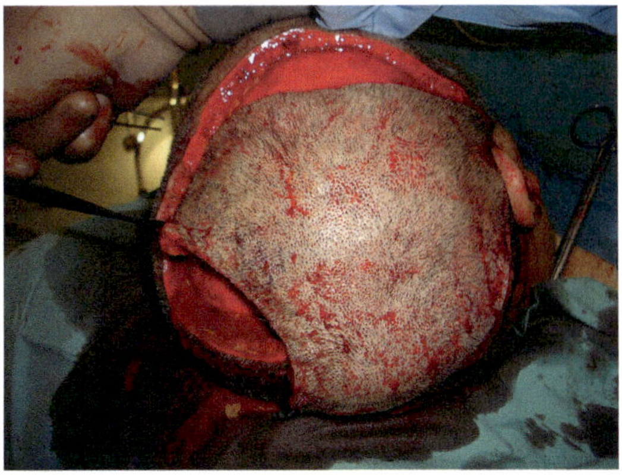

Fig. 1.17 Staged closure sequence

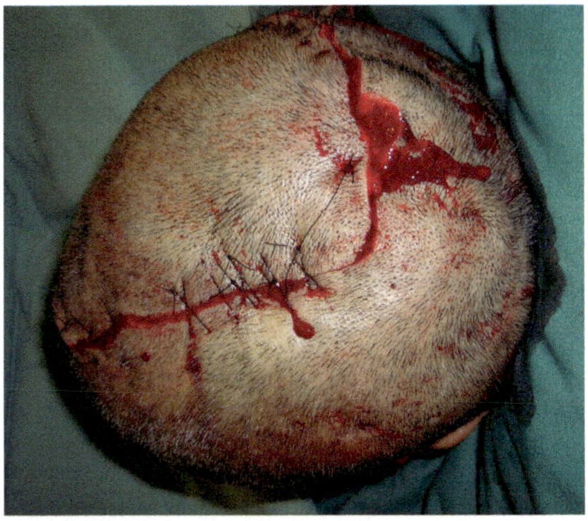

Fig. 1.18 The locking mattress sutures are altered to minimise lines of maximum tension, closing the defect before ordinary mattress sutures produce wound closure

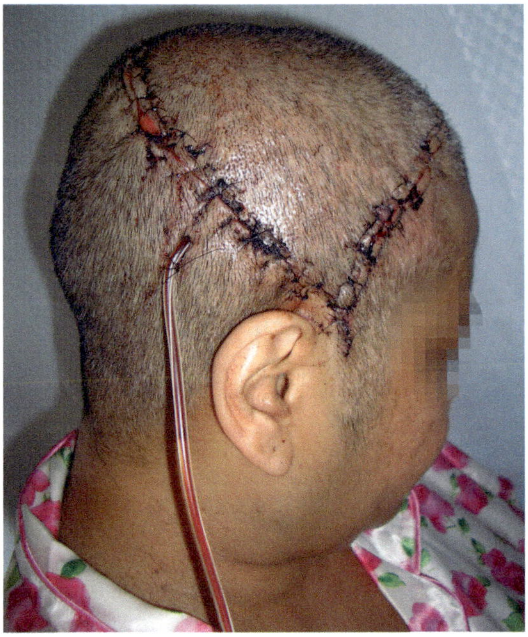

Fig. 1.19 Completion with suction drainage is shown. Note the hyperaemic flare in the island flap compared with the image of the surrounding scalp—this is hypothetically a sympathectomy effect, as explained in the science section

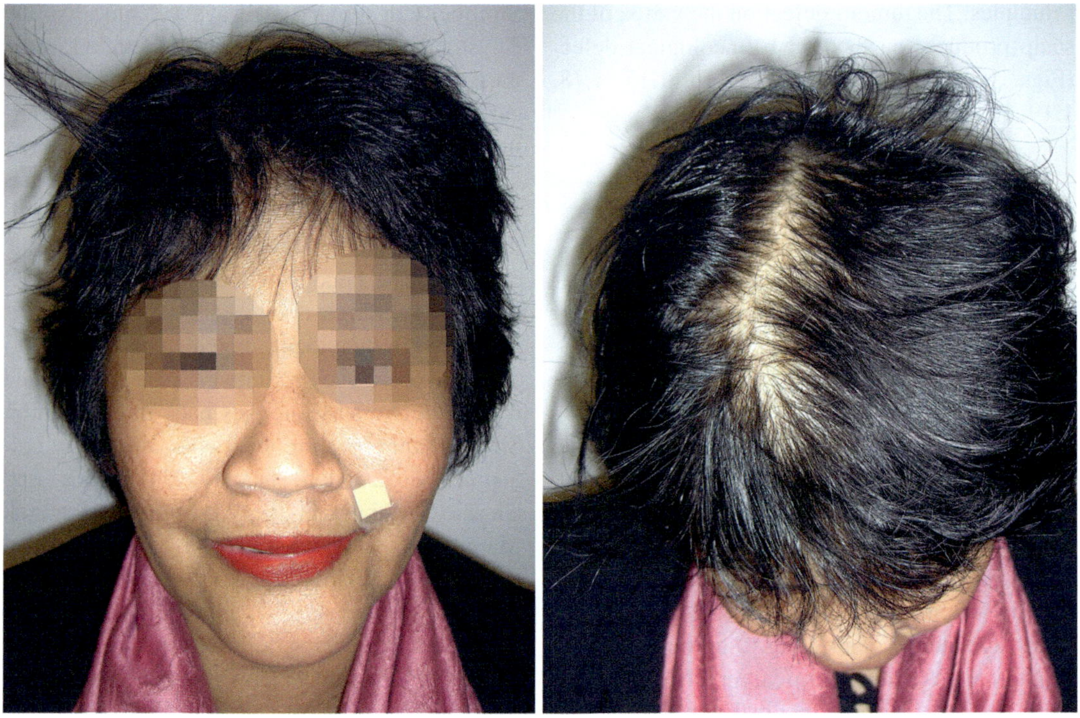

Fig. 1.20 The appearance 6 months later is shown. Note the patient's observation of increased hair growth and density. Again, a clinical outcome aligned along the scar of hypervascularity in the scalp, as seen in Keystone reconstructions

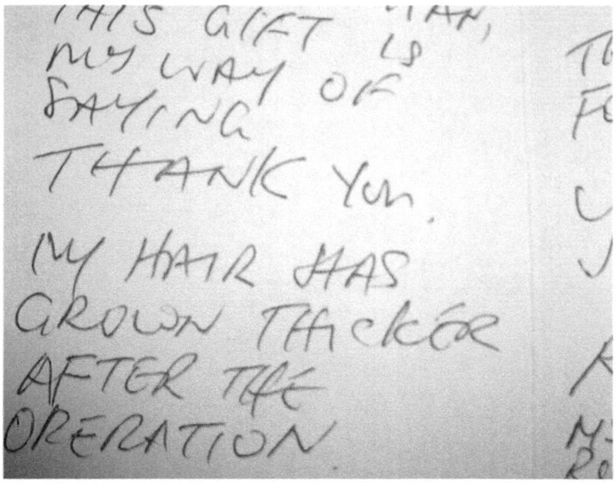

Fig. 1.21 Her Christmas card thanking me for the surgical procedure and stating that her hair is now growing thicker as a result of the surgery, reflecting the Keystone characteric of the hypervascularity of the sympathectomy effect

A case example exemplifying the PACES characteristics is a mitotic lesion of the scalp Merkel cell (the appearance of an amelanotic lesion)—i.e. *malignant fibroxanthoma*—following biopsy clearance and repair using Keystone principles. The tumour defect on the vertex of the scalp produces an 8 × 8 cm oncological defect (Figs. 1.12, 1.13, 1.14, 1.15, 1.16, 1.17, 1.18, 1.19, 1.20 and 1.21).

1.5 The Keystone Technique

The emergence of microvascular surgical repair concepts has played an important role in surgery since Ian Taylor's [31] initial publication in 1973. However, when the Keystone island flap concept is used, cognisant of its listed characteristics, this compares favourably, achieving tissue match. Its low complication rate is noteworthy, contributing to a shorter operative timeframe, and somatic supply in the dermatomal flaps is another benefit, including aesthetic outcomes given that the patients often say that they feel normal again. Thus, its value is continuing to be reassessed as an alternative to microsurgical repair. Thus, clinically, in any applied reconstructive situation, anything that offers the advantages listed above is worthy of consideration.

Acquiring the technique, in the author's experience, takes time, which is why the video supplement of cases explains the background and the reasoning behind the success of the surgical technique, a radical alternative to the established way of treating under the microsurgical domain, which has dominated reconstructive surgery for over 20 years, but repetition is the key note to success. Start small and then work towards larger cases, especially over muscle bellies, which facilitates compressional closure because of the nature of the muscle substrate supplying perforators via the fascia. In the main, the Keystone can cover the majority of soft tissue defects all over the body, including the trunk, as listed in the illustrations.

Various cases have been selected to show the focus and applications of the Keystone concept and how to avoid complications, endeavouring to match the PACES acronym, which is part of any surgical repair. Images from the preoperative to the postoperative phase demonstrate the wide applications, and the Keystone design has become a unifying principle in reconstructive surgery. Simplicity in surgery is always welcome, and the Keystone is simple to apply, once mastered, when these basic principles are followed, and simple cases should be used in the learning process during the initial phases of introduction and can be augmented by additional help from one who has experience in this field. Satisfaction becomes evident at the patient level, including that of the operator. The benefit of looking almost normal has a psychological benefit as well, which is illustrated in the video supplements.

My experience in surgery as a plastic and reconstructive surgeon goes back to my mentor, Sir Benjamin Rank in the 1970s, and to my colleagues in London, namely Ian Wilson and Charlie Westbury at the Westminster Hospital, Marsden Hospital and St George's Hospital, in the fields of melanoma and head and neck cancer repair.

The standard skin grafting technique for major defects led me to develop island flap reconstructions, and based on my research, the Bezier island flap evolved from the V-Y principle (published in 1995), which is a curvilinear ellipsoidal V-Y island flap in the Dieffenbach manner. If larger defects need attention, the size of the V-Y flap can be doubled, and when conjoined with a twin size, based on intercostal random perforators, this was the basis for the design of the Keystone. Geometrically, when one joins the opposite points of the curvilinear Keystone design, it suddenly appears like two conjoined double V-Y flaps with underlying suprafascial and infrafascial perforator support. These design variations (a curvilinear V-Y, a double V-Y flap) can all be used to explain the Keystone concept. It is based on a career of island flap surgery with design variations to cover the topics mentioned above.

DUET surgery is a great contributor that combines the experiences of various surgical minds, one relying on the other when excisions and repairs become difficult. Once the other members realise the beneficial outcome of using the Keystone concept, its applications become widespread. No defect has arisen to date, and no cases have been deemed necessary to revert to microsurgical correction to date. The Keystone can cover most options. Without the input of these combined referrals of complex cases needing complex reconstructions, as illustrated, the range of cases in the text would be insignificant, but no cases that needed microsurgical repair backup were deemed beyond the scope of the Keystone applications. However, repeat Keystone repairs taking the laxity out of facial contours is usually avoided, and we have had one case where a microsurgical repair was deemed necessary.

All photographic illustrations were taken during my own preoperative, intraoperative and postoperative phases, and the advantage of the simple photographic digital camera allowed me to discuss cases during the intraoperative phase. My London experience with Ralph Hutchens, the chief photographer at the Royal College of Surgeons in the early 1970s, was my introduction to photographic expertise. I would routinely clean the wounds with saponified sterilisation solutions, and the clean wounds redraped with fresh theatre garb became a key of my clinical technique, producing good illustrations.

In conclusion, these cases were from the Peter MacCallum Cancer Institute and the Western Hospital in Melbourne, Australia, where the teams all had DUET appointments, so cases could be interchanged depending on the availability of theatre time and could be accommodated with vacancies on any list. Referrals from my surgical colleagues Andrew Sizeland, Stephen Kleid, Michael Henderson and David Speakman and orthopaedic colleagues Ray Crowe, Christopher Haw and Robert Pianta demonstrated that they recognised the value of the expeditious method achievable in reconstructive surgery with a strong focus on Keystone applications. These have all been the basis for this clinical series; hence, the illustrations and the videos become a teaching tool where others less familiar with this technique can see how we have achieved efficient outcomes in surgical repair, even in disadvantaged locations around the world, as recently confirmed by my webinar experiences and the email referrals that followed.

Difficult problems create challenges while observing the principle of Ockham's razor [32]—i.e. rely on the simplest explanations to find a solution. The locoregional Keystone flaps provide attractive aesthetic alternatives with their diverse architectural variations, but they are still constituted of an island flap and random perforator, aligned within the dermatomes and based on suprafascial and infrafascial circulation [33], sourced from regional perforators. They all hark back to and respect the embryological basis of the Keystone repair. In other words, if there is a nerve supply, there must be a blood supply that requires lymphatic drainage support, and the somatic supply is supplemented by autonomic neural supply, the basis of our red dot sign, which is earmarked on almost every case. This is a guarantee of vascular perfusion without harking back to specific perforator sources, which often strip the main input of autonomic and lymphatic support.

Some have asked whether scarless surgery is achievable, and my standard three-phase suture technique, as illustrated, goes some way to achieving such an end, as in the case below of a melanotic lesion in the calf of a 65 year old who was treated with surgical clearance, and a Keystone island flap repair illustrates these

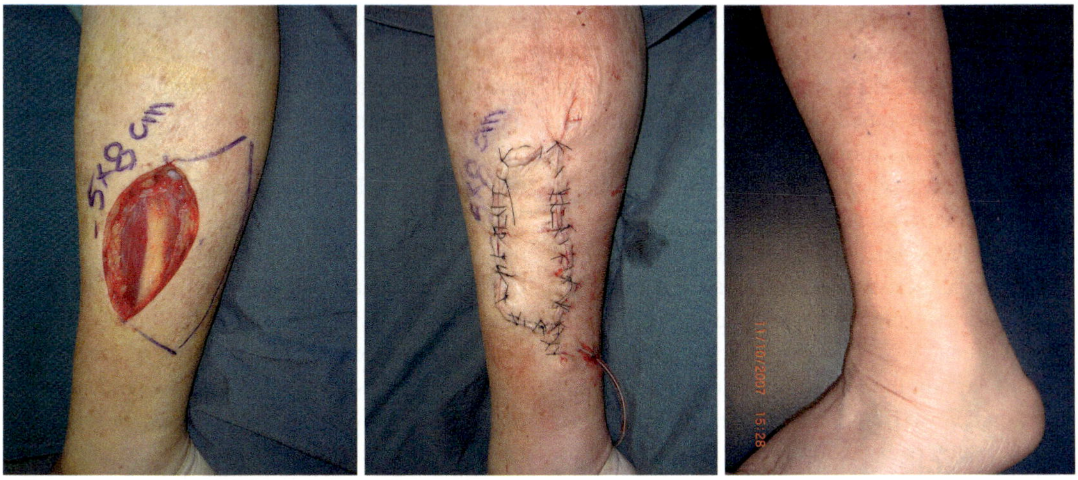

Fig. 1.22 Clearance, closure and conclusion

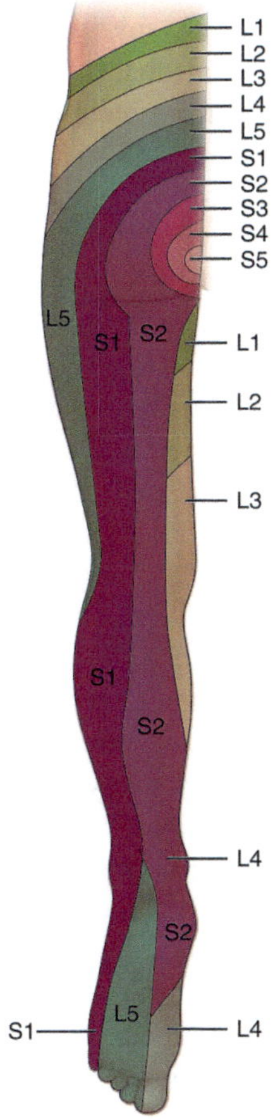

Fig. 1.23 The dermatomal mark out is the guide for the location of the random perforators coming through the fascia in the lower limb. (Reprinted with permission from Atlas, *Reconstructive Technique in Melanoma Management* (p. 137), by Felix Behan, Springer Nature 2023)

principles through the muscles of the peroneal compartment (Figs. 1.22 and 1.23).

As neurovascular island flaps came into prominence in the 1990s and with the introduction of the Keystone concept, first published in the *ANZ Journal of Surgery* in 2003, this island design of reconstruction entered a new phase, avoiding microsurgical repairs. As long as my reconstructive principles apply in raising the Keystone as detailed here, surgeons should have universal success:

1. The dermatome alignment is an absolute prerequisite in the flap location.
2. The standard Keystone repair is a single unit straddling two surgical defects which are closed under tension.
3. With the advancement, rotation and transposition of the fascially based Keystone, it is raised in a distal-to-proximal direction, clipping any fascial perforators, but it leaves one-third of proximal attachment in any therapeutic repair once undermining has been completed at the fascial level.
4. The flap consists of skin/fat/fascia and longitudinal anatomical structures in the vicinity, such as any venous line, and neural structures are all retained in the initial dissection, as deemed appropriate.
5. Two-thirds undermining is a valid technical modification that I have employed to date, with the remaining proximal one-third attached for random perforator perfusional

support as a lifeline allowing distal closure under tension where deemed necessary. The vascular perfusion may be slightly imperilled, but a relocation of sutures on release helps to solve this temporary problem.

6. The cases and their digital images, some with time and date stamps, allow us to be specific about documented data.

The following melanoma/sarcoma case with a 14 × 8 cm defect over the L scapular region will illustrate the principles of the Keystone reconstruction technique, including the source of the intercostal perforators, and the two arms of the Keystone lined with fascia are raised back to the axis of the perforator, allowing them to be turned into the defect because of the laxity of the surrounding tissues, which allows the closure to be shaped as a U or omega symbol—hence the name omega variant (Figs. 1.24, 1.25, 1.26, 1.27, 1.28, 1.29, 1.30, 1.31 and 1.32).

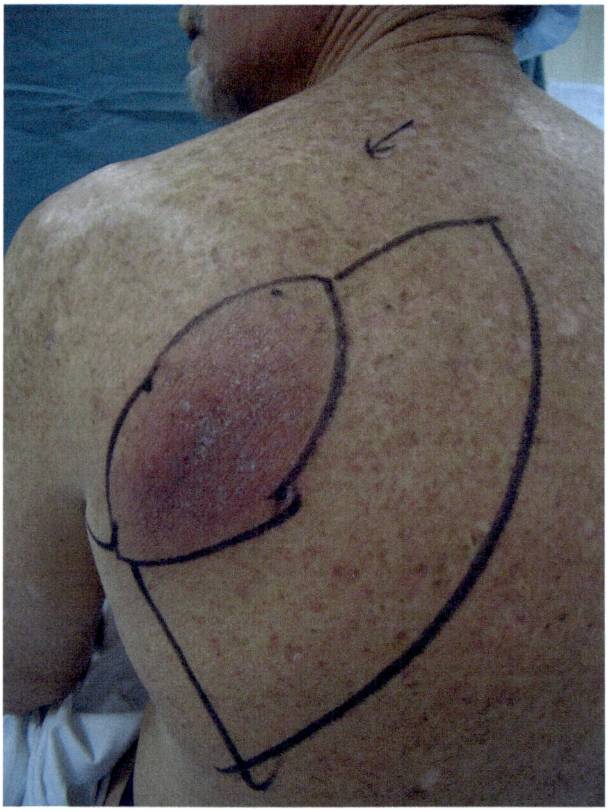

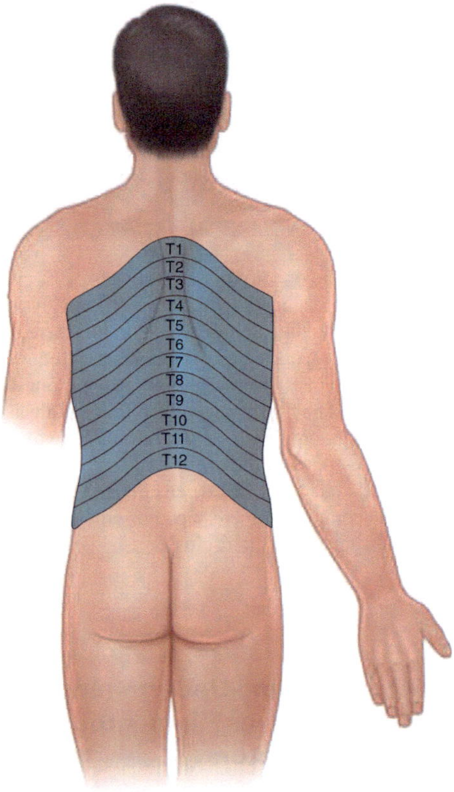

Fig. 1.24 The tumour mass is approximately 14 × 8 cm. Note the Keystone mark out over the T2–T8 intercostal perforators, where the width matches the size of the tumour defect following the clearance of the axillary nodes. (Reprinted with permission from Atlas, *Reconstructive Technique in Melanoma Management* (p. 103), by Felix Behan, Springer Nature 2023)

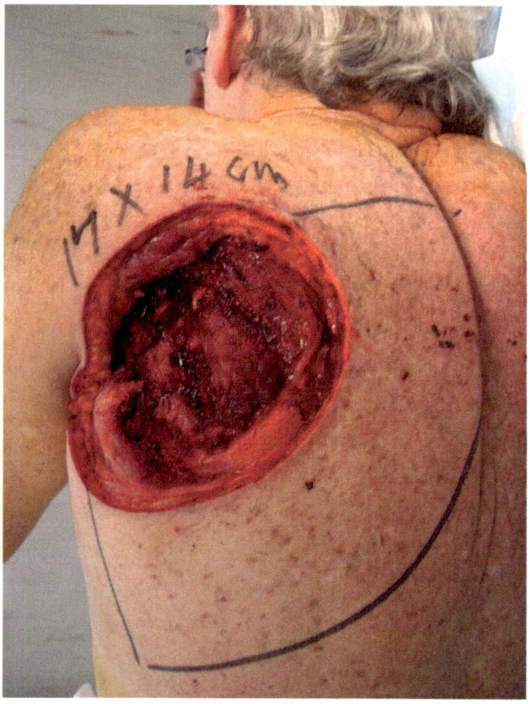

Fig. 1.25 The oncological defect is 14 × 17 cm down to the scapular fascia. The mark out of the Keystone along T2–T8 is along the intercostal perforators raised at the fascial level. My working rule—an essential requirement for flap viability in all Keystones—is leaving one-third deep attachment. The flap is attached in this middle area on the basis of random intercostal perforators which are not defined. In contrast, the upper and lower thirds, both fascial lined and undermined, ensure flap viability for the apices to complete the U-shaped or omega-shaped variant closure when the axilla is closed

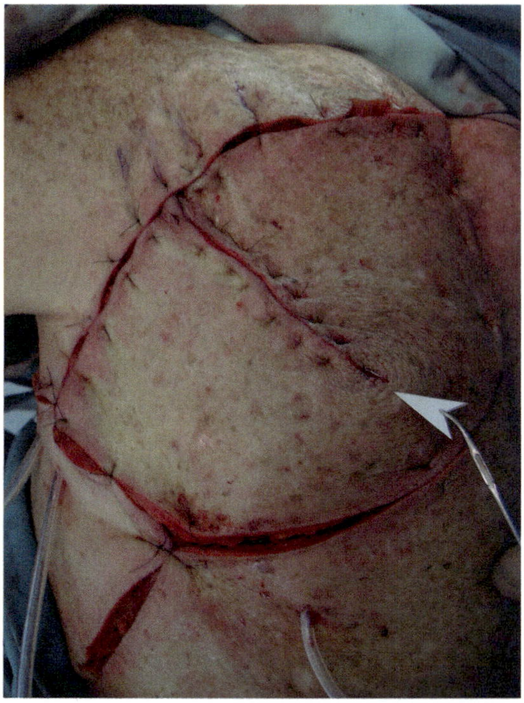

Fig. 1.26 The closure technique under suction drainage separately drains at the two sites and axilla, and the arrow is the site of the intercostal perforator support governing the viability of the flaps, all undermined. Thanks to the reliability and the hyperaemia of this vascular change, the dog ears can be excised in the acute phase down to the limits of the arrow, because the flaps are fascial based and not dermally based. The postoperative appearance confirms this hypothesis, without any need for dog ear correction

1.5.1 Avoiding Undermining Preserves Filamentous Perforators

Undermining the arms of the Keystone is permissible when based on the central intercostal perforators, as illustrated in the case above. This is the source of the random perforators from these embryonic axial sources. Even when undermining is necessary for a locoregional repair, one-third of deep attachment is mandatory, as illustrated here, where the source of infrafascial and suprafascial microfilamentous perforators are not defined as long as they have fascial support [6]. Should undermining be deemed necessary, this will help to facilitate the closure, with the advancement, rotation and transposition of the Keystone island flaps mimicking reconstructive principles, which have all been part of our background as reconstructive surgeons, as illustrated here.

Drainage is an essential prerequisite, and a single drain tube bent into a U shape can drain both surgical defects, the initial surgical problem and the subsequent Keystone flap when discreetly placed beneath the island, avoiding perforators.

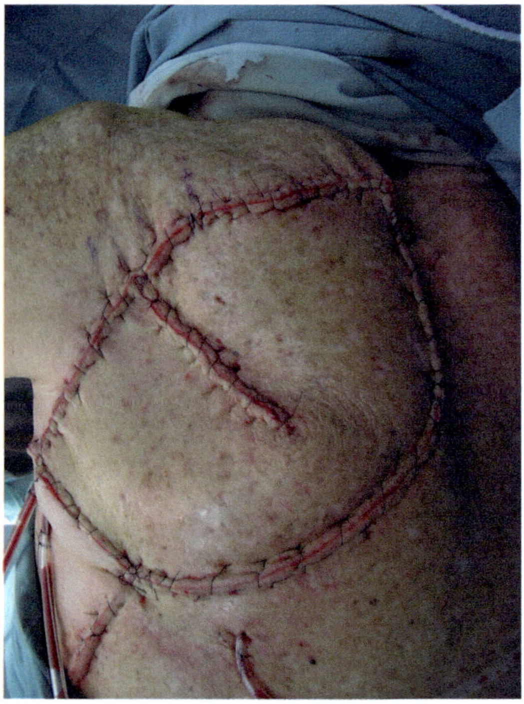

Fig. 1.27 The final specimen with double suction drains in position, one for the axilla and shared between the Keystone flaps. No evidence of cyanosis/necrosis occurred, and the PACES characteristics were all evident

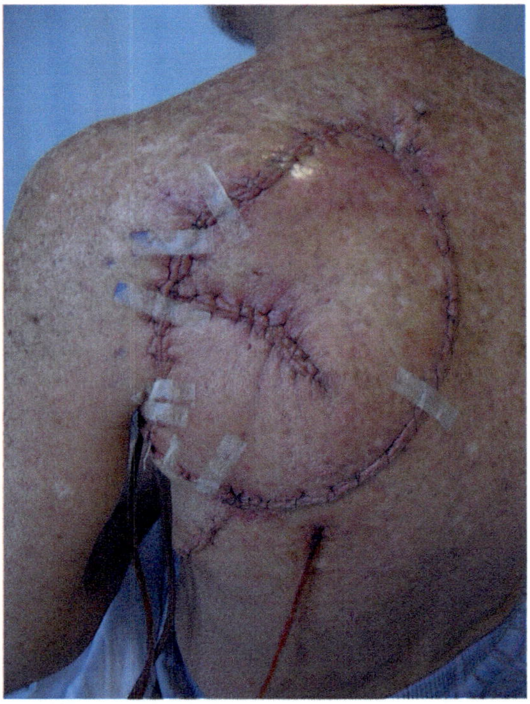

Fig. 1.28 On postoperative day 4, a re-exploration of the axillary collection became necessary following the removal of a drain tube and the reaccumulation of fluid

1.5.2 The Dermatomal Mark Out Avoids Angiography

The original dermatome mark out published in 1900 [34] used virus infiltration by Herpes Zoster to establish the dermatomal mark outs because viruses follow the nerve patterns (Fig. 1.33). Through extrapolation from this on an embryological basis, if there is a nerve supply, there must be a blood supply, and arterial flows create their own venous exit as they expand into the final developmental design. The vessels that grow with the nerves must also have autonomic supply to control their dilatation, and likewise, a somatic input allows their tactile sensation to be retained and recover after surgical intervention. In other words, the flap somatic sensation recovers. Historically, the traditional lumbar sympathectomy for any vascular impedance is followed the next morning by arterial flares and the foot is pink, reflecting increased vascular perfusion, and removing the restrictions of slow wound healing in any trophic ulceration reflects this hypervascularity. Clinically, a lesion pressing on the L1 root of the spinal cord creates an anaesthetic patch below the inguinal ligament on the anterior thigh, again according to embryological principles.

The dermatomal mark out avoiding angiography has cost-saving implications in the present world of cost containment in reconstructive microsurgery. The Keystone flap technique is useful in avoiding individual perforator flaps and sometimes in avoiding the difficulties in finding such units for reconstructive purposes locally or distant, whereas the Keystone, if the flaps are dermatomally aligned, is based merely on filamentous circulatory input as long as one-third of the flap remains attached to its fascial substrate. The clinical angiography is thus not always necessary—another cost-saving factor—because the Keystone technique avoids hunting for specific perforator supply. Undoubtedly, stripping the adventitial tissue away may interfere with the

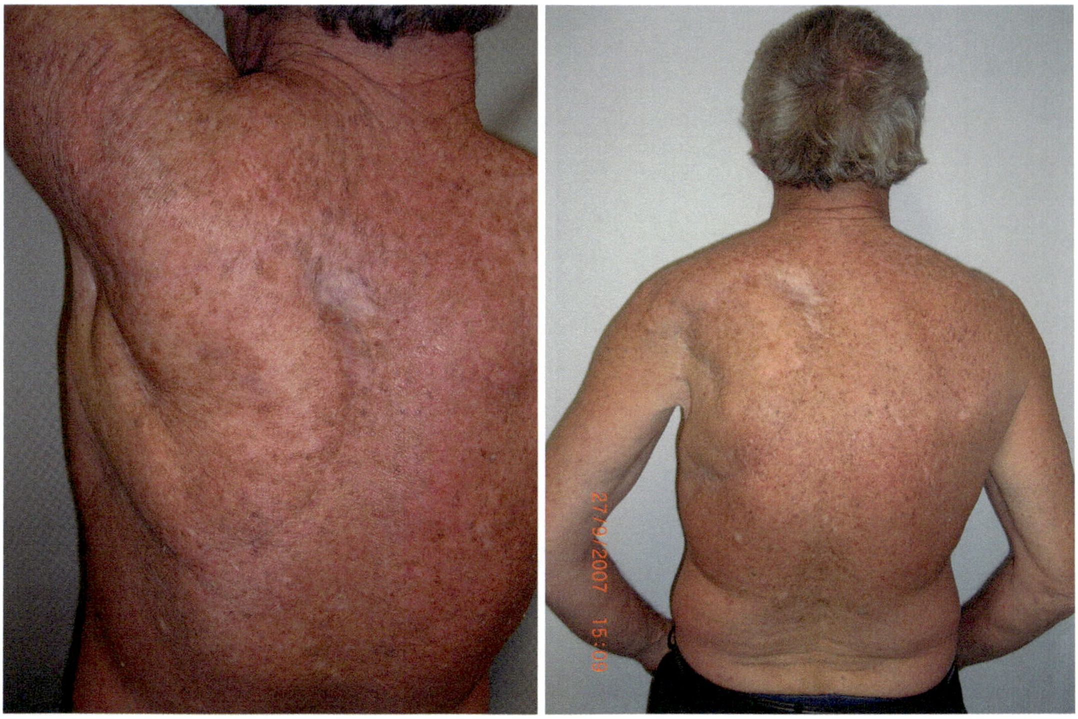

Fig. 1.29 Full functional rotation of the shoulder girdle without any pain or limitations of range of movement (ROM) after 6 weeks was achieved, and this was an important contribution to the patient's mental stability given that he had mental health problems in the past. He was pain-free and preparing to mountaineer up the Himalayas

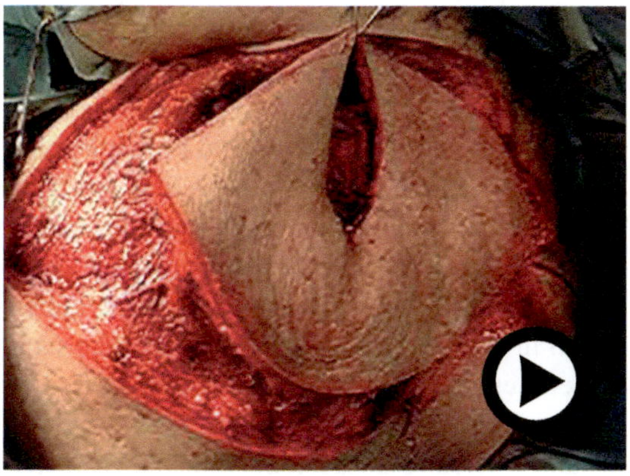

Fig. 1.30 Video 1.1 The operative sequence and the laxity of the surrounding tissues facilitate the closure turning into wound apposition (▶ https://doi.org/10.1007/000-k5w)

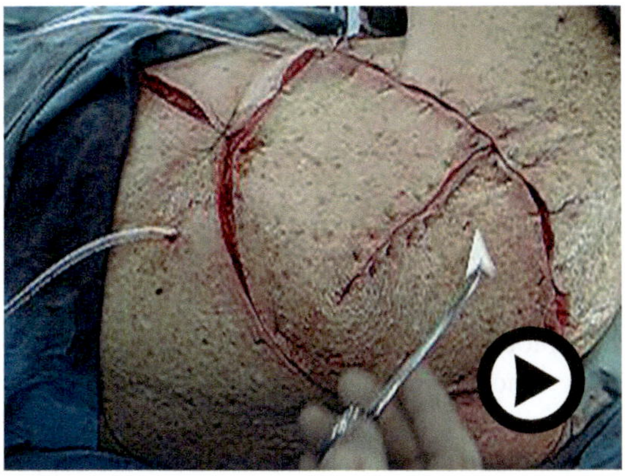

Fig. 1.31 Video 1.2 The standard three-phase locking mattress suture technique was used throughout, and post-operatively, wound care followed the standard method (▶ https://doi.org/10.1007/000-k5v)

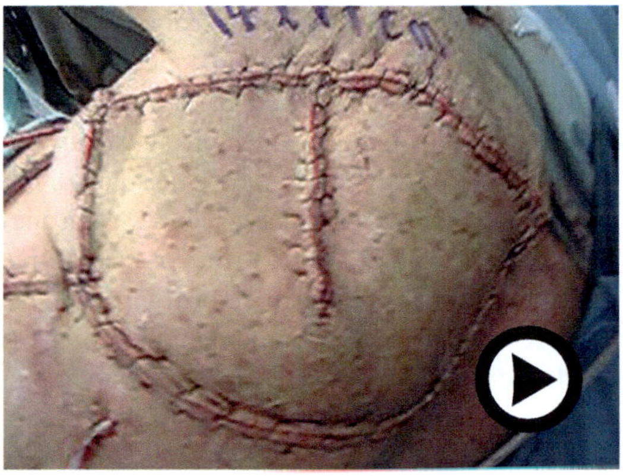

Fig. 1.32 Video 1.3 The operative sequence technique (▶ https://doi.org/10.1007/000-k5x)

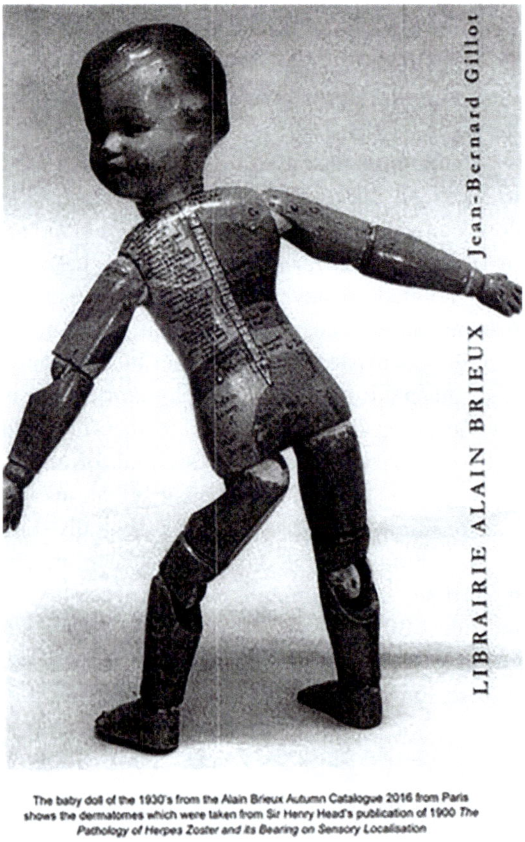

Fig. 1.33 Sir Henry Head's dermatome doll

neurovascular supply of the flap and is economically applicable in routine Keystone closure. In routine closure, the random circulation is based on the following assumption: If there is a nerve supply, there must be a blood supply. None of the nerves needs to be defined; instead, the mark out of the dermatome can be used, which, embryologically, must contain vascular support for its neural development as an overview.

1.5.3 The Keystone Simplifies Reconstructive Surgery

Fascial lining is an absolute prerequisite to line the deep surface of the Keystone mark out for safety purposes and a prerequisite for the source of the perforator supply, including neurovascular support and the accompanying autonomic, somatic and lymphatic input. The division of the deep fascia allows the unit to swing in a collateral way, and this single integumentary Keystone flap closes this double defect (the lesion and the flap) under tension—two for the price of one with drainage.

The dermatome roadmap is a random source of vascular guidance without defining perforators specifically. Thus, the Keystone is designated within the dermatomal mark out and an axiomatic rule applies as random perforators embryologically follow the neural patterns of the dermatome, thus ensuring viability with arterial, venous and lympho-venular anastomoses.

The *three-phase single-layer suturing technique* for closure avoids exerting inadvertent pressure on the microvascular perforators and has been adopted throughout, and we use a standard three-phase suturing technique to achieve a satisfactory closure. Locking mattress nylon sutures at the points of tension stay in situ for 3 weeks and are used on almost every occasion in most cases. The ordinary mattress sutures used to complete the wound closure stay in situ for 2 weeks. And the epidermal running suture closure is done with a continuous 3/0 nylon to provide perfect epidermal alignment and a perfect seal, and these sutures can even be cut after a 7-day period to achieve a satisfactory aesthetic outcome. Absorbable subcutaneous sutures, used as a layered closure technique, are thus avoided, allowing the locking mattress suture to compensate for any deeper defect. Additionally, the absorbable sutures often leave a subcutaneous line of wound-healing reactions, and these lumps tend to be permanent, an observed clinical finding that contradicts published material stating that they are absorbable. If these basic principles are followed, as I have developed over my reconstructive career and illustrated in all these cases, then acceptable outcomes that match the aesthetic developments and appearances are achievable.

1.6 Arteriovenous, Lymphatic Communications and Angiogenesis Are Supported by the Angiotome Concept

Arteriovenous, lymphatic communications and angiogenesis reflect the success of the Angiotome concept [22]; that is, vessels along the dermatomal alignments always exist anatomically. A vascularised dermatome allows one to use comments on vascular supply, which lead to the initiation of this angiotome concept, which is defined in Dorland's medical dictionary as a vascularised segment. Thus, flaps with a fascio-cutaneous base may well be described as a fascio-cutaneous angiotome. This is defined as a system of linked axial pattern flaps using the dermatomes as an aide-mémoire for alignment and design. This concept developed from my research into flap vascularity at the Royal College of Surgeons in London in 1971 as a Bernard Sunley Research Fellow when the importance of the fascial layer in locoregional flaps became self-evident when doing vascular injection studies. The study of the blood supply of the integument led to certain anatomical conclusions about the importance of this fascial layer concept in locoregional repairs. This was presented to the Sixth International Congress of Plastic and Reconstructive Surgery, in Paris in 1975 [3], which gained the support of the international surgical community, including the late Professor John Hueston, Professor William Manchester and Professor Daniel Marchac.

The arteriovenous and lymphatic communications with angiogenesis become clinically illustrated by the cases discussed. The clinical cases provide key support and evidence, and they will be discussed in the subsequent parts in Volumes 1 and 2, including the head and neck, the trunk, the upper and lower limbs, including the groin and axillae.

The dermatomes are the aides-mémoire used to facilitate clinical execution. This avoids the costly investigation of angiography—a standard in microsurgical procedures—which has not been applied to any of these Keystone cases, marking another cost-saving benefit. Intact nerve supply is consistent with an intact blood supply. The universal dermatome designs are the basis for Keystone orientation and are then elevated with a fascial substrate. It is essential for undermined flaps when advancement, rotation and transposition are necessary, but essentially, one must cautiously leave one-third of deep attachment if any undermining is deemed necessary, as in Fig. 1.30. However, the epidermal division ensures the island flap design, which is closed directly on completion as a single layer using

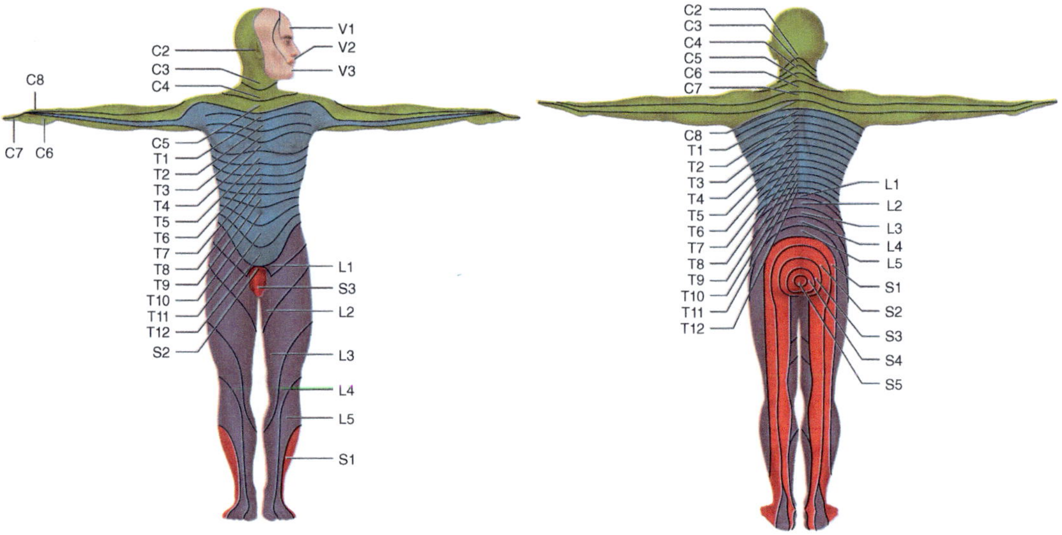

Fig. 1.34 The dermatomal precincts. (Reprinted with permission, *Keystone Flap for Complex Orthopaedic Problems* (p. 13), by Felix Behan, Springer Nature 2024)

locking mattress sutures and a continuous 3/0 nylon for epidermal seal. This ensures the sympathectomy effect of islanding. These dermatome precincts are illustrated in Fig. 1.34, and the Keystone design must lie within the dermatomal mark outs (Fig. 1.34).

1.7 Microvascular Alternatives Are Usually Avoided

Microvascular support has not been found necessary in any of these cases in the event of a recurrence, because the laxity of the tissue is sacrificed, and therefore, any recurrence needs fresh tissue input, which requires microvascular input.

Keystone management has broken certain management rules from a reconstructive perspective, allowing us to continue the Gillies dictum of like for like in any reconstructive saga. The microsurgical dominance now has to be revisited because of cost when one recognises the advantages of the Keystone repair in comparison, its PACES characteristics and helps to avoid such criticisms. Governed by the need for success, let alone aesthetic outcomes, multiple descriptions of techniques plague the literature with various anatomical and architectural variations. The value of pedicle flaps, evolving from microsurgical repair, has been in vogue, and the Blondeel perforator book [35] is the latest update summarising such applications in a universal way. The Keystone technique, which features in the Blondeel book thanks to Prof. Geoffrey Hallock, is based on random perforators from the suprafascial and infrafascial layers, which are sourced from deeper perforators that are often from a muscular orientation. This avoids angiographic investigation and thus has cost-saving implications.

We have all been victims of metamorphosis through the reconstructive perspective from Ian Jackson's work with Gwynn Morgan and through the groin flap that led to Taylor and Daniel's initial microsurgical publication. Aesthetics and function can be found wanting, which applies to many microsurgical applications, as illustrated in Figs. 2.336, 3.10, 3.11 and 3.12. None of the cases in this series, except one, needed microsurgical reconstructive support as a final compromise seeking a solution. Another plastic surgical edict that has been questioned is the use of the Keystone in irradiated tissue, which features frequently in head and neck cases and is the domain for microsurgical repair in most units. In Volume 2, three microsurgical procedures—lat dorsi, radial forearm and gracilis—failed when basic surgical principles were ignored, and they were the victims of having dead space in the bone that was not corrected with any filler. The Keystone technique allows bone graft to fill the dead space with drainage even though orthopaedically bone grafts are not done in infected tissue; however, we succeeded thanks to the hypervascularity of the Keystone, as discussed above.

The Lamberty [36] classification of vascular perfusion may need to be revamped because of these ongoing clinical experiences and not on the basis of latex injection studies on cadavers. Again, the success of the Keystone reconstructive technique is based on ongoing clinical successes revealed through patients' personal responses on video, all of whom are grateful. Reassessing the Keystone is an emerging development, and the Keystone's wider acceptance as an alternative to microsurgical procedures is slowing being re-evaluated. I should add that it is used by units around the world because of its clinical usefulness and has proved its clinical value by not skeletonising perforators, presumably stripping them of somatic, autonomic and lymphatic support. The Keystone preserves the integrity of all these random perforators in a suprafascial and infrafascial orientation. As I stated above, the Keystone's success is based on fascial support as long as one-third of deep attachment remains to supply the epidermal cover as a lifeline and as a means to avoid necrosis. If any release is necessary for advancement or rotation, the variations on the Keystone design will help to rectify the problem as long as the fascia is retained. This respects the integrity of the random perforators.

As the possibility of long-term satisfactory outcome and respecting the patient's wish for an aesthetic outcome, this is where the Keystone seems to unify all the variables, and as described above, the PACES acronym is synoptic. Another advantage of this expeditious means of reconstruction is governed by the patient's comorbidity status, and concerns with complications from mismanagement aggravate the morbidity factor in elderly patients. Thus, if the radical removal of a groin mass or access to the neck or the femur that is comparable to a groin clearance procedure for an open reduction and internal fixation (ORIF) can be done by using this simplified technique, this is where the Keystone application becomes pre-eminently successful. The simplified closure using the L1 dermatome from the anterior thigh, moving upwards and inwards with division of the tensor fascia lata and the fascia down the medial side of the thigh, is described in Volume 2. Distally, the island design is mandatory after creating a division in the epidermis across the suprapatellar region to ensure that the hypervascularity factors of the Keystone are retained to ensure expeditious healing.

References

1. Behan FC, Terrill PJ, Ashton MW. Fasciocutaneous island flaps for orthopaedic management in lower limb reconstruction using dermatomal precincts. ANZ J Surg. 1994;64(3):155–66.
2. Behan FC. The keystone design perforator island flap in reconstructive surgery. ANZ J Surg. 2003;73:112–20.
3. Behan F. Evolution of the fascio-cutaneous island flap leading to the keystone flap principle in lower limb reconstruction. ANZ J Surg. 2008;78:116–7.
4. Behan FC, Lo CH, Shayan R. Perforator territory of the keystone flap – use of the dermatomal roadmap. J Plast Reconstr Aesthet Surg. 2009;62:551–3. https://doi.org/10.1016/j.bjps.2008.08.078.
5. Behan F, Sizeland A, Gilmour F, Hui A, Seel M, Lo CH. Use of the keystone island flap for advanced head and neck cancer in the elderly. J Plast Reconstr Aesthet Surg. 2010;63:739–45.
6. Behan FC, Rozen WM, Tan S. Yin-Yang flaps: the mathematics of two keystone island flaps for reconstructing increasingly large defects. ANZ J Surg. 2011;81:574–5.
7. Behan FC, Rozen WM, Lo CH, Findlay M. The omega – Ω – variant designs (types A and B) of the keystone perforator island flap. ANZ J Surg. 2011;81:650–2.
8. Behan F, Findlay M, Lo CH. The keystone perforator island flap concept. Sydney: Elsevier Textbook Churchill Livingstone; 2012.
9. Behan FC, Rozen WM, Azer S, Gran P. Perineal keystone design perforator island flap for perineal and vulval reconstruction. ANZ J Surg. 2012;82:381–2.
10. Behan FC, Paddle A, Rozen WM, et al. Quadriceps keystone island flap for radical inguinal lymphad-

enectomy: a reliable locoregional island flap for large groin defects. ANZ J Surg. 2013;83:942–7.
11. Behan F. Surgical tips and skills illustrating the keystone principle. Sydney: Elsevier Textbook Churchill Livingstone; 2014.
12. Behan FC, Sizeland A. Keystone perforator island flaps in major head and neck surgery – the P.A.C.E. perspectives. World J Surg Surg Res. 2021;4:1293.
13. Behan FC. Keystone perforator island flap in lower limb reconstruction. Aust J Plast Surg. 2021;4(2):105–7. https://doi.org/10.34239/ajops.v4n2.341.
14. Behan FC. Atlas of keystone reconstructive technique in the management of Melanoma. Springer International; 2023.
15. Behan FC. Keystone flap for complex orthopaedic problems. Springer International; 2024.
16. Fede C, Petrelli L, Pirri C, Neuhuber W, Tiengo C, Biz C, De Caro R, Schleip R, Stecco C. Innervation of human superficial fascia. Front Neuroanat. 2022;16:981426. https://doi.org/10.3389/fnana.2022.981426.
17. Pirri C, Petrelli L, Fede C, Guidolin D, Tiengo C, De Caro R, Stecco C. Blood supply to the superficial fascia of the abdomen: an anatomical study. Clin Anat. 2023;36(4):570–80.
18. Behrbohm H. History of facial plastic surgery in Europe. The European Academy of Facial Plastic Surgery.
19. Esser JF. Studies in plastic surgery of the face: I use of skin from the neck to replace face defects. II. Plastic operations about the mouth. III. The epidermic inlay. Ann Surg. 1917;65(3):297–315.
20. Behan F, et al. Island flaps, including the Bezier type in the treatment of malignant melanoma. ANZ J Surg. 1995;65:870–80.
21. Limberg AA. The planning of local plastic operations on the body surface. Toronto: Collamore Press; 1984.
22. Behan FC, Wilson JSP. The principle of the angiotome a system of linked axial pattern flaps. In: Transactions of the 6th international congress on plastic and reconstructive surgery. Paris: Masson; 1975.
23. Neuman C. The expansion of an area of skin by progressive distention of a subcutaneous balloon. Use of the method for securing skin for subtotal reconstruction of the ear. Plast Reconstr Surg. 1957;19:124–30.
24. Pelissier P, Casoli V, Bakhach J, Martin D, Baudet J. Reverse dorsal digital and metacarpal flaps: a review of 27 cases. Plast Reconstr Surg. 1999;103(1):159–65.
25. Royle JP. A history of sympathectomy. ANZ J Surg. 1999;69:302–7.
26. Coventry B, Walsh J. Cutaneous innervation in man before and after lumbar sympathectomy: evidence for interruption of both sensory and vasomotor nerve fibres. ANZ J Surg. 2003;73:14–1827.
27. Quote Investigator. Absence of evidence is not evidence of absence, 17 Sept 2019.
28. Lo C, Nottle T, Mills J. Keystone island flap: effects of islanding on vascularity. Plast Reconstr Surg Glob Open. 2016;4(2):e617.
29. Behan F, et al. Oncologic clearance with preservation of reconstructive options: literature review and the 'delayed reconstruction after pathology evaluation (DRAPE)' technique. ANZ J Surg. 2012;82(11):780–5.
30. Barron J, Emmett A. Subcutaneous pedicle flaps. Br J Plast Surg. 1965;18:51–78.
31. Taylor I, Daniel R. The free flap: composite tissue transfer by vascular anastomosis. ANZ J Surg. 1973;43(1):1–3.
32. Ockham W. Stanford encyclopedia of philosophy. Archived from the original on 7 Oct 2019. Retrieved 24 Feb 2016.
33. Rodriguez-Unda N, Abraham J, Saint-Cyr M. Keystone and perforator flaps in reconstruction. Clin Plast Surg. 2020;47(4):635–48. Elsevier.
34. Head H, Campbell AW. The pathology of herpes zoster and its bearing on sensory localisation. BRAIN Part III; 1900.
35. Blondeel P, et al. Perforator flaps: anatomy, technique and clinical applications. Missouri: Quality Medical Publishing; 2013.
36. Cormack GC, Lamberty BG. Cadaver studies of correlation between vessel size and anatomical territory of cutaneous supply. Br J Plast Surg. 1986;39(3):300–6.

2 Major Head and Neck Defects

Contents

2.1 Case Presentations

Traditionally, head and neck reconstruction is a formidable challenge [1]—usually involving the domain of microsurgical free flap reconstructions, where tissue from another site is often a poor tissue match.

The Keystone flap allows one to close large soft-tissue defects, even under tension, because they are all random and perforator based and receive no contribution from any input from the subdermal plexus, where islanding creates an umbrella of tissue circumventing tension with contributions from the subdermal plexus, as indicated with the Red Dot Sign and vascular flare, which are valid observations of this reconstructive tool, which has been repetitively seen to avoid necrosis. The neurodermatomal pattern is the basis of the Keystone's success in the design format and of the characteristics of the Keystone, namely pain-free, aesthetic, complication rarity, economical and sensory recovery, or PACES:

Pain-free: Why are they *pain-free?* All surgeons have experienced surgical wounds with a nonsensate area in the healed phase along the links of the incision that takes some weeks to eventually recover sensate supply. The Keystone and its island design follow the same idea that no somatic input at the integumentary level subsequently recovers, which allows the patient to say that they are totally pain-

Supplementary Information The online version contains supplementary material available at https://doi.org/10.1007/978-3-032-21716-5_2. The videos can be accessed individually by clicking the DOI link in the accompanying figure caption or by scanning this link with the SN More Media App.

F. Behan, *Keystone Reconstructive Solutions for Major Surgical Defects*,
https://doi.org/10.1007/978-3-032-21716-5_2

free. Could the cutaneous somatic supply divided around the arc of the Keystone create a temporary anaesthetic surface that takes some weeks to recover, as is characteristic of all linear surgical wounds? The only symptom that the patient notices is a feeling of tightness, which is one of the key features when wounds are closed under such tension. Again, we have broken one of the rules in reconstructive surgery: to not close under tension. But such are the elements of hypervascularity with the Red Dot Sign, where closure under tension is a clinical possibility, and it allows us to trim out dog ears, avoiding a secondary procedure, sometimes indicated for aesthetic reasons. The cases listed illustrate these observations, undermining the criticisms of the uninitiated.

Aesthetics The Gillies principle of using *like for like* is a standard reconstructive principle entrenched in history, one producing outcomes that are most satisfying to the patient, particularly on exposed sites. The normal attractive appearance of the integument is lost when large defects are grafted or when microvascular free flaps, without tissue matching, are used to fill the soft-tissue contour defects out of surgical necessity.

Complications Complications and adverse outcomes are not common in vascular repair, because of the hyperaemic effect achieved in the island flap based on suprafascial and infrafascial circulation. Sometimes sutures need to be realigned to eliminate any lines of tension in the flap repair, but the major wound breakdown occurs when dressings are done at an outside clinic with the premature removal of sutures and when the principles of closure with the Keystone have not been respected. Again, the surgical repair is a standard three-phase locking mattress suture technique, as illustrated throughout all the cases, and conceivably, if wound dressing is delegated to an inexperienced operator, the single layer of the locking mattress suture could lead to wound breakdown. My 3-week rule for points of tension is applied routinely, and when the locking mattress loop is cut, the suture is easily delivered, without having to look for hours for the buried knot in the deep mattress suture. Vascular complications do occur, particularly in diabetic patients and those with vascular impendence, because these flaps are not based on a singular perforator but rather a filamentous collection, which becomes defined only with blunt dissection and the teasing apart of the tissues to achieve closure. Perforators are not precisely defined, because the reliance on the filamentous network helps to overcome the problem of blood supply. Skeletonising for perforators may strip away the filamentous autonomic, somatic and lymphatic supports along the axial channels of such vascular perforators at suprafascial and infrafascial locations. Irradiated tissue is not a contraindication in the use of Keystone applications, because of the hypervascularity principles already discussed. In a type II diabetic patient's lower limb, where microcirculation is the focus of pathology, the elements of partial necrosis have occurred, and as a consequence, closure must be done without tension, and a generous use of skin grafting is an alternative fallback position, particularly in patients aged 50-95 when located in the lower limb.

Expeditious execution 'Time is money' is a Benjamin Franklin quote from Fisher's book of 1748. If one can operate in a reduced timeframe, this has benefits for all modalities in the treatment and care of patients, particularly elderly patients. It also has an economic factor and affects theatre throughput, whereas long reconstructive sagas continue to produce adverse alternatives. Microsurgical team procedures have cost implications and time implications, particularly for staff allocation and the availability of theatre time. We all have experiences of umpteen cases being cancelled because microsurgical reconstructions are still continuing in spite of inadvertent or intermittent setbacks. The Keystone cases illustrated here will go some way to overcoming this setback, and the audiovisual account helps to facilitate the teaching process.

Somatic recovery with the resolution of oedema These final outcome characteristics go hand in hand with surgical success, and we have tried to elaborate on certain areas to bypass any incidental complications, such as wound breakdown with any premature removal of sutures (staples are not used). As in any surgical wound, the division of the filamentous cutaneous branches creates a temporary anaesthetic field around the operative site. This may recover in the weeks that follow when the integument has healed and the scar is maturing. A final characteristic under observation is the resolution of swelling and oedema, which occurs during a recovery period of up to 8 weeks. My observational suggestion is that when the sympathectomy effect of the island fascial flap is evident with vascular flare and Red Dot Signs, it could simply be transferred to the lymphatic network as a means of explaining why swellings at the surgical site seem to resolve spontaneously.

Reconstruction utilising the principles of subunits does not apply, because the Keystone allows one to reconstruct the surgical defect on the basis of the surgical site and the region-preserving function. Also, the facial grimace lines are all respected, and that adds to the approximation to a normal appearance from the scalp, forehead, nose, cheeks and the periorbital and perioral regions, which meets the patient's desires for aesthetics. What some specialists [2, 3] call subunits, I term *neurodermatomal alignments* in Keystone reconstruction.

Locoregional flaps, parts of the standard plastic surgical repertoire, are listed in every textbook on reconstructive techniques. The Keystone embraces all these variables, and its success, even closing under tension, is due to the characteristic of its applications.

Lip: Some of these locoregional principles go back to the time of Gillies [4] and the Karapandzic flap [5] with its retained innervation, particularly in lip reconstruction. My Keystone variant of the lip in an oncological case shows the value of dermatomal alignments, which are based on embryological mark outs. The value of such a system is an example of fulfilling the Gillies edict of creating a reconstruction using 'like for like'.

The *suturing technique* employs the standard three-phase single-layer elements of the following:

- Locking mattress sutures with deep fascial involvement at the points of tension stay in for 3 weeks.
- Ordinary locking mattress sutures close the wound to align the epidermis and avoid a subcutaneous cat gut, and the nylon closes all layers all in anatomical alignment. These stay in for 1–2 weeks.
- The continuous surface nylon suture is used to achieve an epidermal seal, which are cut at 7 days to perfect wound healing.
- Absorbable sutures are avoided because of their unreliability in closing under tension, and wound breakdown is a more common occurrence when they are used. Additionally, the absorbable sutures often leave a subcutaneous line of wound-healing reactions, which often lead to subcutaneous lumps, lumps that prevent a completely aesthetic presentation and tend to be permanent.

Every case illustrated here is repaired by this standard three-phase suture technique, which avoids deep dermal sutures because they might interfere with or impede fine filamentous circulation, the basis of the Keystone circulation support and the Keystone's success. Skin grafts are rarely used, though they are used in sites of *extreme tension*, such as in cases of nasal reconstruction; for example, a full-thickness graft was used in Case 38.

Locoregional flaps, including bilobed flaps [6], rhomboidal flaps [7], transpositional flaps [8] and hatchet flaps [9], have been superseded by this Keystone reconstructive design because island flaps are safer when deep attachment leaves only one-third of the dissected base. The design of the Keystone can be schematically likened to two conjoined V-Y flaps, which yields larger flap coverage areas while retaining *vascular perfusion* (Fig 2.1).

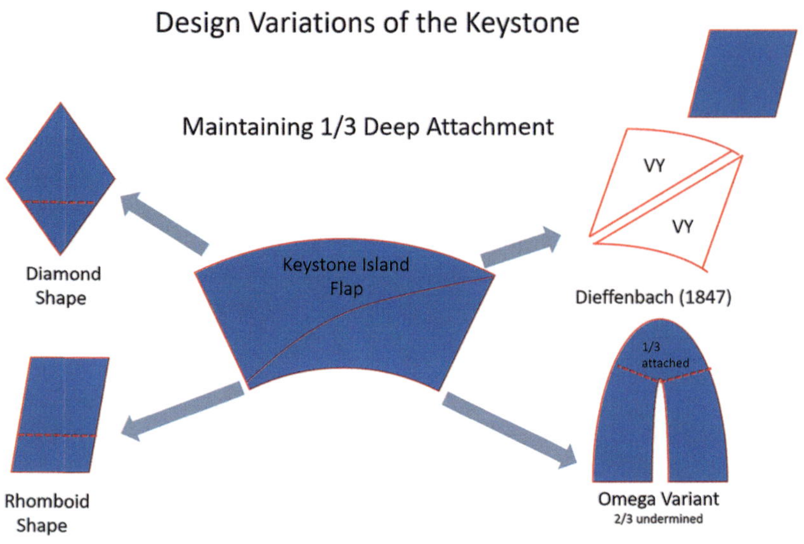

Fig. 2.1 Design variations of the Keystone flap are governed by the surgical defect needed for repair

Free tissue transfer is not part of the design requirements with the Keystone, except where large scalp defects preclude its effectiveness, and in that case, the use of a latissimus dorsi free flap becomes necessary.

Jaw reconstruction cover: The Keystone flap may play a part in the facial contour soft-tissue reconstruction overlying any microvascular jaw replacement. No cases in this series relate to this application; that is, no microsurgery was previously performed.

For bony defects of the face, such as in the vicinity of the ethmoid complex (Case 40) or lateral maxilla (Case 57), standard teaching creates mucosal replacement via skin grafting the deep surface of any reconstruction flap. Such techniques can be avoided given that the mucosal lining from the sinuses advances over the deep surface of the Keystone. As we know, mucosa 'grows like grass', and using a mucosal replacement over an exposed sinus avoids the crusting problems of skin grafting the deep surface of the flap, which has been the standard in plastic surgery teaching.

In the scalp melanoma case (Case 64) illustrated using the island flap, which was not quite Keystone in design but which reflected the Keystone characteristics without skeletonising the posterior occipital artery, which was advanced into the defect while retaining all the periadventitial components of the neurovascular stalk. We see the outcome of tightness in the postoperative phase without pain, aesthetic match, no complications, an expeditious operating timeframe and the return of sensory function. All the defects in the major defect series were repaired around those specific axes of named vessels, but again, skeletonising them for ease of mobilisation detracts from its overall usefulness and is not necessary.

Multiple other variations, such as bilobe flaps, rotational flaps and pinwheel flaps, are just named flaps that incorporate design variations.

Forehead and temple reconstruction, as in Case 32, shows the value of the island flap reconstruction that is based on the V2 area of the infraorbital neurovascular structure but that has been turned into an island to embrace the Keystone principles of hypervascularity in a tissue plane on a single neurovascular stalk—the infraorbital neurovascular complex. Advancement and rotation techniques are parts of the island flap, which can adopt the Keystone characteristics to optimise closure and repair.

The Keystone application in ear reconstruction relates to complex issues like reconstructing the conchal fossa. The cases illustrated here show the advantage of the C2 and C3 cervico-submental flap from the neck, undermined containing cervical fascia but leaving one-third of the proximal area attached over sternomastoid to retain random perforators, which are not defined. The Keystone island flap closes the conchal defect with a de-epithelialised bridge, allowing the reconstruction of the conchal defect and allowing the helix margin to be reinserted, reflecting the hypervascularity and thus the safety of such a repair.

The Keystone closure of parotid defects has made a valuable contribution in this area of reconstruction, normally the province of free flap repair. It needs no elaboration on the aesthetic outcome using locoregional repair when compared with microvascular tissue borrowed from an external source. The aesthetic outcome reflects the patient's satisfaction, whereas at clinics that have not used this Keystone reconstructive method, the constant story of the patient's dissatisfaction is not unique. Patients have become social outcasts hiding from society and wearing clothing as a disguise for any public appearance. The Keystone provides an alternative option, and the technique is easily mastered when the regulations are followed: dermatomal alignment, fascially based, totally islanded, leaving one-third deep attachment at the point of rotation and retaining all venous links.

Nasal reconstruction: The aesthetic units of the nose are respected, and the applications of the Keystone and its variants at three sites facilitates nasal repair. The side of the nose and a V-Y island flap (the hemisection of a Keystone) provides skin closure that is pain-free, with an aesthetic appearance, without complications, within an expeditious timeframe and with full sensory recovery. This V-Y principle based inferiorly adjacent to the lobule can be advanced, rotated and transposed to reconstruct nasal tips by advancing the tissue without skeletonising vascular axes to reach the nasal tip.

The nasal tip procedure using a collateral Keystone is advanced from the side of the nose and teased with blunt dissection with random branches from the facial artery, and the nerve supply stems from the infraorbital complex used to cover the defect.

The Keystone variant for total nasal cover reconstruction employs a forehead flap principle using a Keystone variant design that is placed along the bridge of the nose to meet the nasal tip, avoiding tension, and grafting the forehead should it be deemed necessary, as revealed in Case 38. It is based on supraorbital and supratrochlear neurovascular axes, which achieve soft-tissue cover. The lateral side of the nose is covered with a full-thickness graft to yield an acceptable aesthetic outcome.

Keystone application in cheek reconstruction is a fairly simple procedure, as detailed in the cases below. An example can be found in one of the malar eminence cases, where the procedure extends down to the mid-section and over the angle of the mandible in a 97-year-old, and a massive 6 × 5 cm reconstruction is an example of a Hutchinson melanotic freckle in a 76-year-old. The aesthetic balance in the reconstruction of the cheek is evident, and the Keystone characteristics are fully visualised in all that flaps that close the wound aesthetically:

Pain-free postoperative outcome
Aesthetically acceptable method of reconstruction
Complication rarity in wound problems
Expeditious execution and favourably comparable to microsurgical sagas
Somatic recovery and rapidly resolved swelling, confirming lymphatic drainage and presumably the dilation of the lymphatic trunks in a similar way to that of the vascular trunks

In *irradiated fields*, which usually preclude standard forms of reconstruction because of the subdermal vascular insufficiency created by radiation treatment, the Keystone reconstruction overcomes any restriction because it becomes hypervascularised. In Case 42, the slightly variable appearance of the hyperaemic phase is noticeable with the predominant circulation in the flare over the posterior margin adjacent to the auricular temporal perforators, with facial artery branches involved. The anterior section of the Keystone is supplied by the collateral circulation branches, and the predominant flare is evident along the line of the artery. This healed without necrotic complications.

Finally, the Keystone has sound applications in elderly patients when the expeditious repair is of paramount importance, especially for anaesthetic safety.

The *lip reconstruction* for a Hutchinson's Melanotic Freckleinvolving 2–3 cm along the vermilion margin is a simple surgical exercise when direct closure is standard practice. This avoids the complication of the shaving margin along the vermilion. If it is closed directly without a Keystone, the margins of the vermilion become close to the hair-bearing tissue of the lip. This simple technique of doing a mucosal island flap from the inner surface of the lower lip in a Keystone design and with blunt dissection can refashion the lower lip and returns the lip to normal function, and the mucosal defect in the buccal sulcus is allowed to mucosalise, healing through secondary intention without any surgical closure of the secondary defect. Otherwise, the vermilion inversion would occur with hair-bearing tissue along the margin. The two-thirds excision of the lower lip in Case 36 and its subsequent closure using the V3 dermatome for the external repair and a mucosal island at the region of the L modiolus creates normal lip apposition without any effect on mastication, articulation or drinking.

In the *neck*, the applications of the Keystone along clavicular perforators and intercostal perforators are all random. Leaving one-third of the Keystone attached ensures viability, hyperaemia and an aesthetic match in like-for-like closure, without complications, which is expeditiously sound in principle with full sensory recovery. Again, we achieve these outcomes on the basis of using embryological mark outs, avoiding microsurgical free flaps on such an exposed site.

Each of the cases below substantiates my findings and is accompanied by photographic images with video supplements in the operative procedure. The achieved outcome is explained, and the basis of our clinical observational findings, which have been repeated, is evident.

In summary, the Keystone is a universal technique with applications in most sites of the body, and for major head and neck defects, it seems to supersede all the eponymous names of locoregional designs over the years. This simple idea in terminology—the Keystone—is based on embryological principles, with dermatomal alignments and wide applications.

2.1.1 Parotid/Ear

Surgical defects in the region of the *parotid* are usually associated with the excision of primary or secondary lesions and the underlying *parotid mass* as an oncological principle, with or without neck dissection, usually indicating levels II, III and IV and usually excised as one mass.

This case series extends in age from 35 to 97 years. But the Keystone reconstructive principle can embrace all age groups, and the speed and efficiency of reconstruction are always welcomed by the anaesthetic team thanks to the rapid exit off the operating table despite age and morbidity concerns. This case series covers simple reconstructions and complex reconstructions depending on the location and whether the pathology is recurrent. Additionally, all the Keystone clinical characteristics, as summarised in the PACES acronym, can be visualised and have been recorded, including patients' responses. The closure under tension avoids any facial nerve reconstruction, and this static rather than dynamic method increases speed and efficiency with no drawbacks from the patient's point of view.

The size of the oncological defect is not a contraindication for the Keystone application, as in Case 1, even in the case of undermining. Closing under tension yet hypervascularising the perfusion is a guarantee of successful wound closure and sound healing, another edict in surgery that can now be reassessed.

The parotid cases illustrated in my earlier publication, titled 'Atlas of Keystone Reconstructive Technique in the Management of Melanoma' [10], are not repeated here for obvious reasons but can be retrieved separately in the Melanoma Atlas.

The anatomical breakdown of the *ear* with its skin and cartilaginous components is easily repaired when wedge excisions and the like are necessary for melanoma. However, the Keystone is particularly relevant in conchal fossa reconstructions. The postauricular design using random mastoidal and postauricular neurovascular structures can be channelled from the postauricular groove into the conchal defect by using the trapdoor principle. By attaching it to the epidermal lining of the external canal, the helix rim can be aligned back over the Keystone bridge defect, which is de-epithelialised over the helical mark out and repaired surgically to cover exposed tissue and yield anatomical and aesthetic continuity. This is a new concept in conchal fossa reconstruction.

2.1.1.1 Case 1—Massive 10 × 9 cm Parotid Defect with Neck Dissection Levels II, III and IV, Where the Continuity is Closed with a Cervico-submental Keystone

Level III melanoma over the R parotid with secondary dissemination into the R neck is involved. The clearance of the tumour includes levels II, III and IV neck dissection. Cervical undermining is indicated by the digital elevation of the cervical skin, fascia and neck tissue in this 70-year-old woman (Figs. 2.2, 2.3, 2.4, 2.5, 2.6, 2.7, 2.8, 2.9, 2.10 and 2.11).

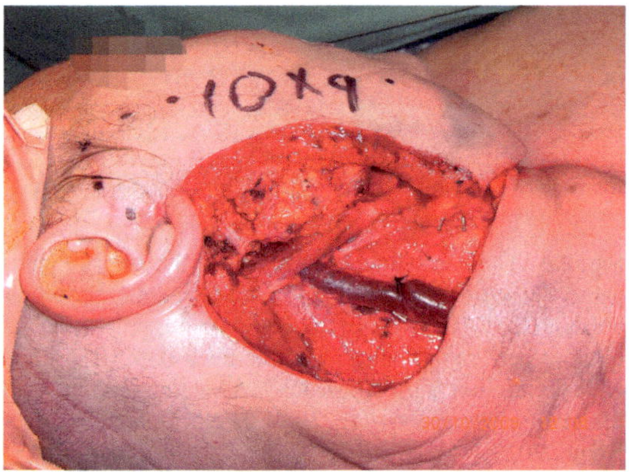

Fig. 2.2 The defect size is 10 × 9 cm. Facial nerve function has been preserved. The external jugular vein has been preserved and repaired if necessary for any tributary rupture. This ensures adequate venous drainage, a prerequisite for healthy flap survival. A McGregor [11] edict of our past training always stipulated that flap necrosis is usually a consequence of venous stasis and not necessarily arterial insufficiency

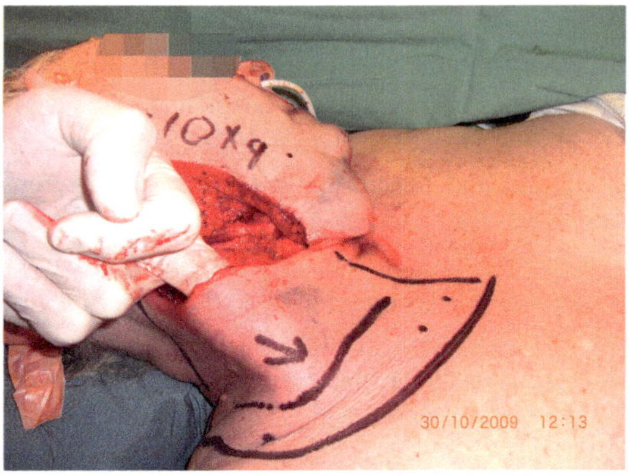

Fig. 2.3 The extent of undermining in the neck tissue for cervical nodal clearance levels II and III from the neck dissection would be a contraindication and constitute a different form of reconstruction. Yet the Keystone principle overcomes this potential problem with its hypervascularity. The working rule for the design of the infra-supraclavicular circulatory perforator support is that circulatory healing can be maintained as long as one-third of deep flap attachment remains distal to the undermined section. The dots constitute a guide to the random supraclavicular perforators, which are randomly located and not individually sited

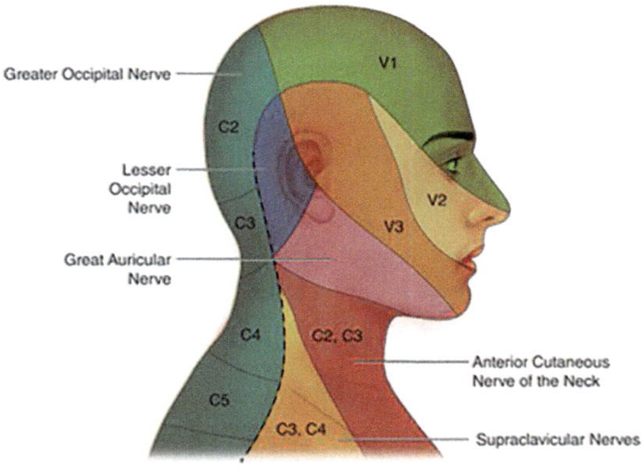

Fig. 2.4 The dermatomal mark outs of the anterior cutaneous nerve of the neck (C2, C3) and the supraclavicular nerves (C3, C4) designate the compass alignment for the random perforator support for this neck flap. (Reprinted with permission from Atlas, *Reconstructive Technique in Melanoma Management* (p. 19), by Felix Behan, Springer Nature 2023)

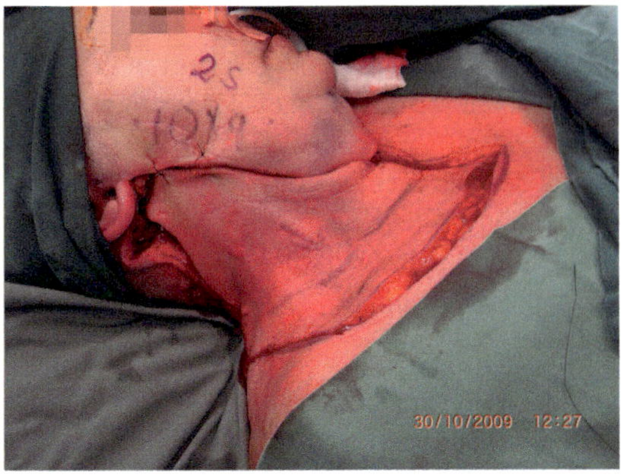

Fig. 2.5 Islanding creates hyperaemia, indicating flap viability. The closure is achieved with a neck tilt with some tension when using the apical three-phase standard locking mattress suture technique. The island flap mark out ensures Keystone hyperaemia, guaranteeing successful closure under tension and a pain-free postoperative phase

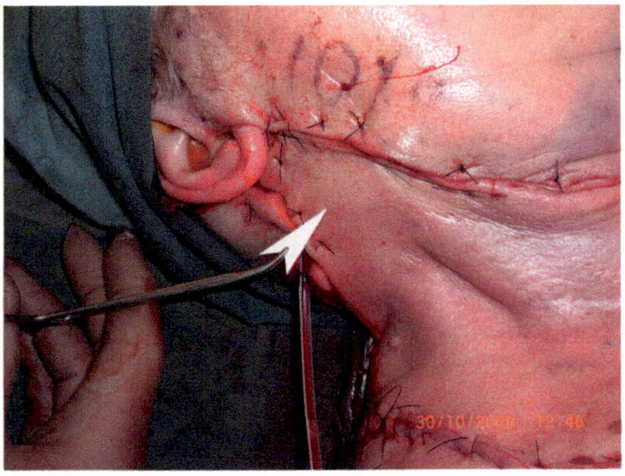

Fig. 2.6 This staged closure of a wound and the apex of the flap (arrowed) show no sign of vascular insufficiency, once more confirming the Keystone characteristic of hypervascularity. The standard three-phase single-layer suture technique is employed: (1) locking mattress sutures are introduced at the tension points, (2) an interrupted mattress aligns the wound and (3) continuous nylon closes the epidermal level

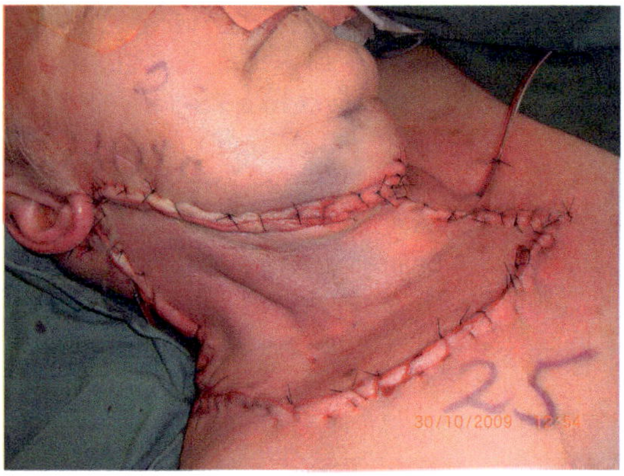

Fig. 2.7 On completion, the timeframe of 25 min relates to the second part of the closure; the total time was 50 min. Suction drainage is a necessity following neck clearance

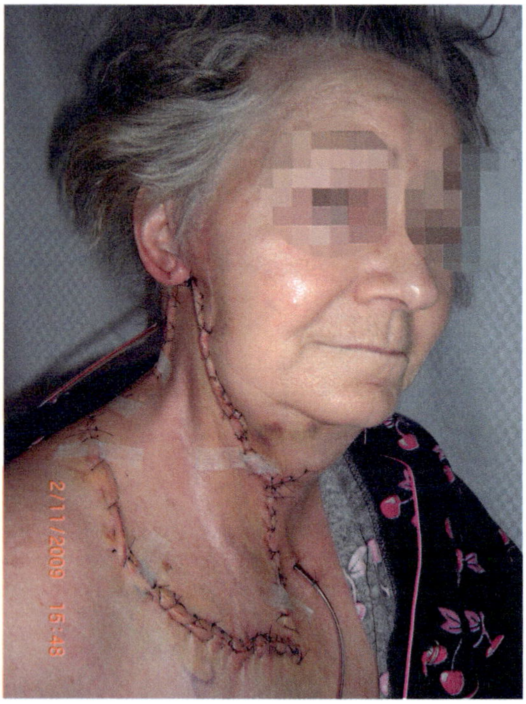

Fig. 2.8 The postoperative ward appears at 3 days from the timestamped images, and the patient has a satisfied appearance, confirming the Keystone characteristic of being pain-free

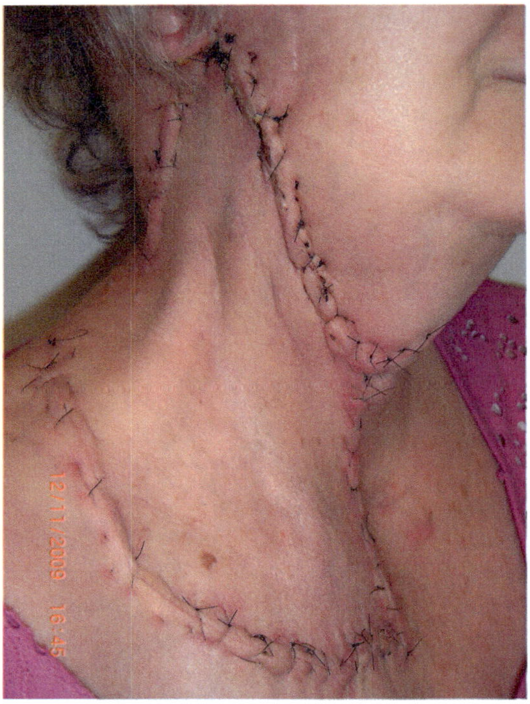

Fig. 2.9 Wound dressing at 10 days shows no evident necrotic complications. The continuous epidermal nylon is released to remove cross hatch marks. The standard mattress sutures are then removed at 2 weeks and locking mattress sutures at 3 weeks

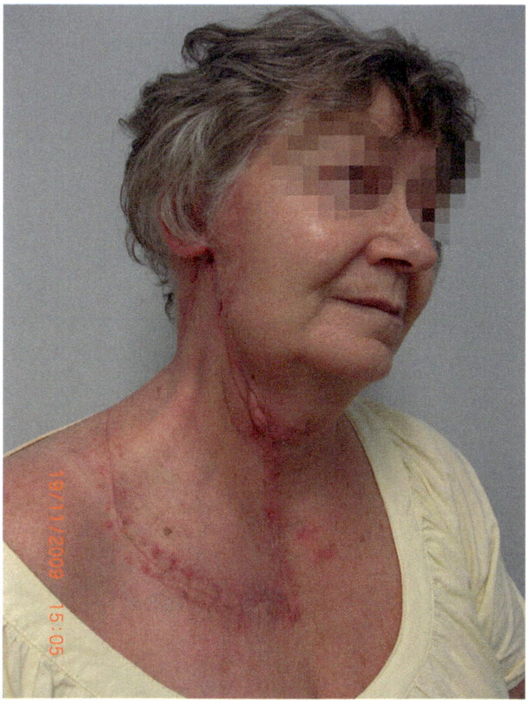

Fig. 2.10 The cross hatchings are released and the sutures left in situ before later removal. The tension sutures stay in for at least 3 weeks. At 3 weeks, note the patient's satisfied appearance

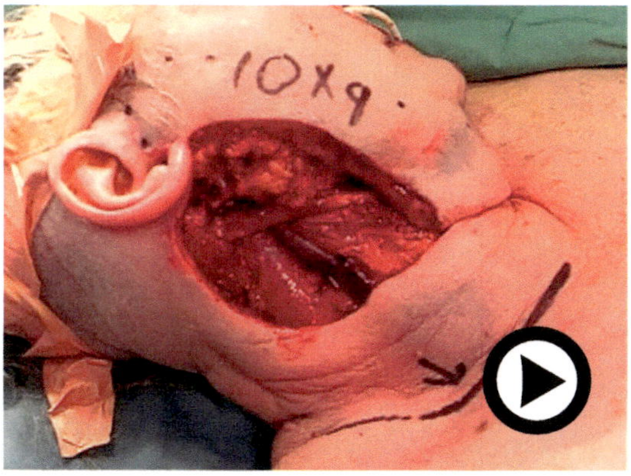

Fig. 2.11 Video 2.1 Operative sequence is shown. The redundant tissue in the posterior cervical region becomes part of the Keystone design to be rotated up into the anterior lobule area of the ear (▶ https://doi.org/10.1007/000-k5y)

The PACES characteristics were all exemplified: pain-free, aesthetic, no vascular no vascular complications, economical in terms of time and sensory recovery with the resolution of the oedema.

2.1.1.2 Case 2—Anterior Cervical Submental Keystone for a Large Parotid Defect in a 75-Year-Old

Melanoma level III and IV over the parotid with R neck clearance and with sentinel node (negative) is shown. A delayed reconstruction awaiting pathology evaluation (DRAPE) procedure was performed (Figs. 2.12, 2.13, 2.14, 2.15, 2.16 and 2.17).

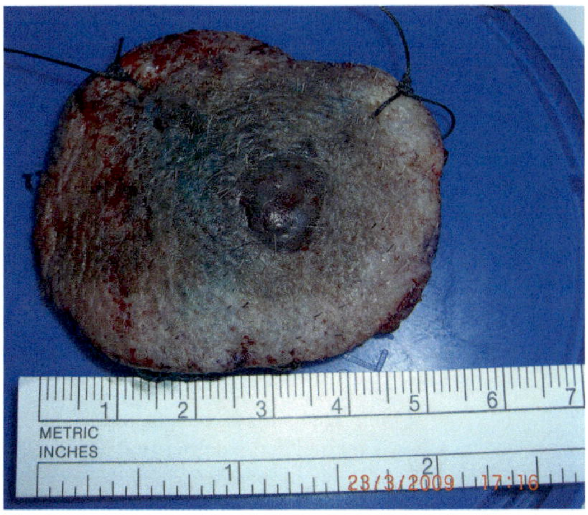

Fig. 2.12 The surgical specimen was 5 × 5 cm with sentinel node staining

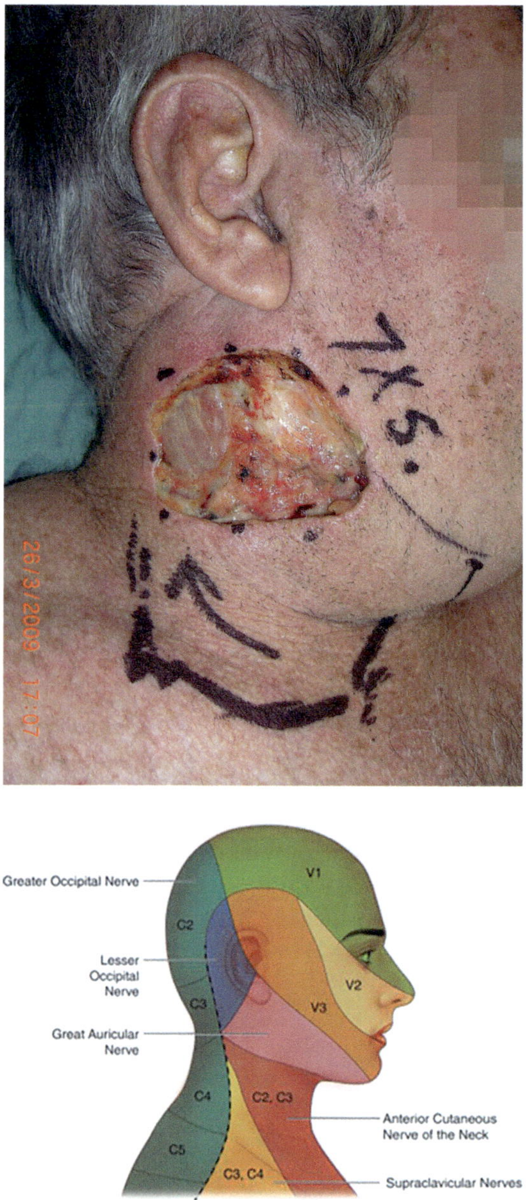

Fig. 2.13 The 7 × 5 cm defect sits over the angle of the mandible. The cervico-submental Keystone (arrowed) is the choice for closing the defect. The excisional defect is shown after tumour removal was closed. The cervico-submental flap from the neck to the point of the chin incorporates anterior cutaneous nerves (C2, C3) from the dermatomal mark out. (Reprinted with permission from Atlas, *Reconstructive Technique in Melanoma Management* (p. 19), by Felix Behan, Springer Nature 2023)

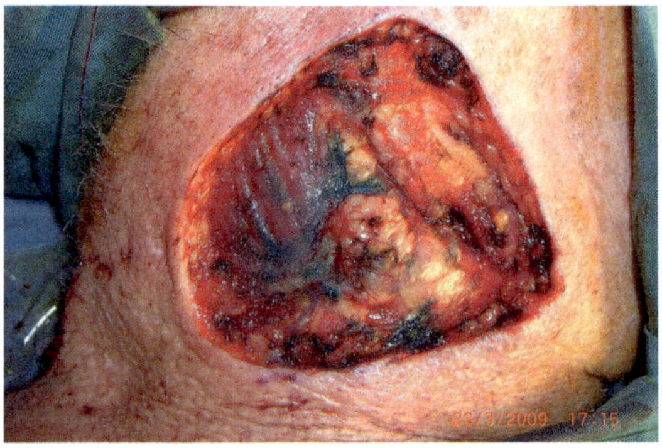

Fig. 2.14 A closeup of the excisional defect

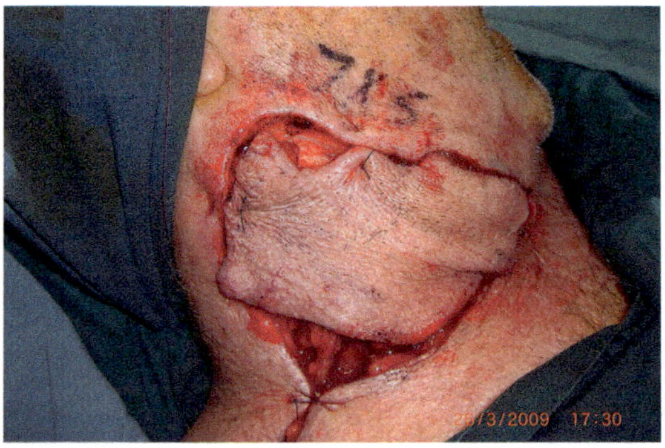

Fig. 2.15 The cervico-submental Keystone, based on cervical fascia and designed within the dermatomes (C2, C3), is two-thirds undermined. The proximal one-third attachment over sternomastoid random perforators ensures viability. Next, the Keystone is rotated into the defect, and then the three-phase single-layer suture technique is employed, using locking mattress sutures in a single layer at the points of maximum tension, an ordinary mattress to close the wound and an epidermal continuous nylon to produce a cutaneous seal. The 30 min timeframe (timestamped) covers the reconstruction, the Keystone insertion and the closure of the secondary defect

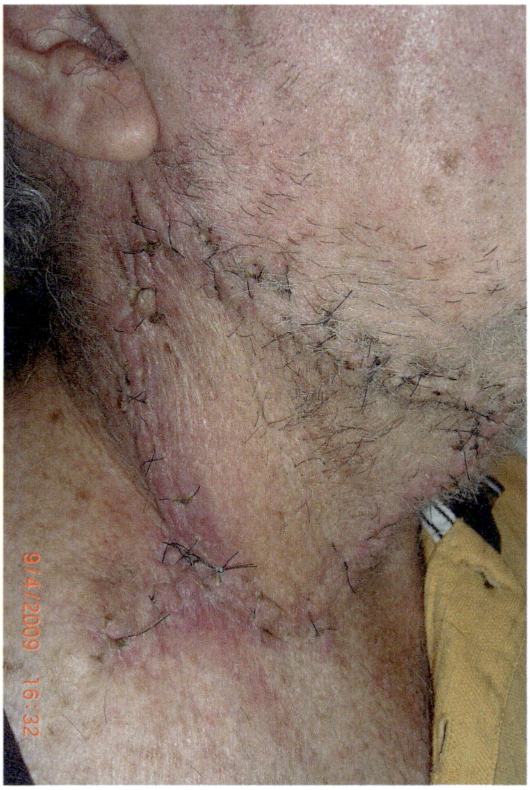

Fig. 2.16 Appearance at 14 days from timestamped image

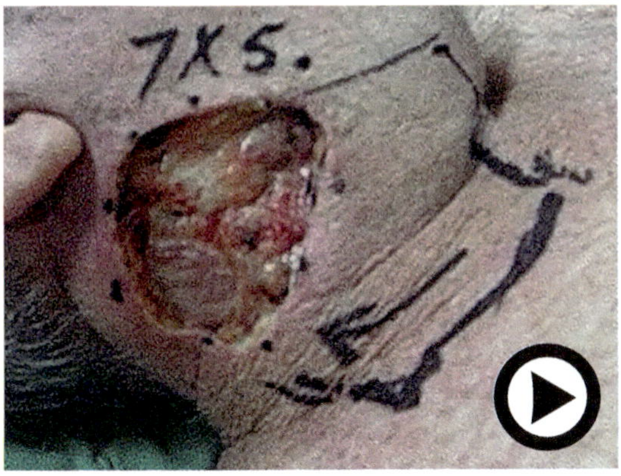

Fig. 2.17 Video 2.2 Planned operative procedure (▶ https://doi.org/10.1007/000-k5z)

The PACES characteristics were all exemplified: pain-free, aesthetic, no vascular complications, economical in terms of time and sensory recovery with the resolution of oedema.

2.1.1.3 Case 3—Parotid and Trimming of the Dog Ear on Dialysis

The parotid and the trimming of the dog ear on dialysis are shown (Figs. 2.18, 2.19, 2.20, 2.21, 2.22, 2.23, 2.24, 2.25, 2.26, 2.27, 2.28, 2.29, 2.30, 2.31 and 2.32).

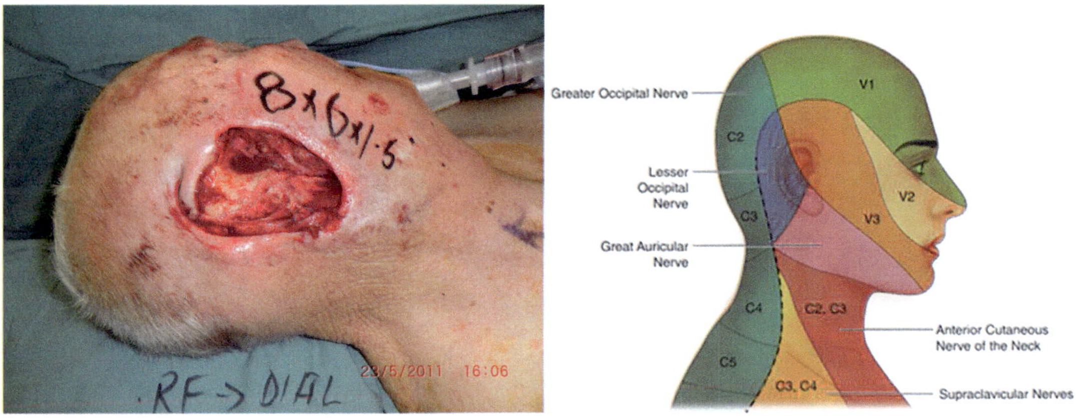

Fig. 2.18 The 8 × 6 × 1.5 cm defect shown over the external auditory canal. The dermatomal mark outs become the line of incision of the dermis and epidermis, ensuring that one-third deeply is attached with only partial undermining to facilitate the closure and vascular integrity of the defect. (Reprinted with permission from Atlas, *Reconstructive Technique in Melanoma Management* (p. 19), by Felix Behan, Springer Nature 2023)

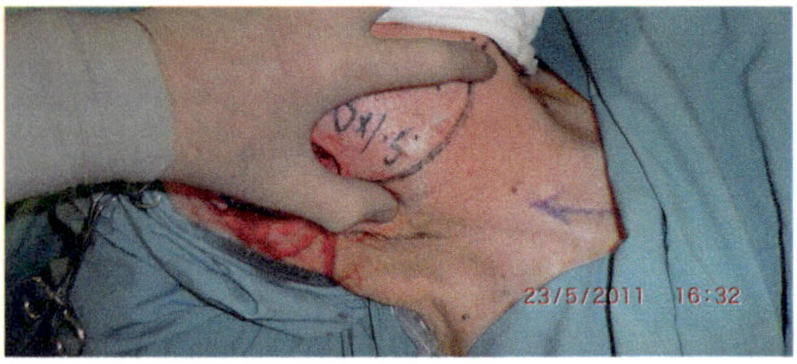

Fig. 2.19 The parotid mass, where the Keystone aligned with cervical fascia hinged on the random perforators at the sternomastoid junction

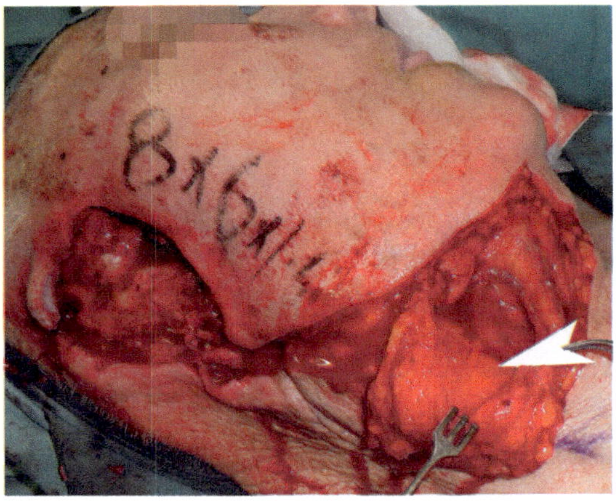

Fig. 2.21 Closeup of Fig. 2.20

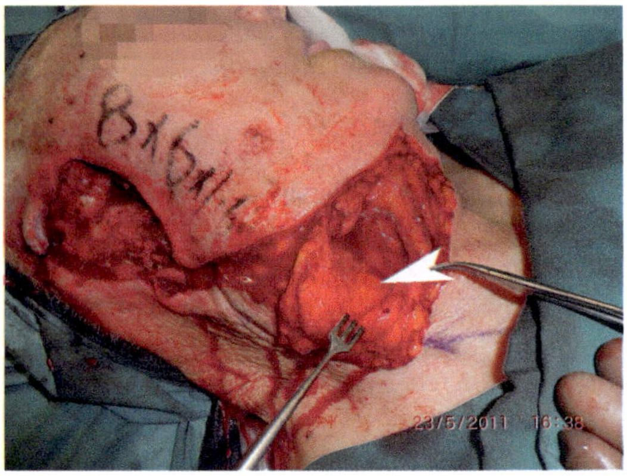

Fig. 2.20 The cervico-submental and the fascial base (white arrowed)

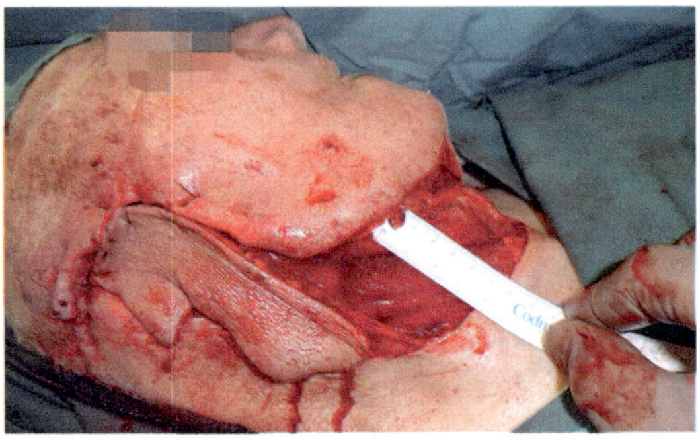

Fig. 2.22 6 cm secondary defect closed directly with locking mattress sutures

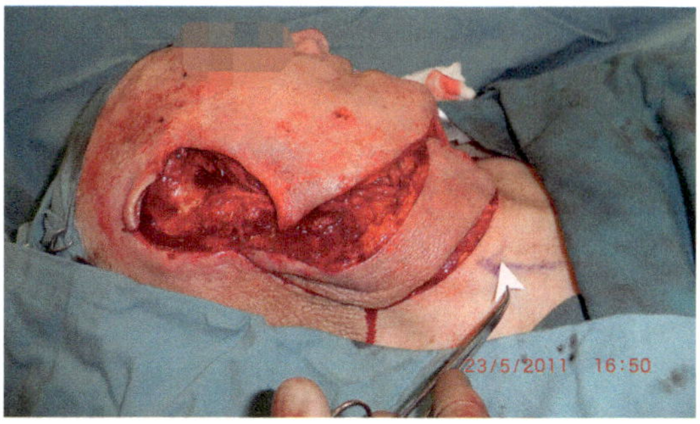

Fig. 2.23 The flap replaced, showing hypervascularity prior to definitive insertion—what we call the pink flare

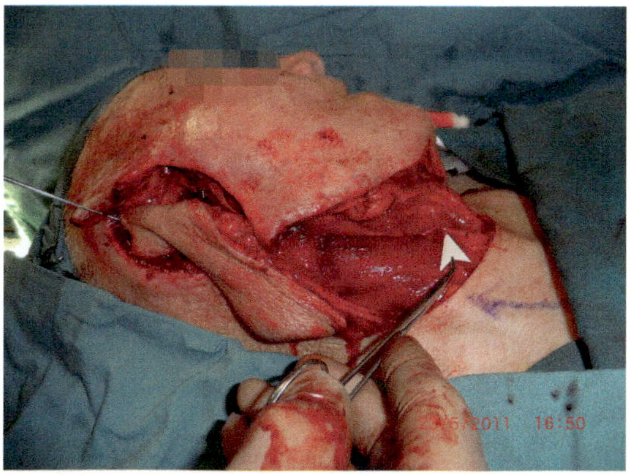

Fig. 2.24 Preservation of the nerves in the block dissection (white arrowed)

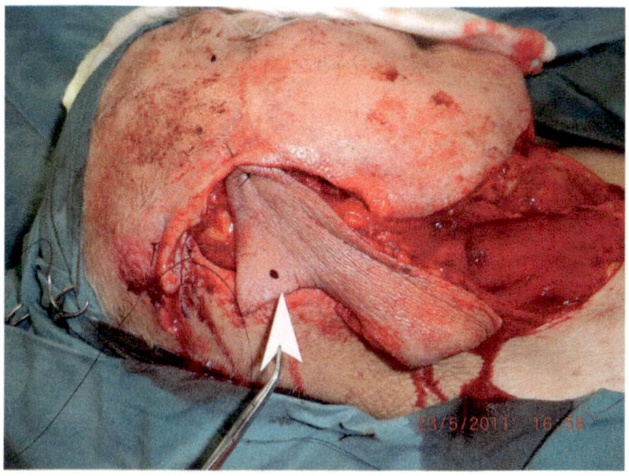

Fig. 2.25 The Red Dot Sign (white arrowed) is the complementary vascular indicator used to accompany the pink flare of the island flap—a sympathectomy effect

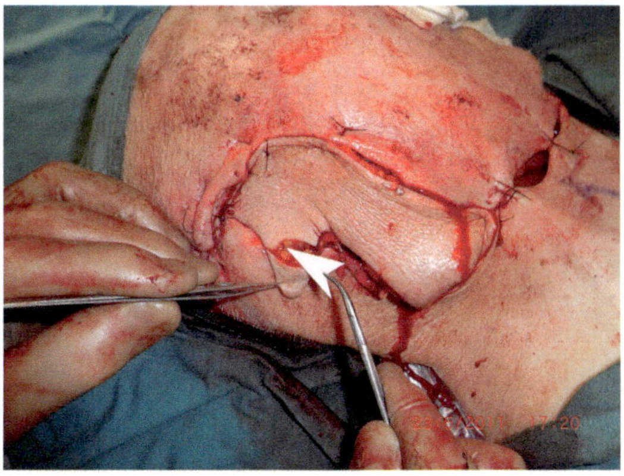

Fig. 2.26 Dog ear excision (white arrowed) is shown, a contraindication in flap surgery, but the suprafascial vascular supply allows one to trim the dog ear in the fresh flap to avoid a readmission

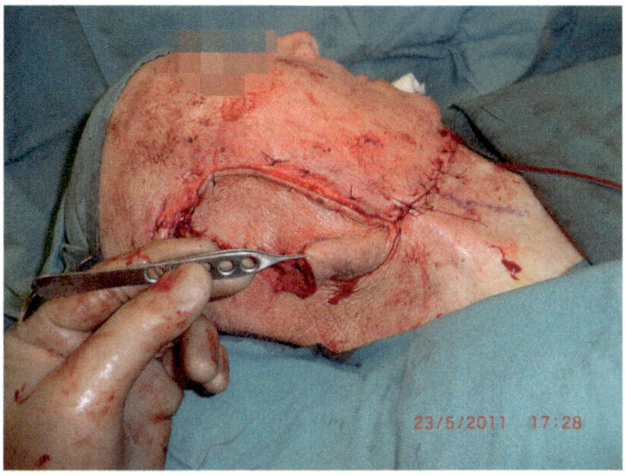

Fig. 2.27 Another dog ear excision is shown, and the timeframe indicated of 8 min is consistent with the sympathetic hypothesis

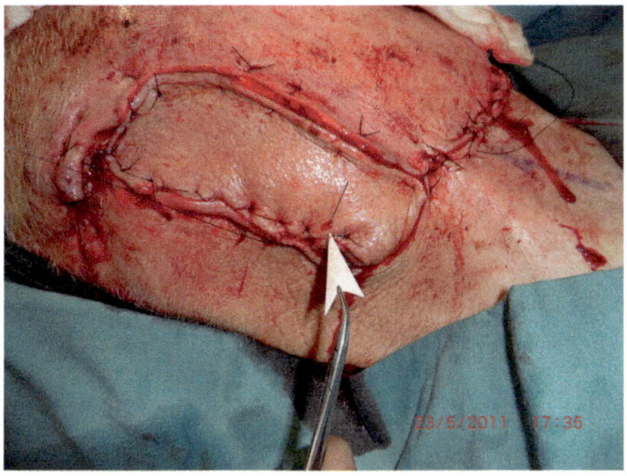

Fig. 2.28 The Red Dot Sign of arterial blood (white arrowed) at the suture point confirms vascular reliability to ensure wound closure

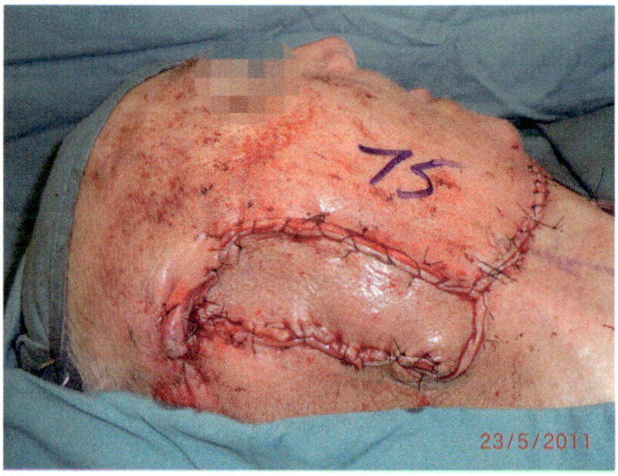

Fig. 2.29 The timeframe for wound closure is stated, and a comparison with the microsurgical alternative yields hours of difference

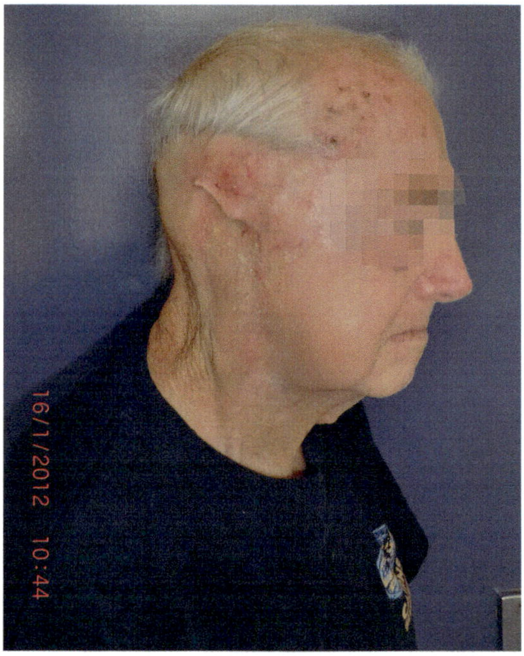

Fig. 2.30 A postoperative appearance 6 months later following a course of external radiation therapy (XRT), again showing no sign of recurrence

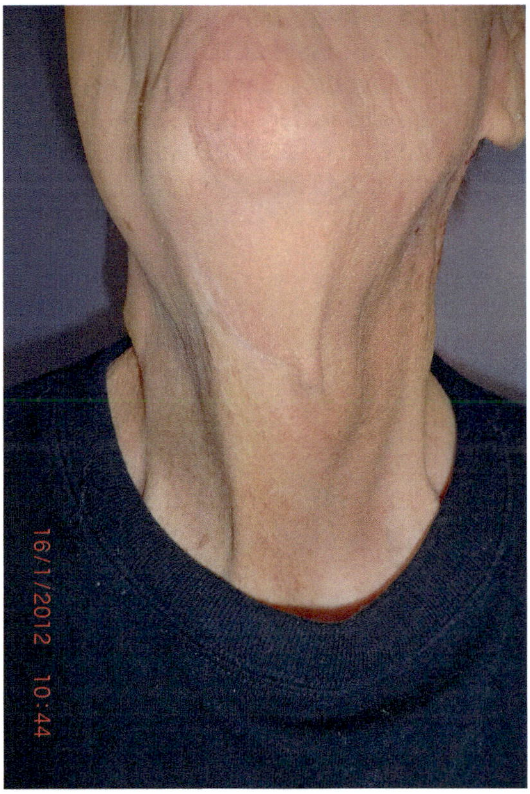

Fig. 2.31 A postoperative appearance of the scar at 6 months following the cervico-submental Keystone

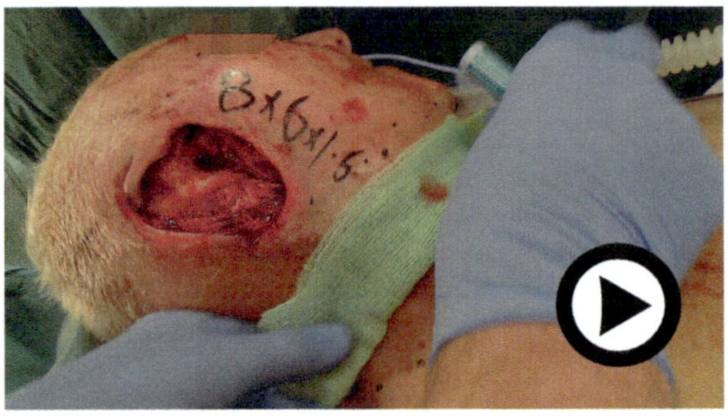

Fig. 2.32 Video 2.3 Planned operative procedure (▶ https://doi.org/10.1007/000-k60)

The PACES characteristics were all exemplified: pain-free, aesthetic, no vascular complications, economical in terms of time and sensory recovery with the resolution of oedema.

2.1.1.4 Case 4—Squamous Cell Carcinoma (SCC) Large Parotid Defect Closed with a Double Keystone (Figs. 2.33, 2.34, 2.35, 2.36, 2.37, 2.38, 2.39, 2.40, 2.41, 2.42, 2.43 and 2.44)

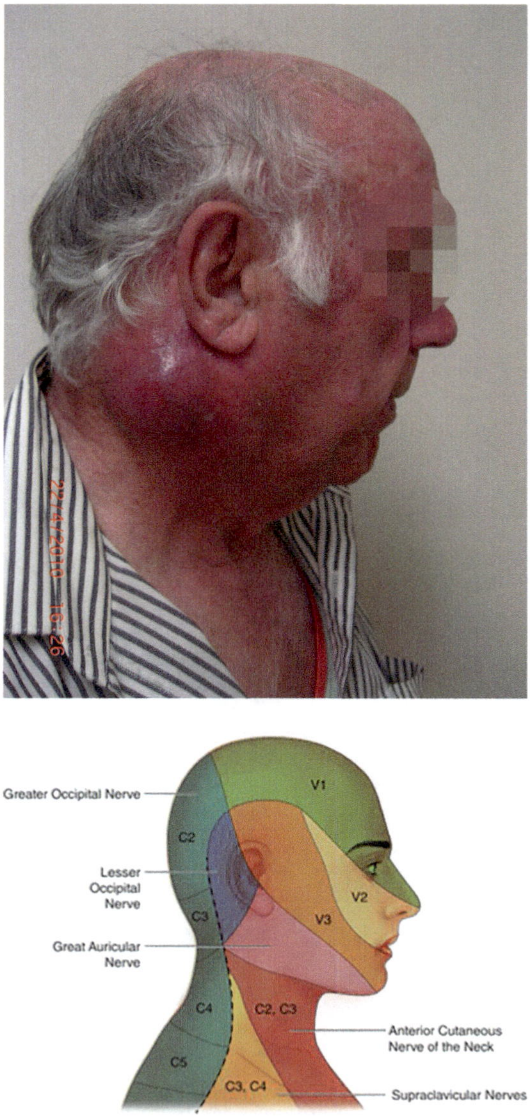

Fig. 2.33 Parotid mass where SCC and the dermatomal mark outs become the line of incision of the dermis and epidermis, ensuring that one-third deeply is attached with only partial undermining to facilitate the closure and vascular integrity of the defect. (Reprinted with permission from Atlas, *Reconstructive Technique in Melanoma Management* (p. 19), by Felix Behan, Springer Nature 2023)

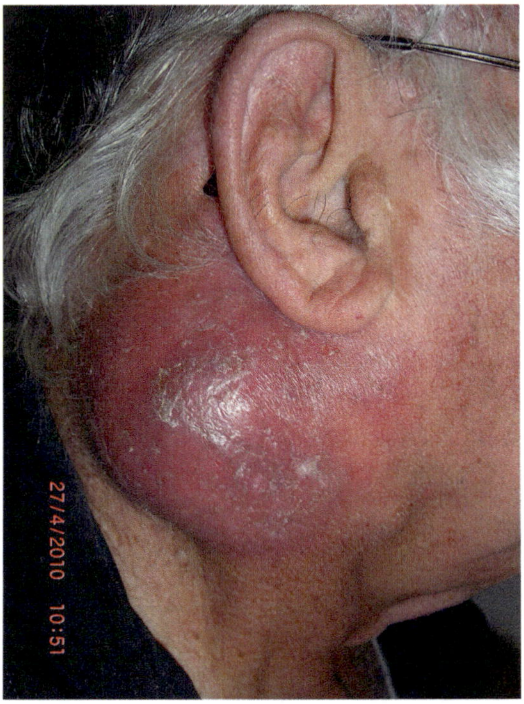

Fig. 2.34 15 × 20 cm parotid mass

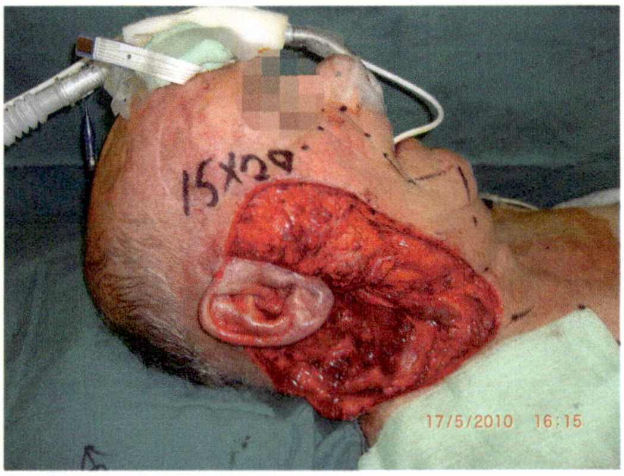

Fig. 2.35 Locoregional double Keystones, facial and supraclavicular

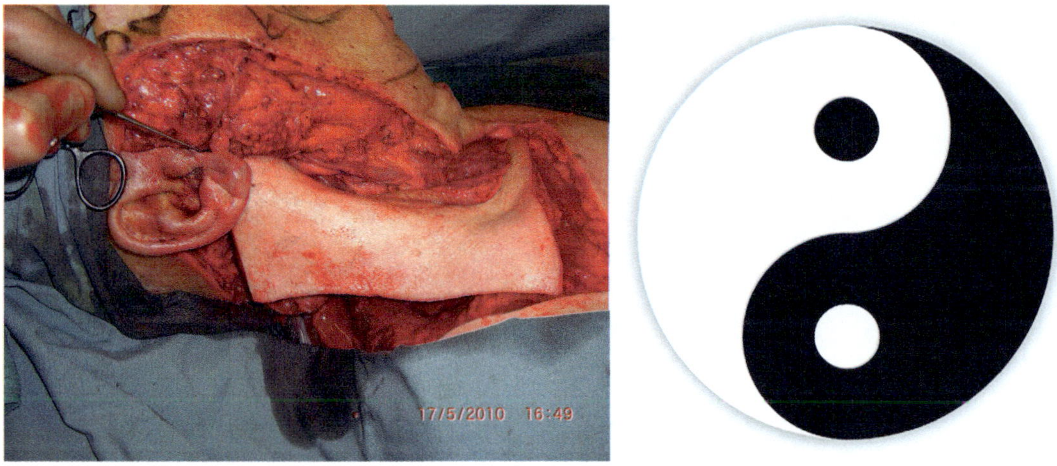

Fig. 2.36 Covering the neck mass with the supraclavicular Keystone and using a facial Keystone in a yin-yang manner

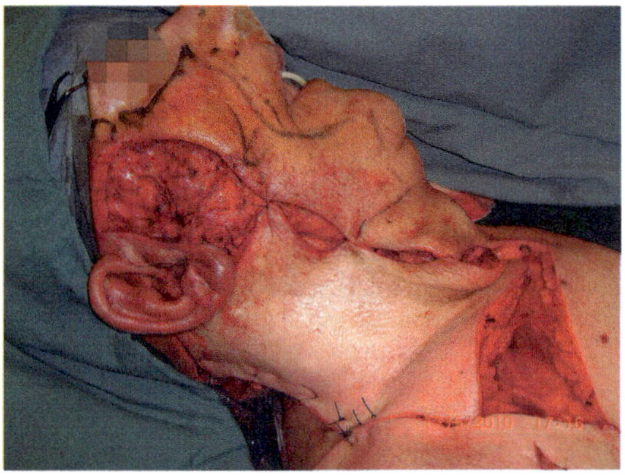

Fig. 2.37 The supraclavicular Keystone before the facial Keystone has been inserted

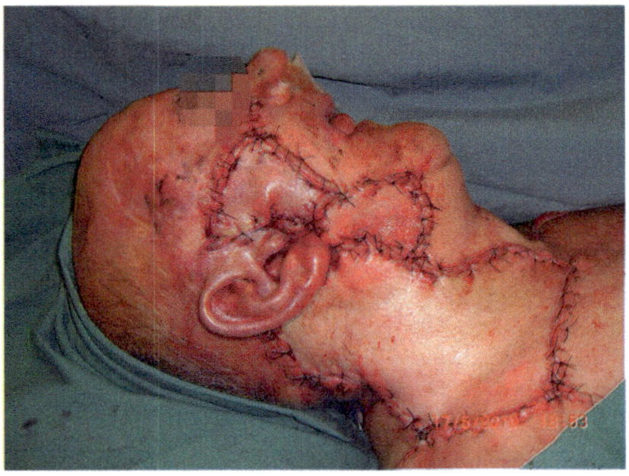

Fig. 2.39 Wound closure with some tension

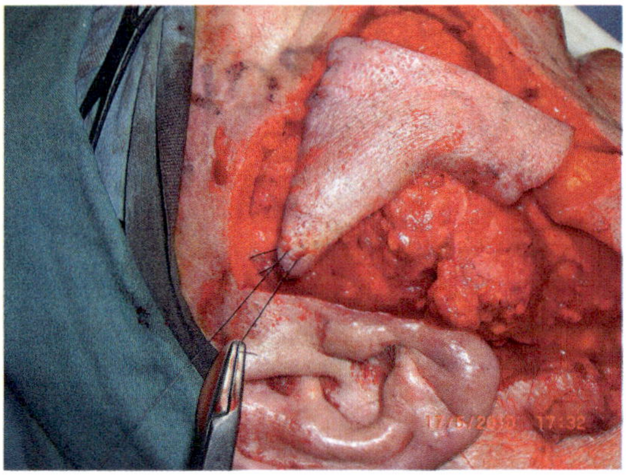

Fig. 2.38 The facial Keystone based on the infraorbital circulation, with a pink flare

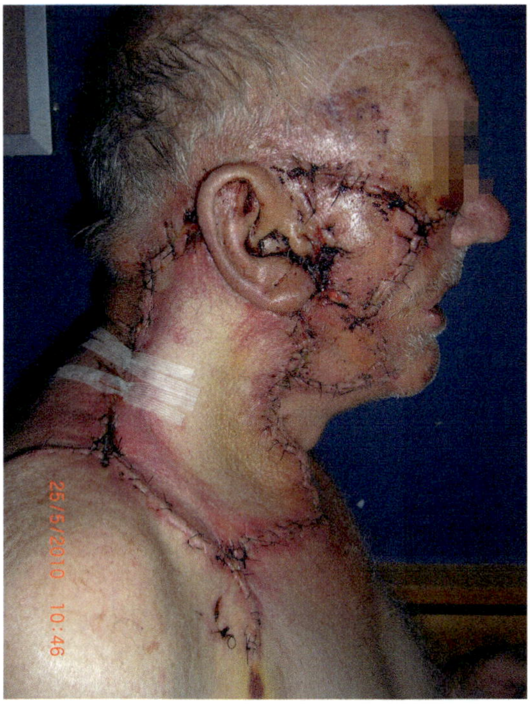

Fig. 2.40 Postoperative appearance at 8 days with no necrosis and the perfusion around the limits of the supraclavicular Keystone flap

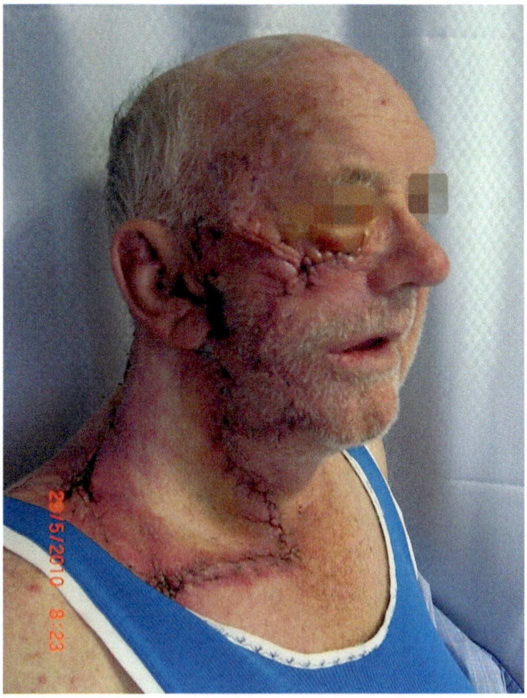

Fig. 2.41 Postoperative appearance at 12 days where the recovery of the vascular perfusion and the central part show ongoing perfusional improvement

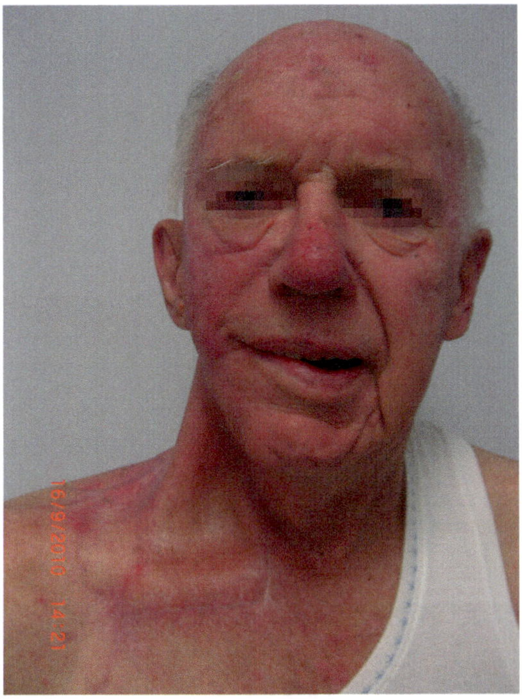

Fig. 2.42 Postoperative appearance at 4 months, showing full recovery with a fully satisfied patient, who even gave me an endearing embrace in the outpatient department, thanking me. The reason for his delay in presentation was that he was wheelchair bound and the expeditious solution with a Keystone added to his satisfaction

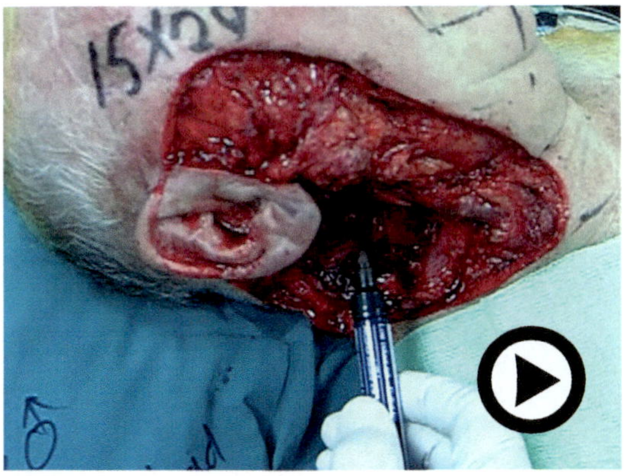

Fig. 2.43 Video 2.4 Planned operative procedure (▶ https://doi.org/10.1007/000-k61)

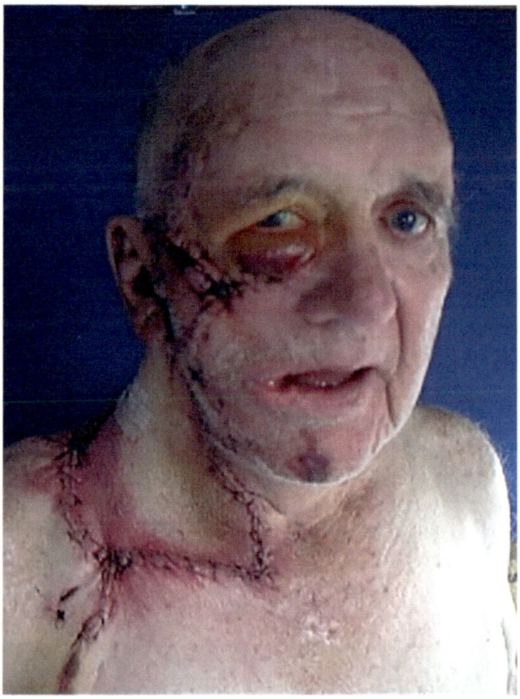

Fig. 2.44 Video 2.5 Postoperative positive patient response (▶ https://doi.org/10.1007/000-k62)

The PACES characteristics were all exemplified: pain-free, aesthetic, no vascular complications, economical in terms of time and sensory recovery with the resolution of oedema.

2.1.1.5 Case 5—Large Periauricular Defect at the Bony Canal in a Diabetic Patient (Figs. 2.45, 2.46, 2.47, 2.48, 2.49, 2.50, 2.51, 2.52, 2.53, 2.54 and 2.55).

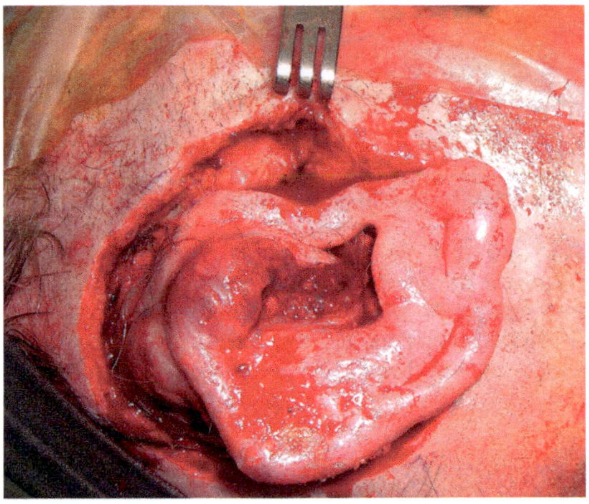

Fig. 2.45 Staged excision by Professor Andrew Sizeland

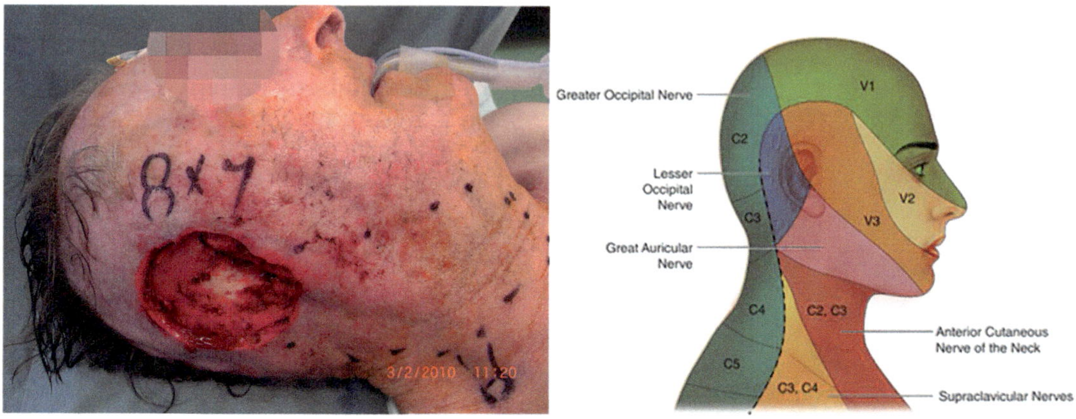

Fig. 2.46 A 8 × 7 cm defect is shown. The cervico-submental Keystone is dotted. The video explains how the repair covers the whole area, including the external canal, which can be left for a later occasion after XRT. The dermatomal mark outs become the line of incision of the dermis and epidermis, ensuring that one-third is deeply attached with only partial undermining to facilitate the closure and vascular integrity of the defect. (Reprinted with permission from Atlas, *Reconstructive Technique in Melanoma Management* (p. 19), by Felix Behan, Springer Nature 2023)

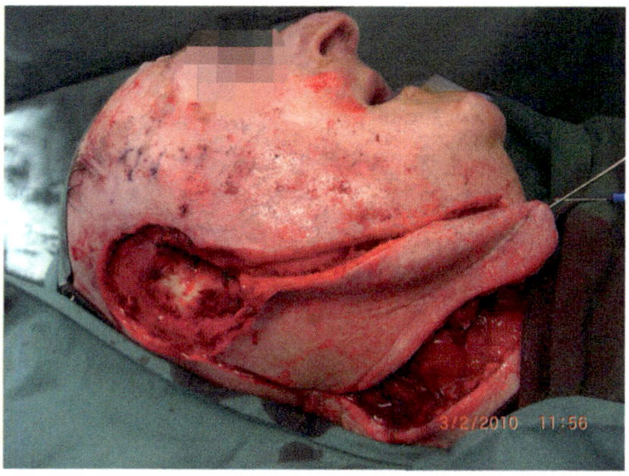

Fig. 2.47 The flare in the flap is aligned along the cervical fascia and is supported with filamentous perforators in the sternomastoid region, which are not skeletonised but left intact as a unit to facilitate the hinging movement to cover the skull defect

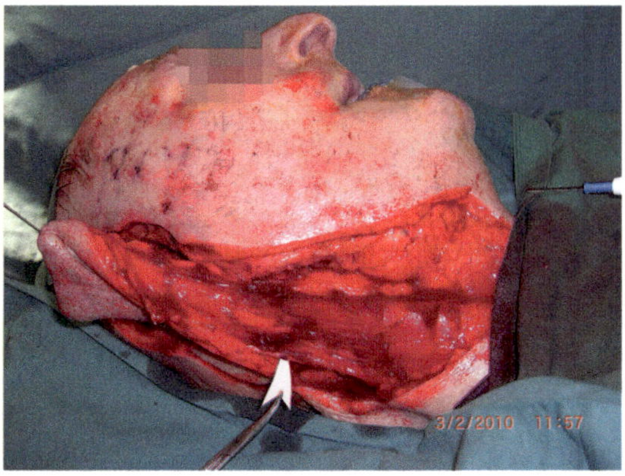

Fig. 2.48 Various nerves in the block dissection indicated

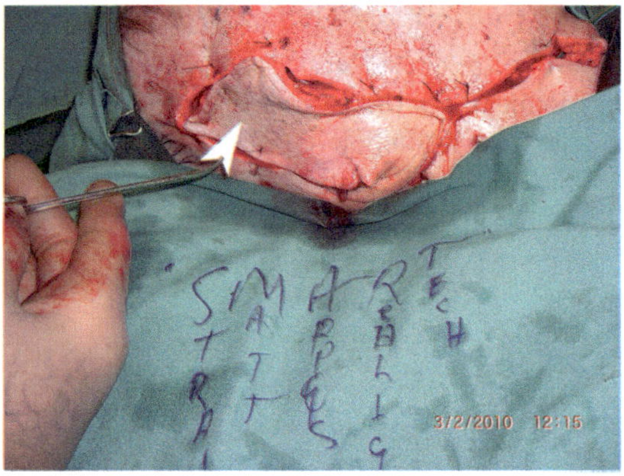

Fig. 2.49 Staged insertion with lines of tension cause some temporary vascular impedance, and with reinsertion, this eliminates the lines of tension

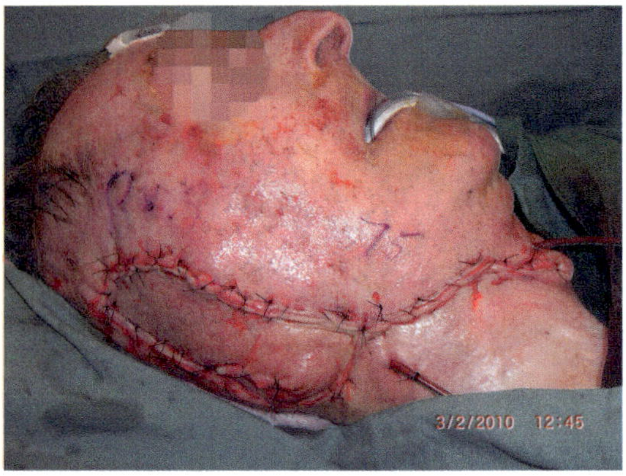

Fig. 2.50 Timeframe of 75 min is noted. The secondary defect in the neck with the locking mattress suture technique shows the wound closure and two drainage sites because of the unpredictable nature of the ooze from the deep surface

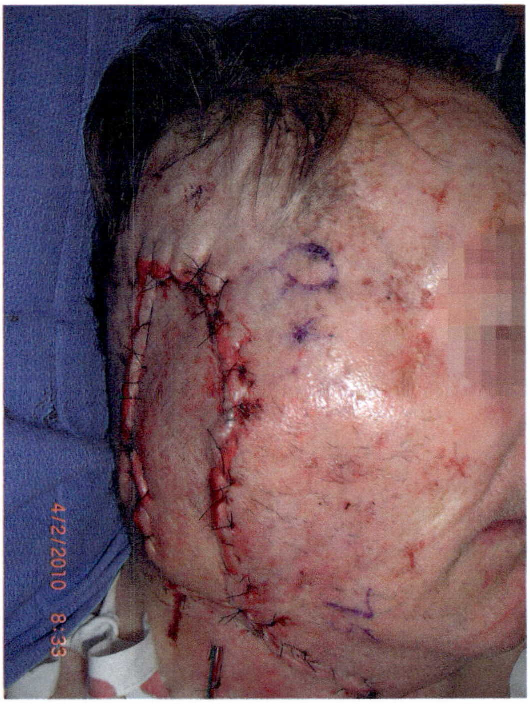

Fig. 2.51 Postoperative appearance at 24 h

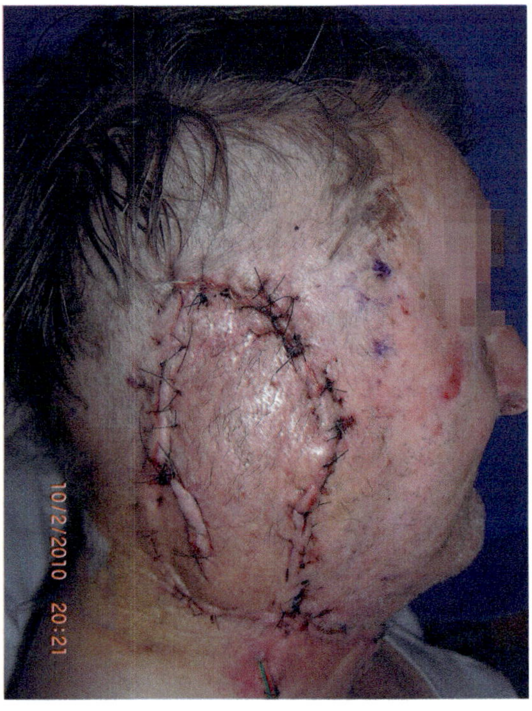

Fig. 2.52 Postoperative appearance at 7 days

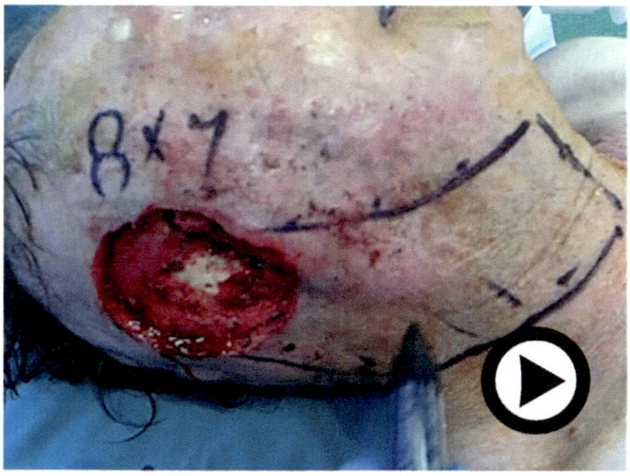

Fig. 2.53 Video 2.6 The planned operative procedure (▶ https://doi.org/10.1007/000-k63)

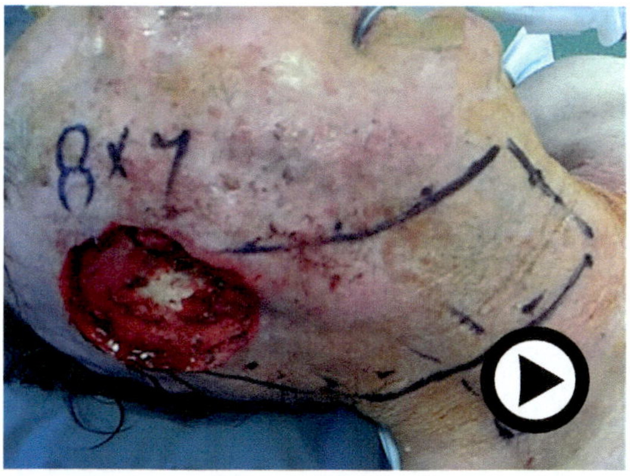

Fig. 2.54 Video 2.7 The planned operative procedure (▶ https://doi.org/10.1007/000-k64)

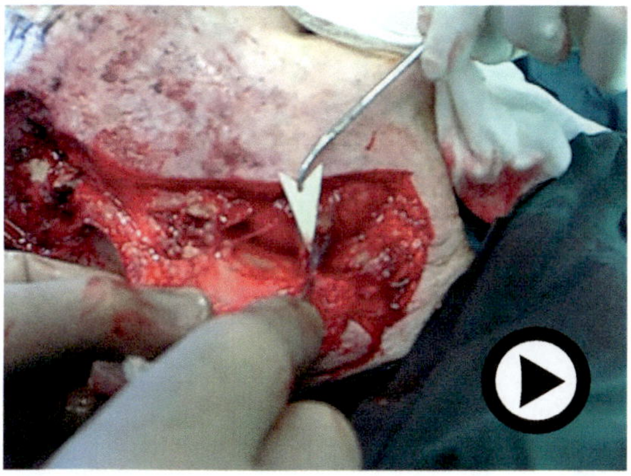

Fig. 2.55 Video 2.8 Developing the plane of the cervical fascia using blunt dissection, which helps to preserve the microperforators and repairing any damaged veins (▶ https://doi.org/10.1007/000-k65)

The PACES characteristics were all exemplified: pain-free, aesthetic, no vascular complications, economical in terms of time and sensory recovery with the resolution of oedema.

2.1.1.6 Case 6—SCC of the Periparotid Region in a 94-Year-Old—Age Is No Major Hindrance for Keystone Reconstruction (Figs. 2.56, 2.57, 2.58, 2.59, 2.60, 2.61, 2.62, 2.63, 2.64, 2.65, 2.66, 2.67, 2.68, 2.69, 2.70 and 2.71).

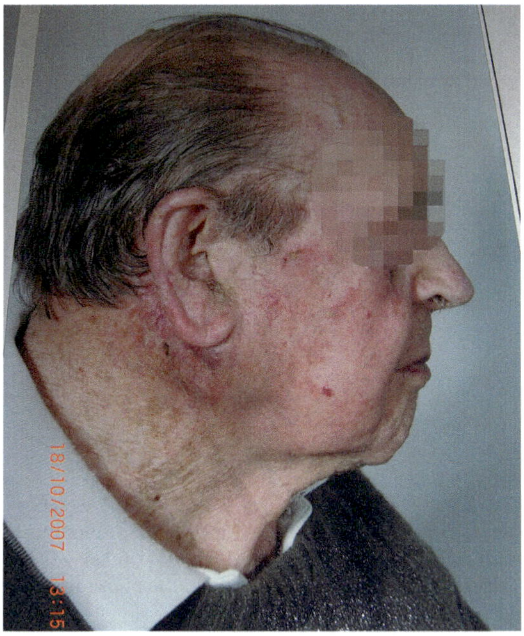

Fig. 2.56 The SCC in the infralobular location

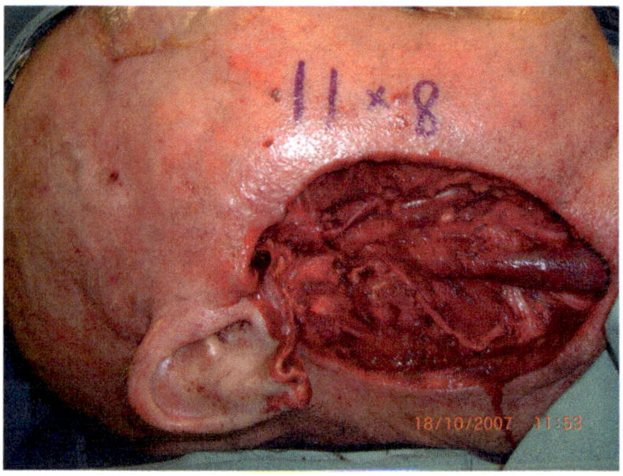

Fig. 2.57 The 11 × 8 cm defect up to the zygomatic arch is shown. The preservation of all venous networks, including the internal jugular in the block dissection, is used to assist in the revascularisation and healing

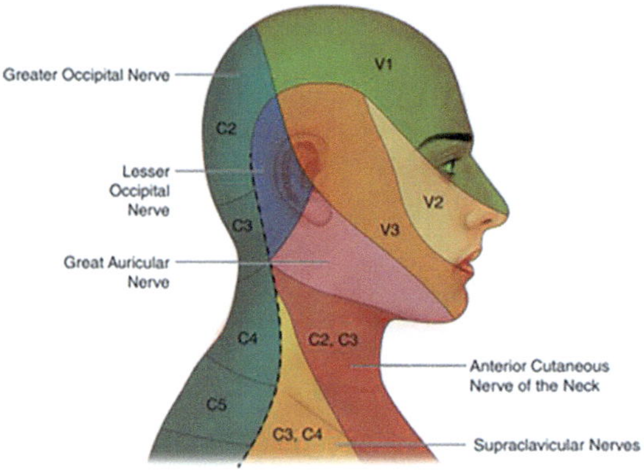

Fig. 2.58 The dermatomal mark outs become the line of incision of the dermis and epidermis, ensuring that one-third deeply is attached with only partial undermining to facilitate the closure and vascular integrity of the defect. (Reprinted with permission from Atlas, *Reconstructive Technique in Melanoma Management* (p. 19), by Felix Behan, Springer Nature 2023)

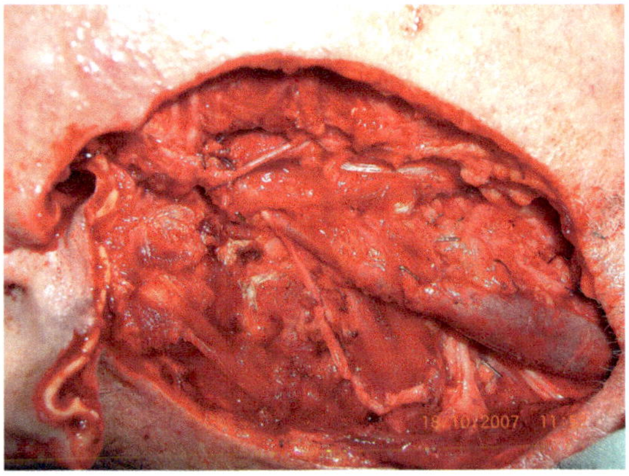

Fig. 2.59 Preservation of the vascular network, internal jugular and cranial nerve accessory

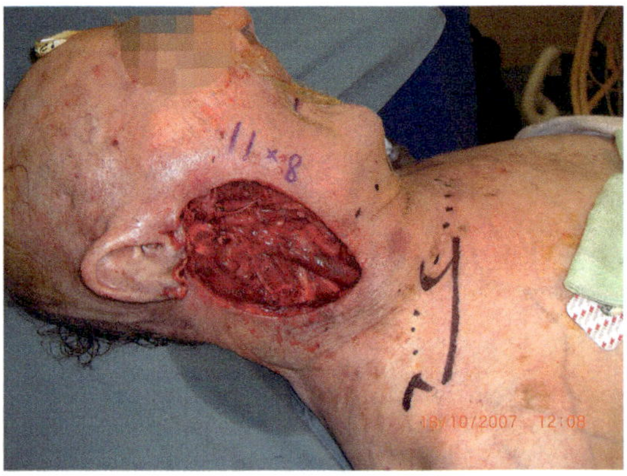

Fig. 2.60 The supraclavicular mark out for a supplementary Keystone

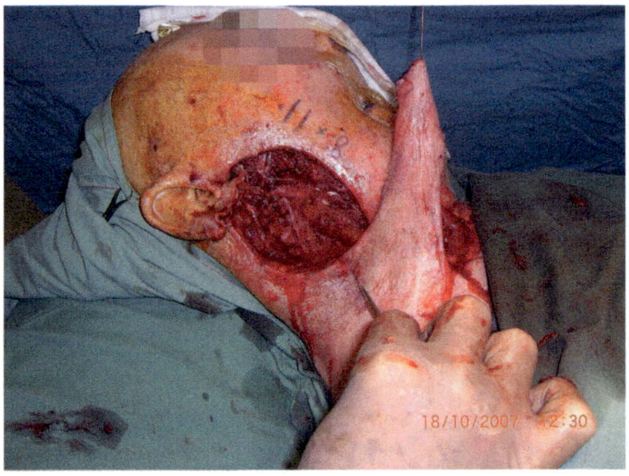

Fig. 2.61 The cervico-submental Keystone hypervascularised on the basis of the sternomastoid insertion site

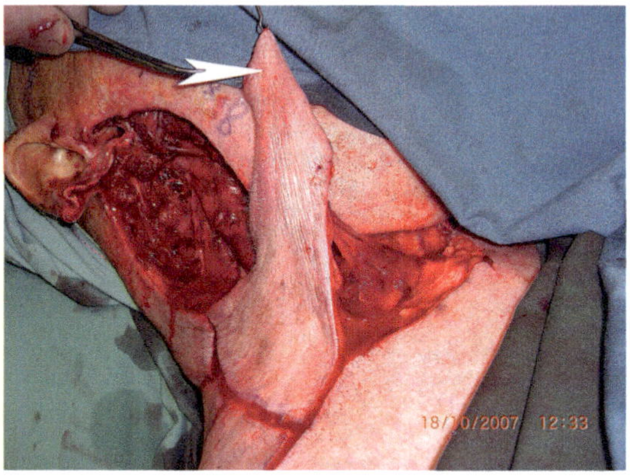

Fig. 2.62 The hypervascularised island flap reflecting the sympathectomy effect as a simple explanation when designed within the dermatome

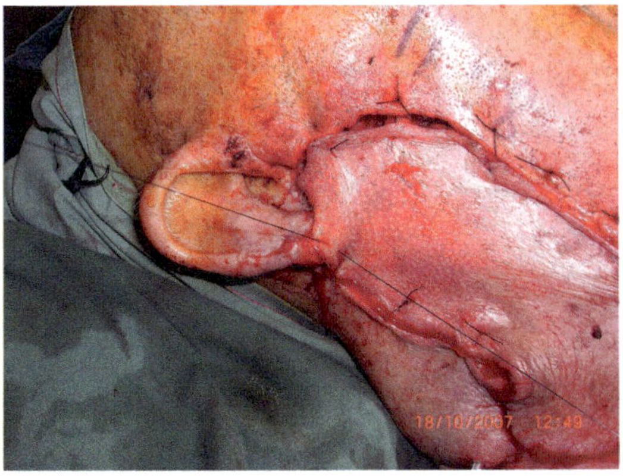

Fig. 2.65 Tension locking mattress sutures are inserted at the key points, and then a continuous epidermal suture seals the wound

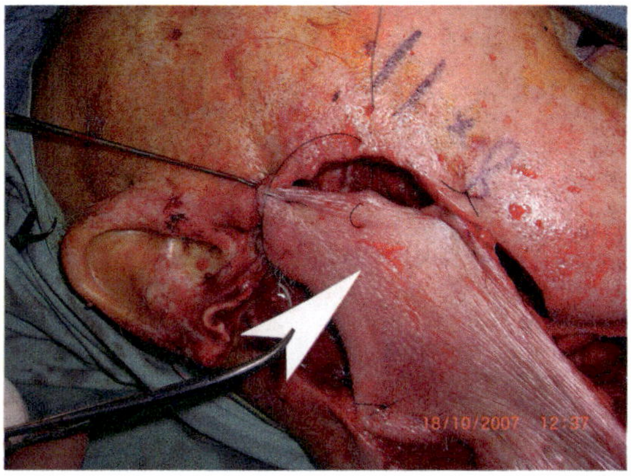

Fig. 2.63 The hypervascularisation was achieved in 4 min

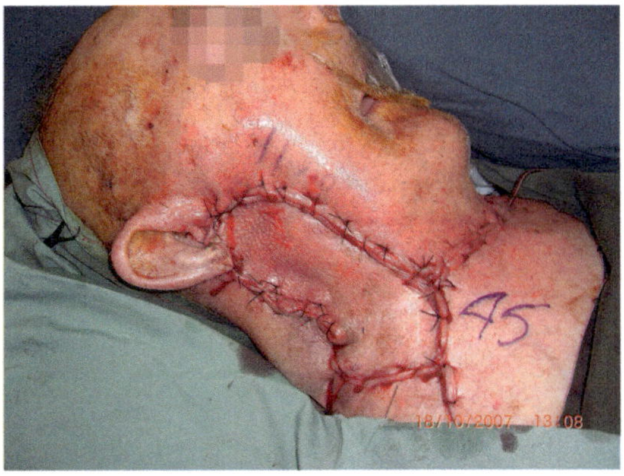

Fig. 2.66 Expeditious completion and off the operating table for elderly patients in the shortest, safest timeframe

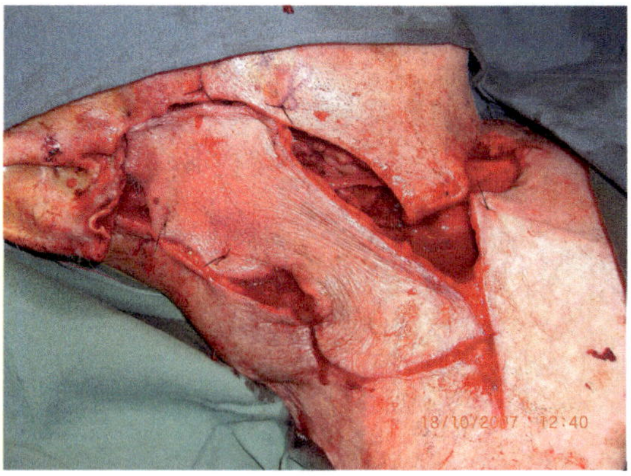

Fig. 2.64 The staged insertion of the hypervascularised flap

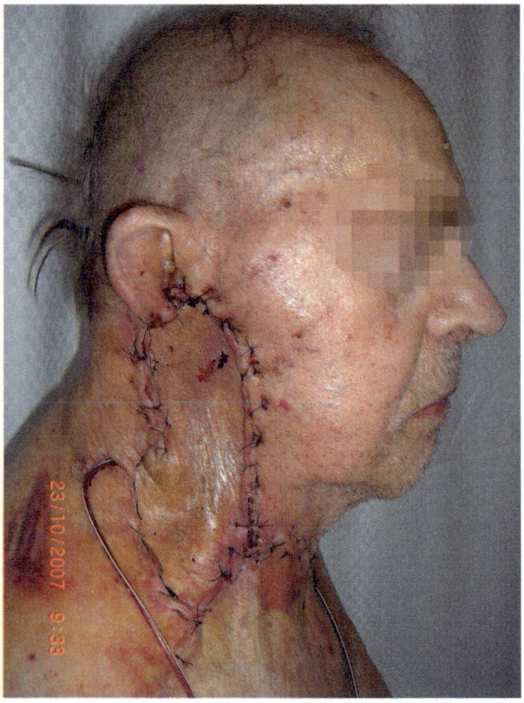

Fig. 2.67 Postoperative appearance at 5 days, where the key locking suture for the closure of the cervical defect must stay in for 2–3 weeks

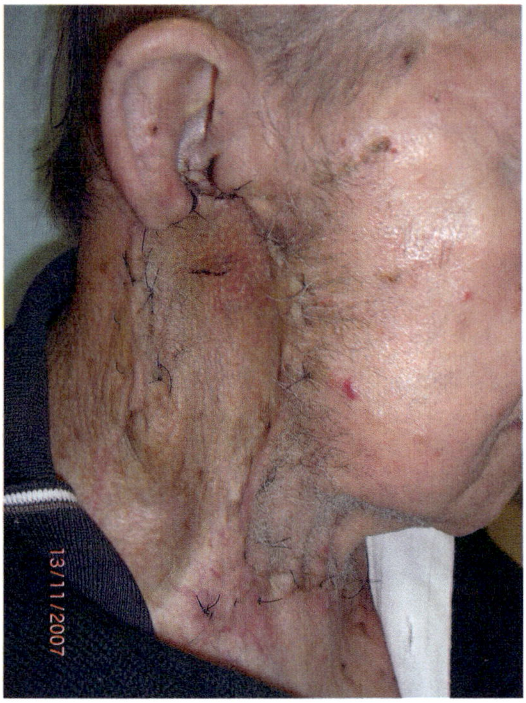

Fig. 2.68 Postoperative appearance at 4 weeks

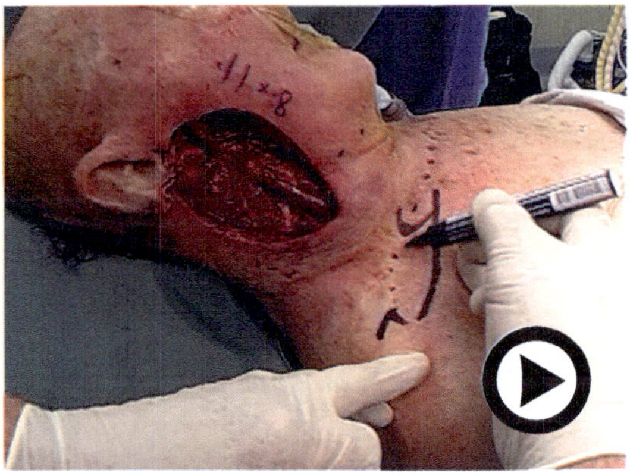

Fig. 2.69 Video 2.9 The technique of raising the cervico-submental Keystone (▶ https://doi.org/10.1007/000-k66)

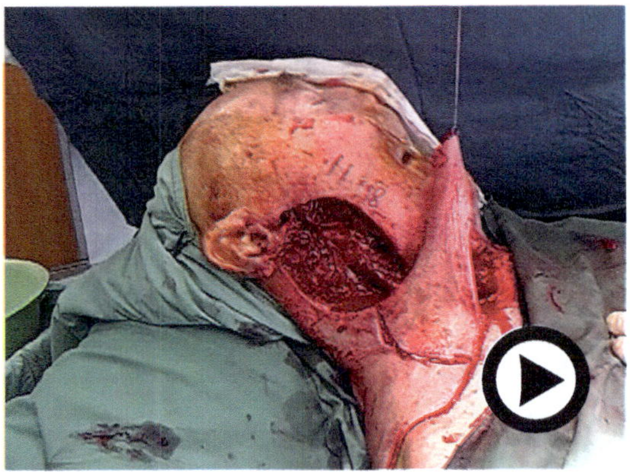

Fig. 2.70 Video 2.10 Creating the island in the cervico-submental flap by incising the dermal-epidermal mark out to create hypervascularity to optimise healing (▶ https://doi.org/10.1007/000-k67)

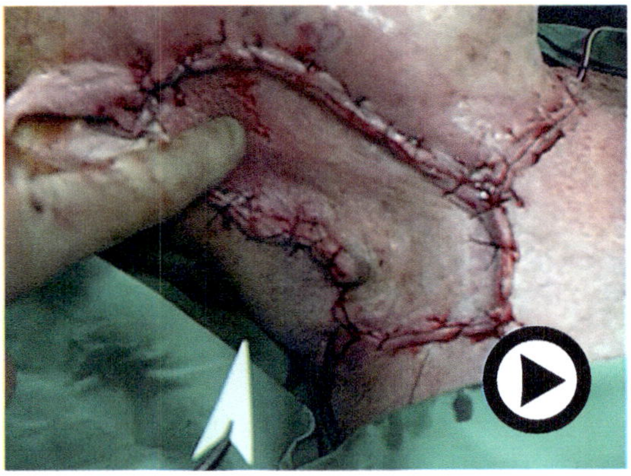

Fig. 2.71 Video 2.11 Hypervascularisation at the suture points of tension (▶ https://doi.org/10.1007/000-k68)

The PACES characteristics were all exemplified: pain-free, aesthetic, no vascular complications, economical in terms of time and sensory recovery with the resolution of oedema.

2.1.1.7 Case 7—Parotid Mass with External Protrusion Extending into the Cheek (Figs. 2.72, 2.73, 2.74, 2.75, 2.76, 2.77, 2.78, 2.79, 2.80, 2.81, 2.82, 2.83, 2.84, 2.85, 2.86 and 2.87).

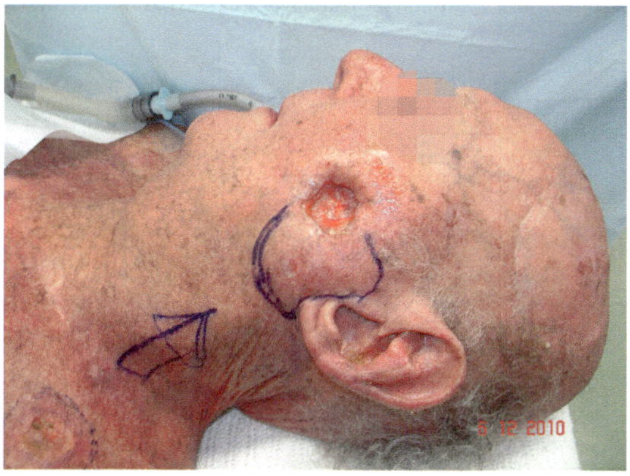

Fig. 2.72 A large parotid defect

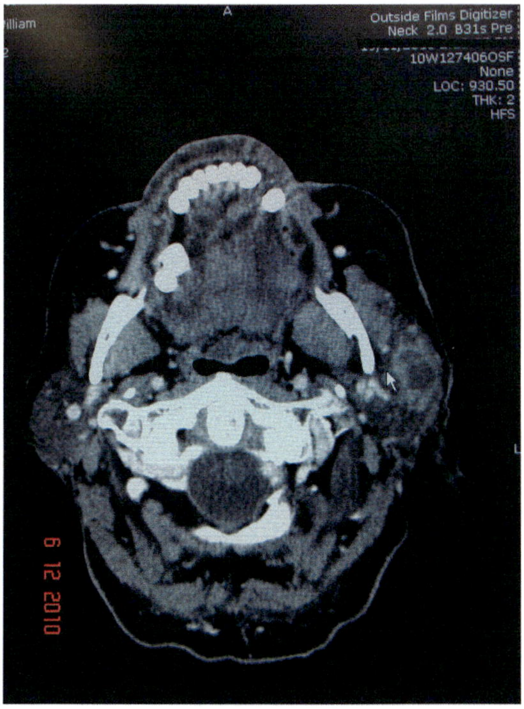

Fig. 2.73 Computed tomography (CT) image

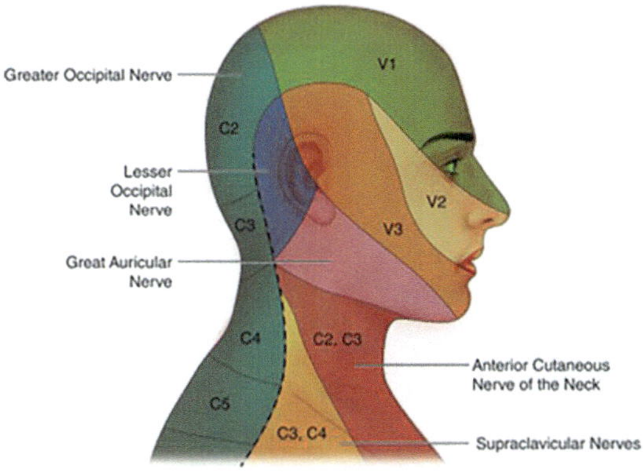

Fig. 2.74 The dermatomal mark outs become the line of incision of the dermis and epidermis, ensuring that one-third deeply is attached with only partial undermining to facilitate the closure and vascular integrity of the defect. (Reprinted with permission from Atlas, *Reconstructive Technique in Melanoma Management* (p. 19), by Felix Behan, Springer Nature 2023)

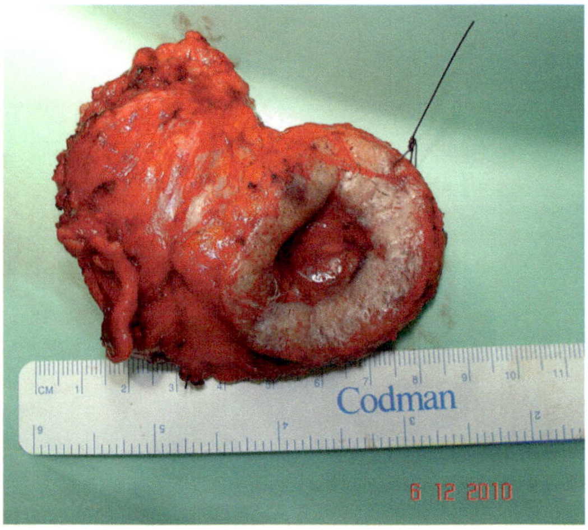

Fig. 2.75 The tumour mass creating the large surgical defect after excision

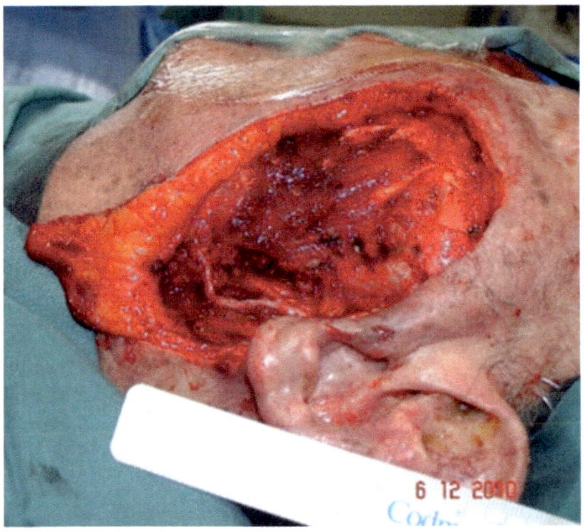

Fig. 2.77 The exposed facial nerve, which has been retained to maintain muscle tone and function

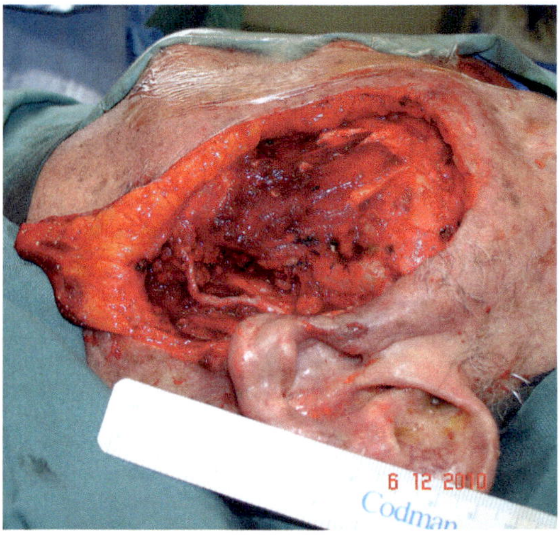

Fig. 2.76 The large 8 × 7 cm defect over the zygomatic arch

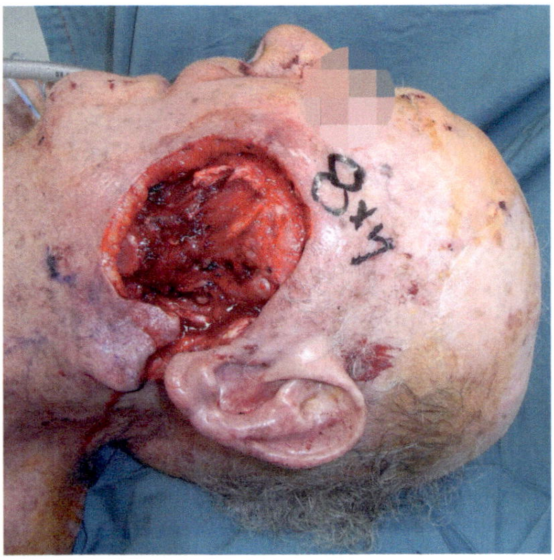

Fig. 2.78 Defect of 8 × 7 cm, including the parotid

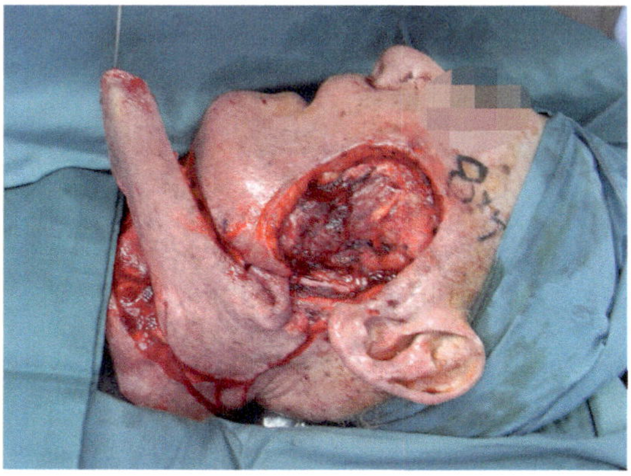

Fig. 2.79 The cervico-submental flap based on sternomastoid perforators is raised, creating its pink flare from the sympathectomy effect when raised within the dermatome mark out

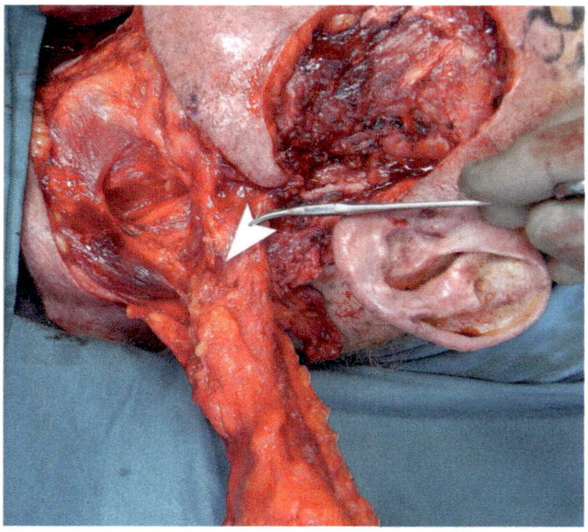

Fig. 2.80 Areas of the filamentous perforators at the base of the sternomastoid, the hinge site for the rotation of the flap

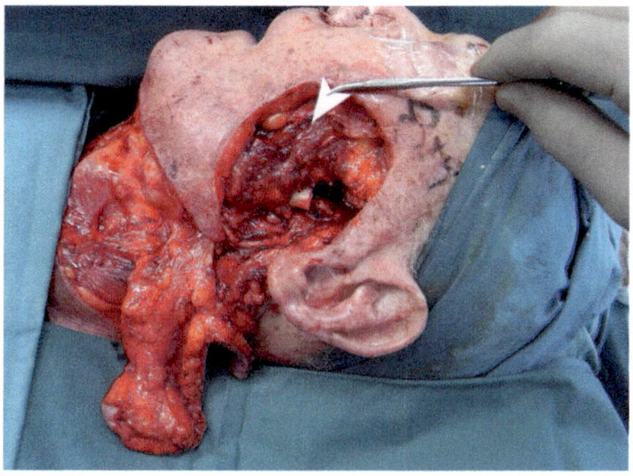

Fig. 2.81 Branch of the facial nerve preserved

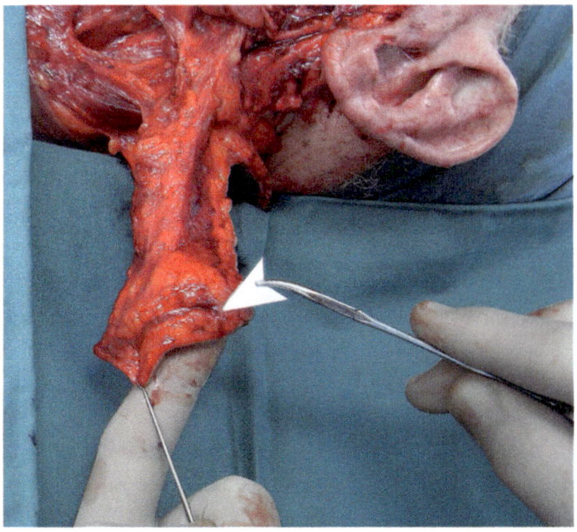

Fig. 2.82 Microcirculation perfusion at the distal limit of the flap—length not a hindrance

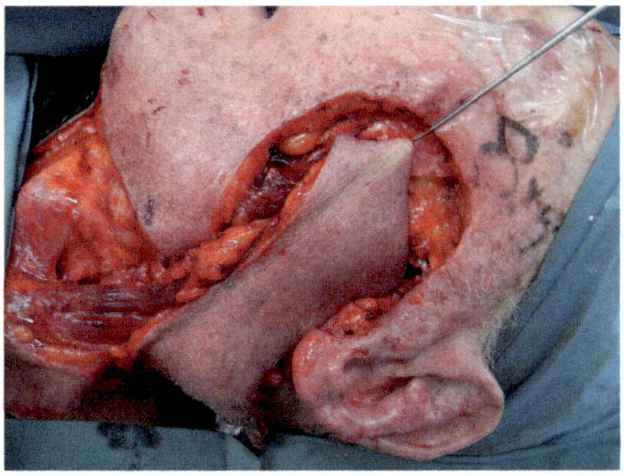

Fig. 2.83 Staged insertion, where the line of tension disappears with tissue rearrangement after a short period

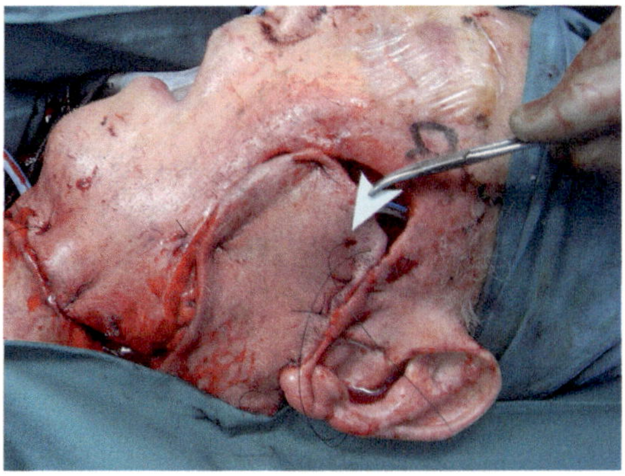

Fig. 2.84 Staged insertion of the flap and the arrow on a red dot site of the nylon suture exit point

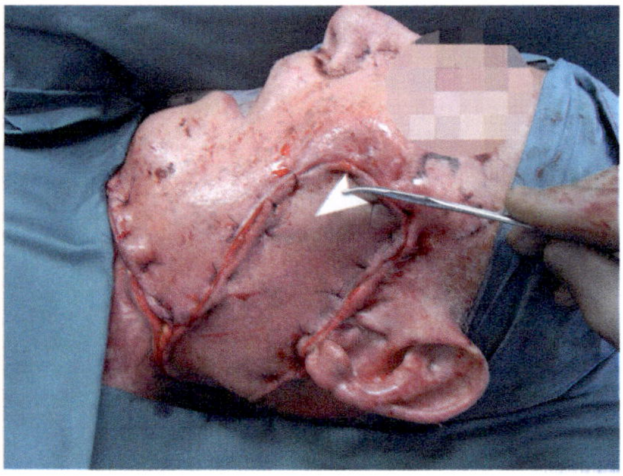

Fig. 2.85 Complete closure here used the three-phase locking mattress suture technique. The vascular flare confirms the vascular integrity; however, this is supported by redivac drainage

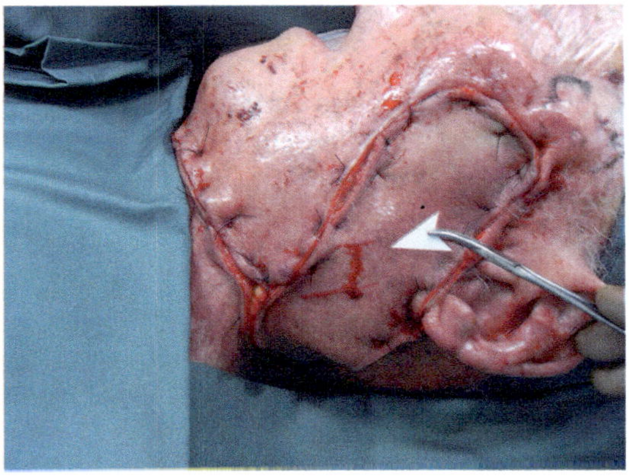

Fig. 2.86 Another red dot sign is shown. Note the arterialised blood appearance

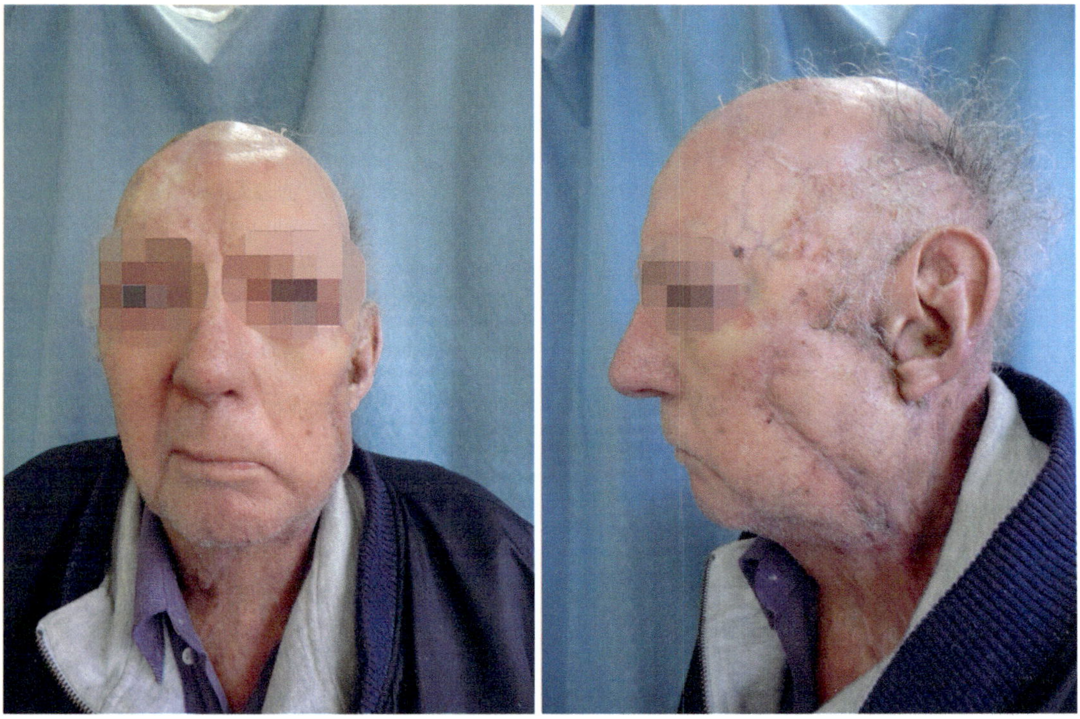

Fig. 2.87 The appearance at 12 months shows the ectropion fully corrected. Sometimes the oedema and the weight of the Keystone tend to precipitate ophthalmic problems like ectropion, and this is the correction done with a graft. Notice the Keystone and the slight dragging effect with the resolution of oedema in the flap, which compares favourably when a microvascular free flap is used

The PACES characteristics were all exemplified: pain-free, aesthetic, no vascular complications, economical in terms of time and sensory recovery with the resolution of oedema.

2.1.1.8 Case 8—Recurrent SCC in a 78-Year-Old Following XRT for SCC of the Tonsil, Presenting as a Supraclavicular Mass (Figs. 2.88, 2.89, 2.90, 2.91, 2.92, 2.93, 2.94, 2.95, 2.96 and 2.97)

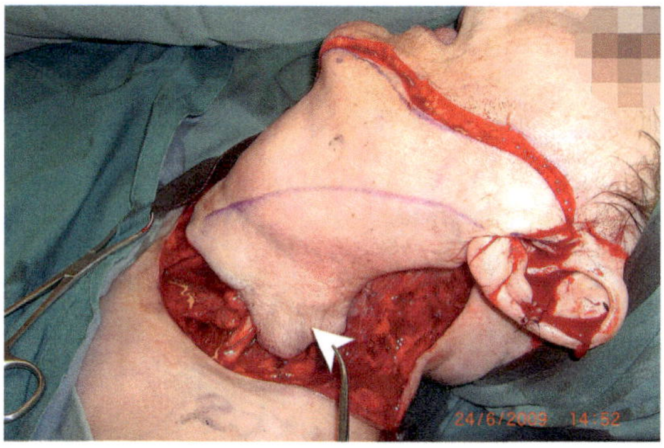

Fig. 2.88 The blue line marks the extent of the undermining of the flap, used to facilitate nodal clearance. The white arrow shows the relative sluggishness of the circulation to the top of the flap, which is hypervascularised, by outlining the dermatomal mark out

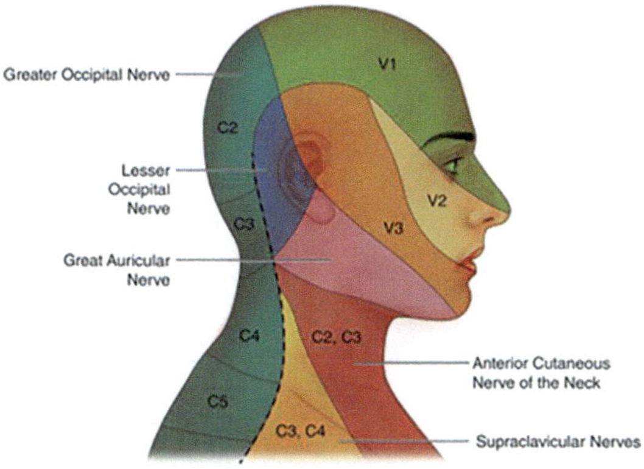

Fig. 2.89 The dermatomal mark outs become the line of incision of the dermis and epidermis, ensuring that one-third deeply is attached with only partial undermining to facilitate the closure and vascular integrity of the defect. (Reprinted with permission from Atlas, *Reconstructive Technique in Melanoma Management* (p. 19), by Felix Behan, Springer Nature 2023)

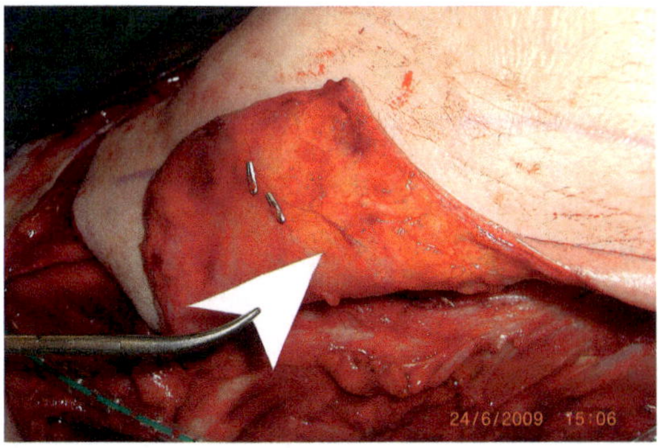

Fig. 2.90 The suprafascial and infrafascial circulation in an irradiated field is at the point of the arrow, and micro clips are used for haemostasis

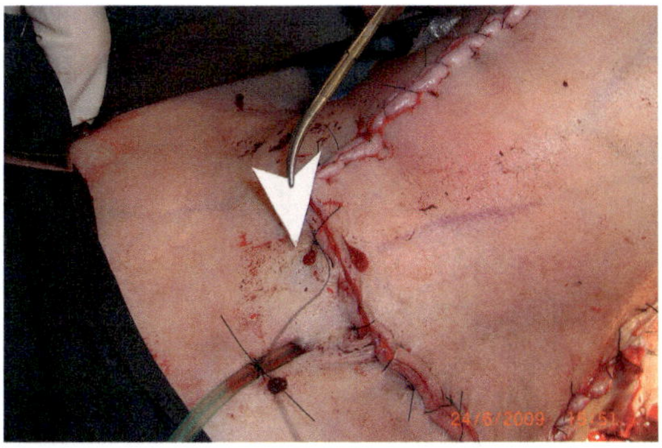

Fig. 2.91 The red dot sign on wound closure is ongoing evidence of the hyperaemic phase of the sympathectomy effect when the dermatomal mark out is surgically delineated

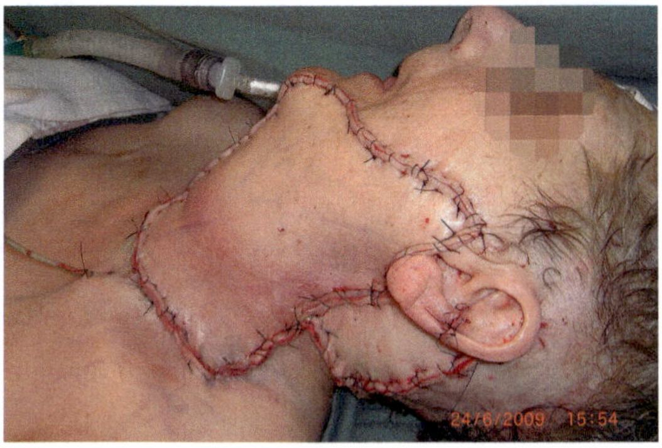

Fig. 2.92 The wound on closure with the standard three-phase suture technique is shown, without evidence of vascular impedance in the flap, and to save tension, an additional infra-auricular Keystone was raised to produce this effect

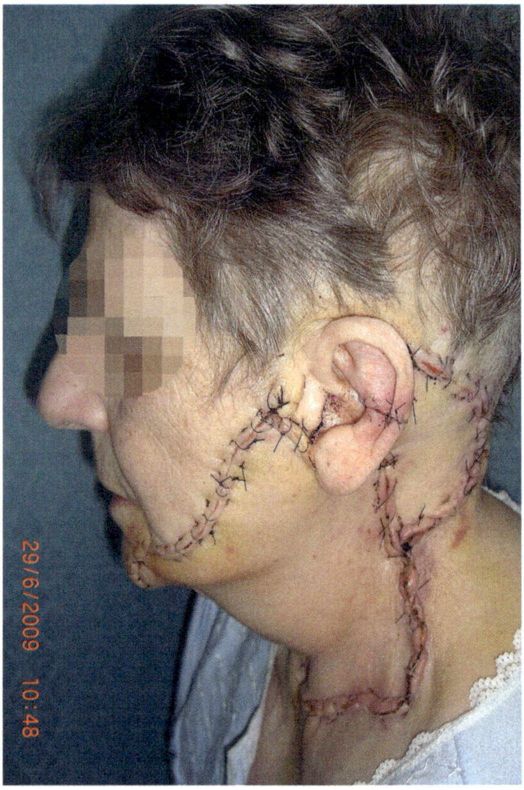

Fig. 2.93 Postoperative appearance at 5 days is shown, and the patient on video will describe their level of comfort and desire to go home pain-free

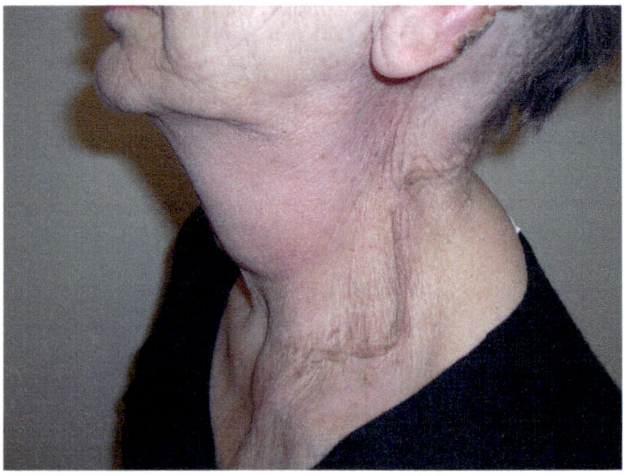

Fig. 2.94 Appearance at 1 month, where the video records the patient's satisfaction

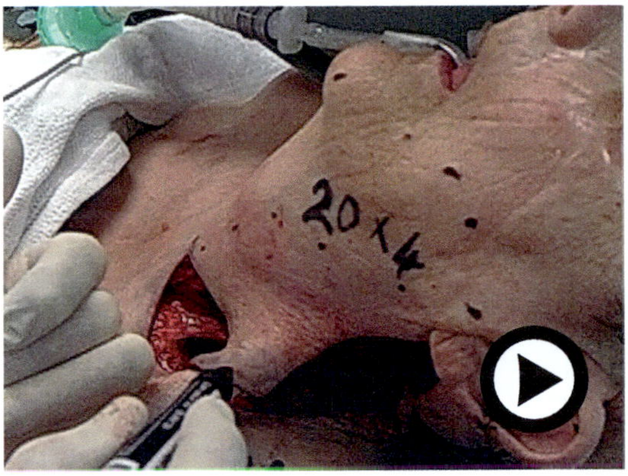

Fig. 2.95 Video 2.12 The cyanotic tip in an irradiated tissue flap salvaged by Keystone delineation, creating hypervascularity (▶ https://doi.org/10.1007/000-k69)

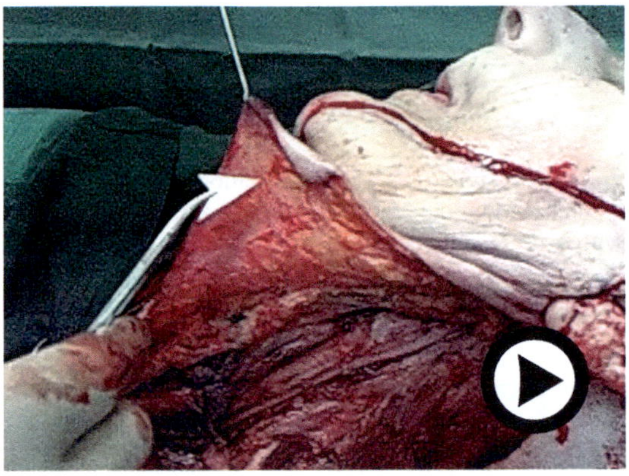

Fig. 2.96 Video 2.13 The microcirculation in the depths of the flap from the cervical fascia (▶ https://doi.org/10.1007/000-k6a)

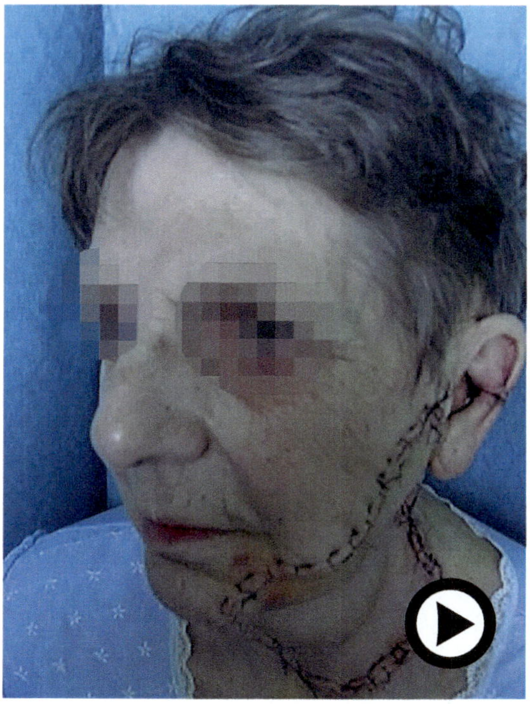

Fig. 2.97 Video 2.14 The patient's postoperative response about the procedure in an irradiated field solved with the Keystone concept (▶ https://doi.org/10.1007/000-k6b)

The PACES characteristics were all exemplified: pain-free, aesthetic, no vascular complications, economical in terms of time and sensory recovery with the resolution of oedema.

2.1.1.9 Case 9—The Closure of a Large Parotid Defect Using a Combined Keystone Approach (Figs. 2.98, 2.99, 2.100, 2.101, 2.102, 2.103, 2.104 and 2.105)

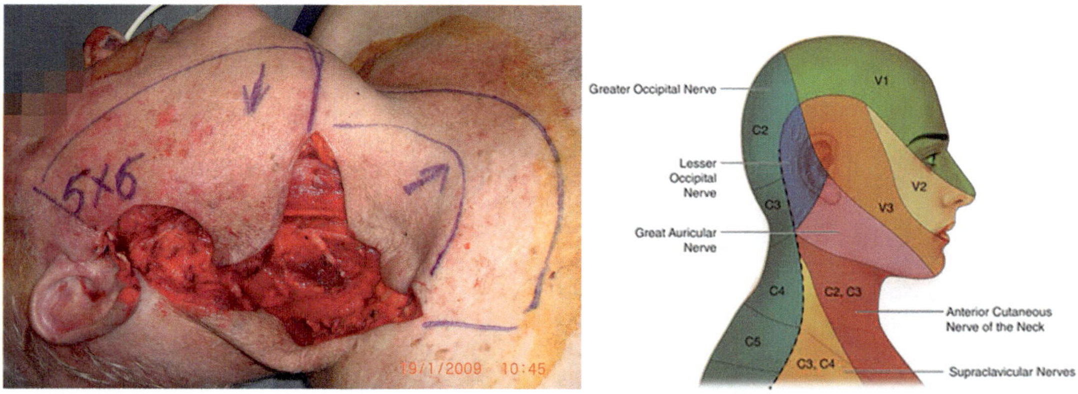

Fig. 2.98 The 5 × 6 cm parotid defect is shown, and the neck clearance of levels II, III and IV cover the vital structures. The dermatomal mark outs become the line of incision of the dermis and epidermis, ensuring that one-third deeply is attached with only partial undermining to facilitate the closure and vascular integrity of the defect. (Reprinted with permission from Atlas, *Reconstructive Technique in Melanoma Management* (p. 19), by Felix Behan, Springer Nature 2023)

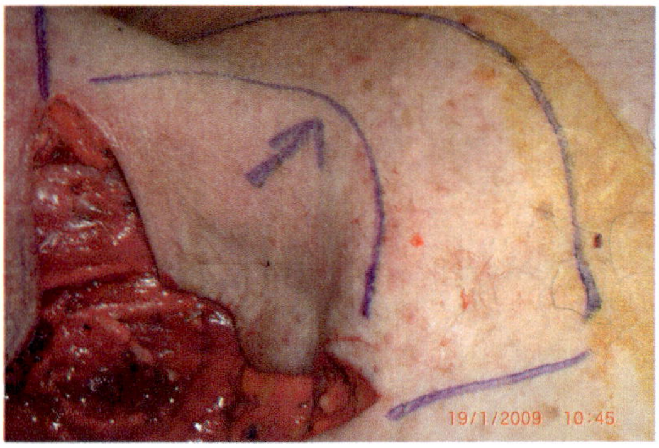

Fig. 2.99 The island of the flap design is indicated by the arrow. This creates the hypervascularity phase that ensures flap perfusion, with arterialised blood helping to close the wounds under tension with drainage

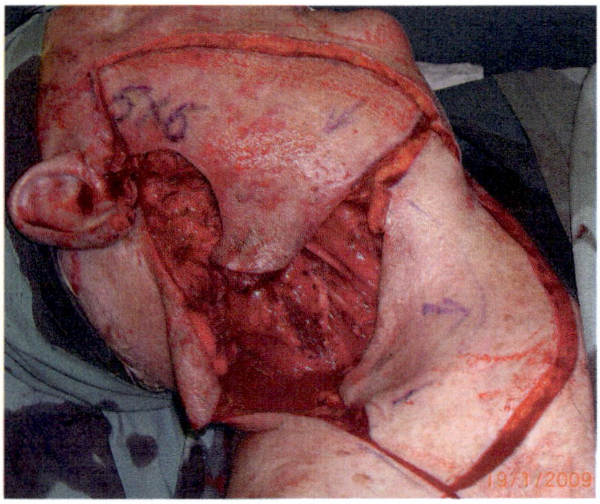

Fig. 2.100 The island flap with one-third deep attachment creates the hypervascularity at the suture point and helps to eliminate the cyanotic phase in the flap survival before it becomes hypervascularised in 15 min

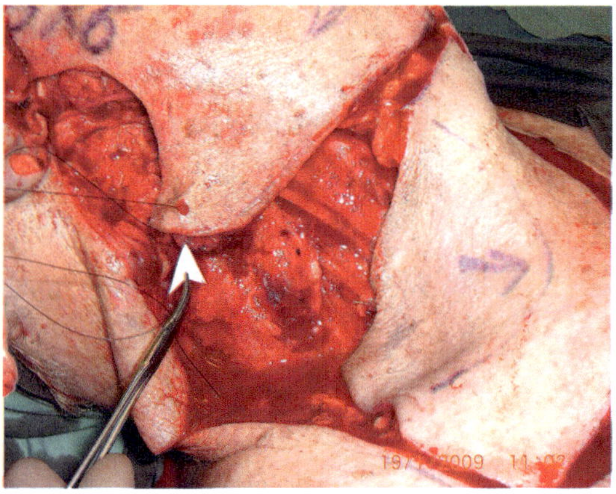

Fig. 2.101 The red dot sign at the extreme point of the island flap, which is now hypervascularised and guaranteeing this perfusional improvement, will contribute to successful healing

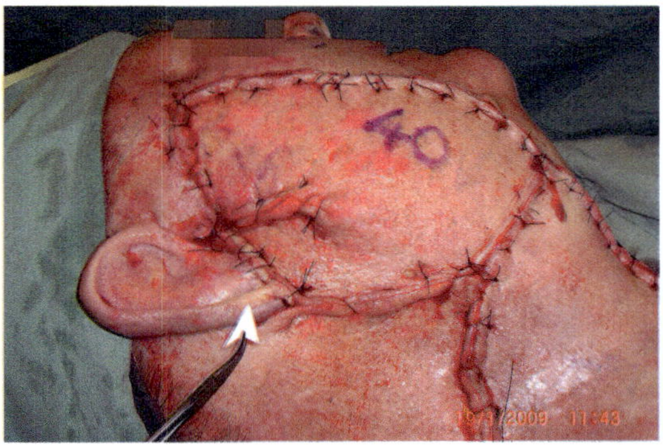

Fig. 2.102 The timeframe of 40 min is evident, and the dog ear excess tissue in the infralobular region can be trimmed because reliance on perfusion allows this secondary additional adjustment in the closure of the wound at the initial period of repair

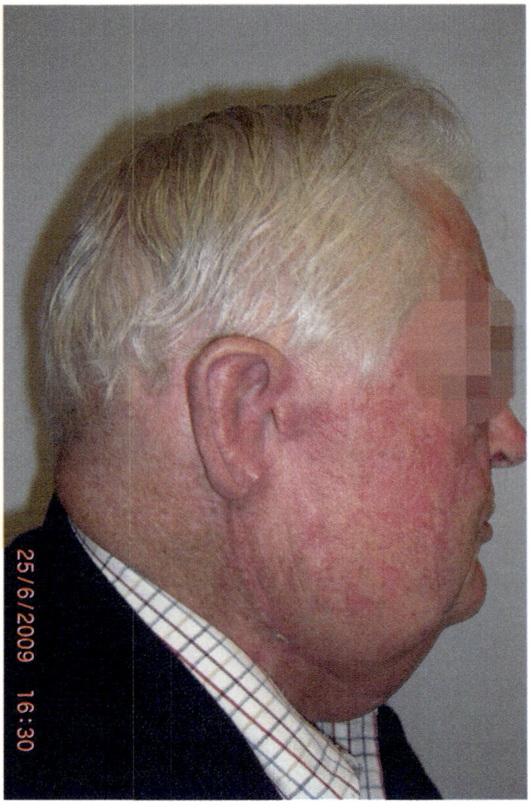

Fig. 2.103 Appearance at 6 months, showing all the characteristics of the Keystone (PACES)

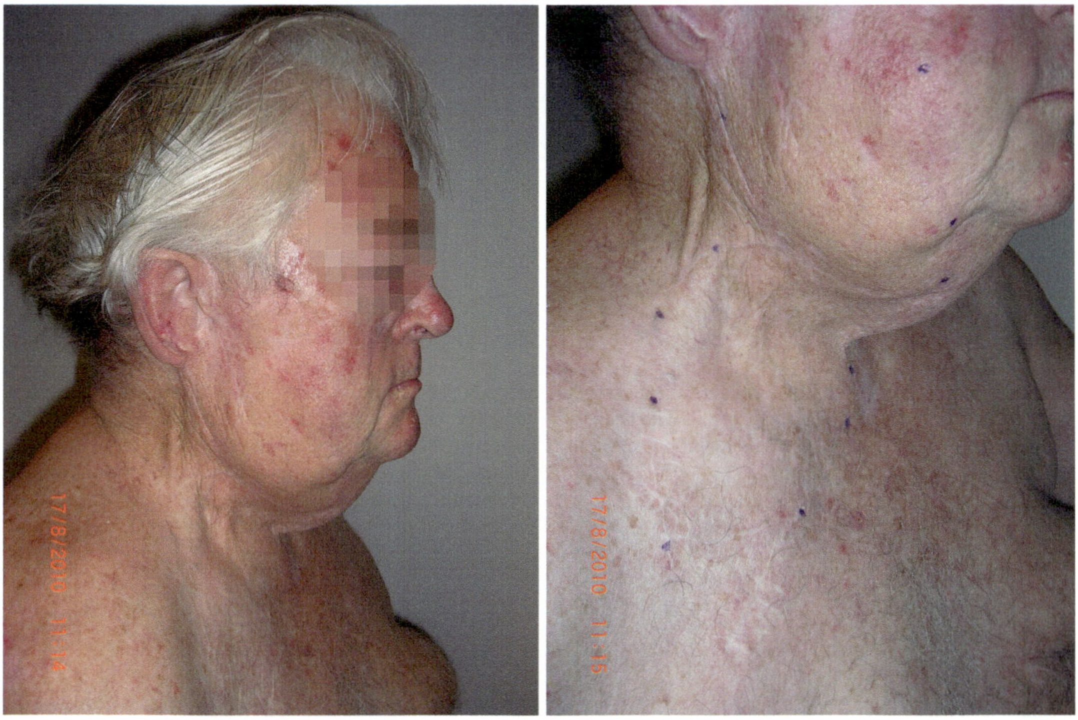

Fig. 2.104 The patient has achieved total comfort and is completely satisfied with the outcome. The indiscernible scarring of the neck reinforces the value of epidermal incisions to hypervascularise flaps with deep attachment. The wounds are closed directly, but any vascular necrosis tends to be bypassed

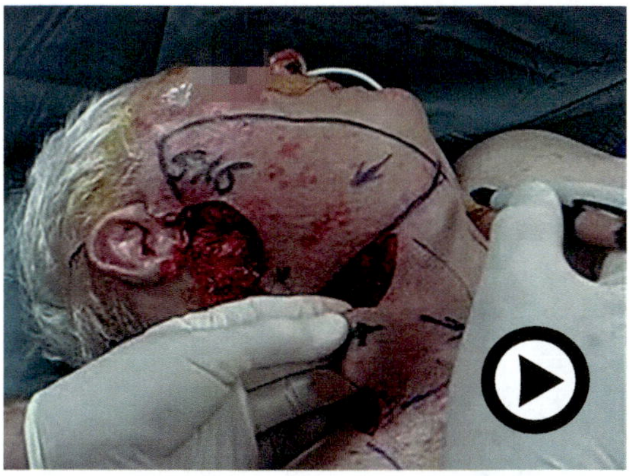

Fig. 2.105 Video 2.15 Salvaging an undermined flap using Keystone principles in an irradiated field (▶ https://doi.org/10.1007/000-k6c)

The PACES characteristics were all exemplified: pain-free, aesthetic, no vascular complications, economical in terms of time and sensory recovery with the resolution of oedema.

2.1.1.10 Case 10—7 × 6 × 3 cm Defect from a Melanoma over the L Parotid (Figs. 2.106, 2.107, 2.108, 2.109, 2.110, 2.111, 2.112 and 2.113)

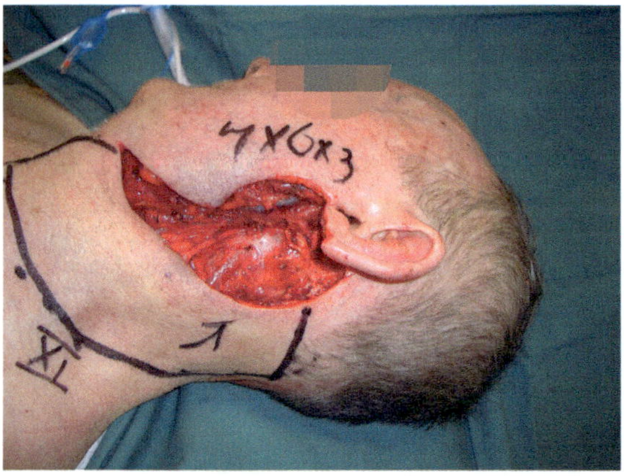

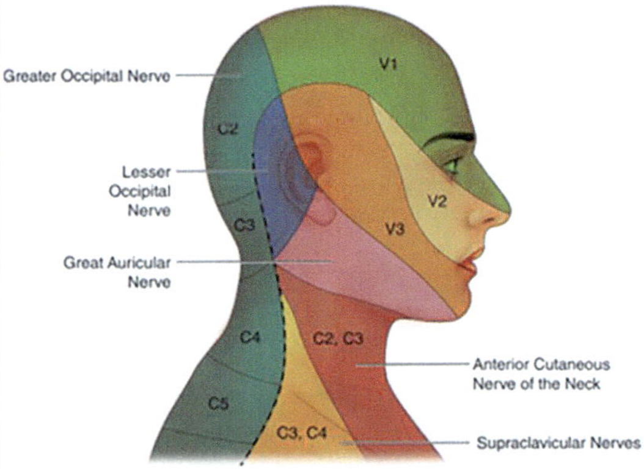

Fig. 2.106 A postoperative 7 × 6 × 3 cm parotid defect from a melanoma is shown. The delineation of the flaps of the Keystone are incised only along the margins, leaving one-third deep attachment without extensive undermining before rotation and advancement. The dermatomal mark outs become the line of incision of the dermis and epidermis, ensuring that one-third deeply is attached with only partial undermining to facilitate the closure and vascular integrity of the defect. (Reprinted with permission from Atlas, *Reconstructive Technique in Melanoma Management* (p. 19), by Felix Behan, Springer Nature 2023)

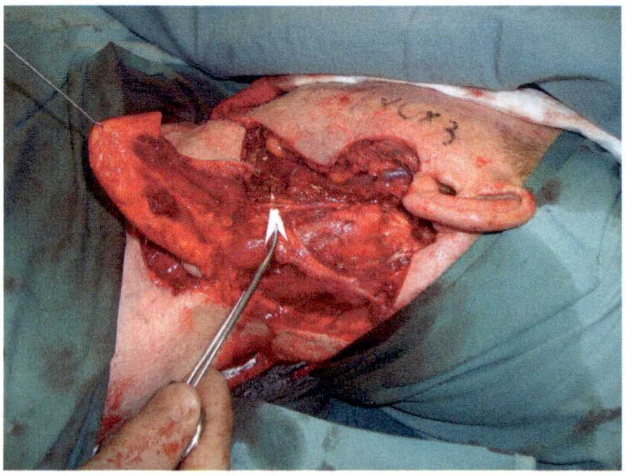

Fig. 2.107 The exposed structures from the neck dissection (arrowed)—accessory nerve

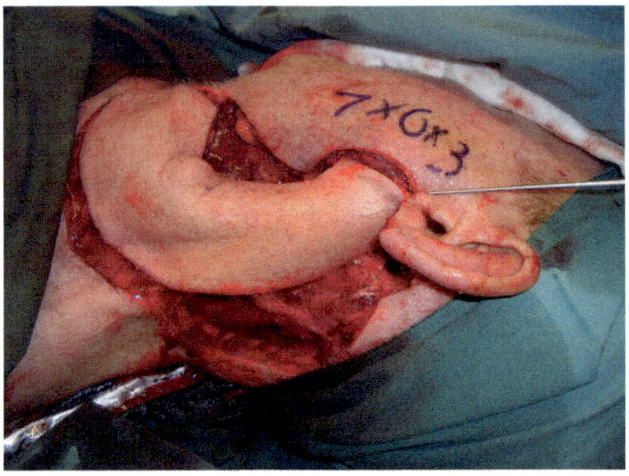

Fig. 2.108 One-third has been undermined to close the excisional defect, and the deep attachment around the sternomastoid is left intact as a source of vascular supply

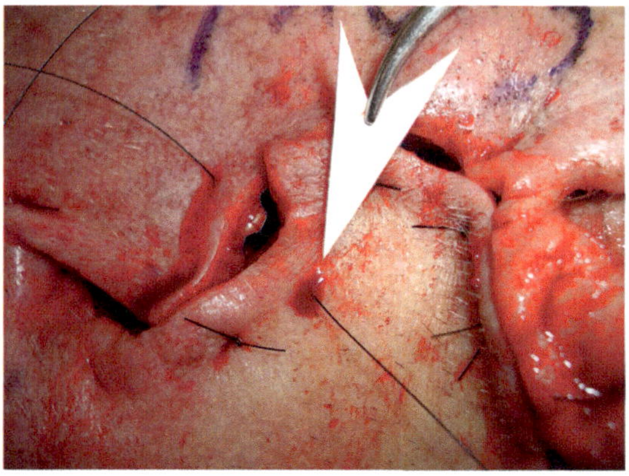

Fig. 2.109 The sequence of closure and the development of hypervascularity is illustrated on the arrow at the suture point by the red dot sign

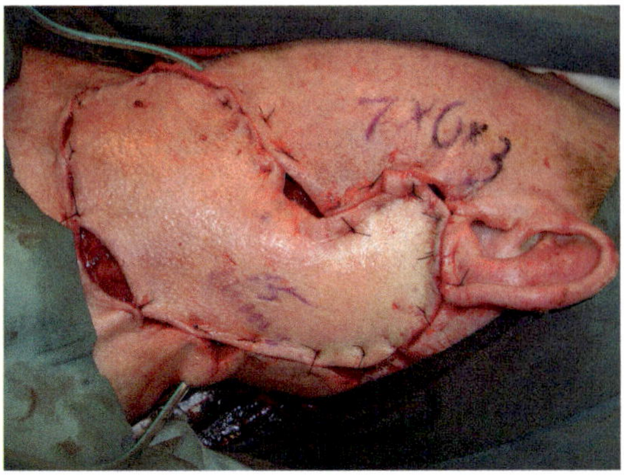

Fig. 2.110 This dermal-epidermal closure has undergone the standard three-phase locking mattress suture technique. The whitish changes in the top disappear at 15 min, as indicated

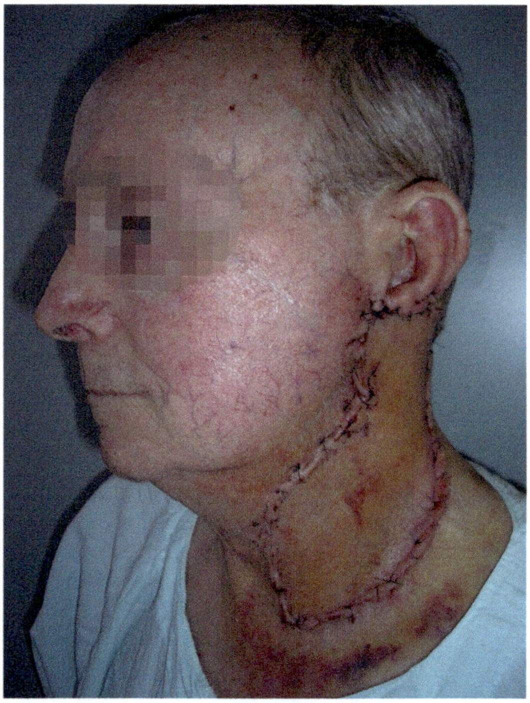

Fig. 2.111 Appearance at 7 days, showing no necrosis and satisfactory wound healing, with a totally pain-free patient

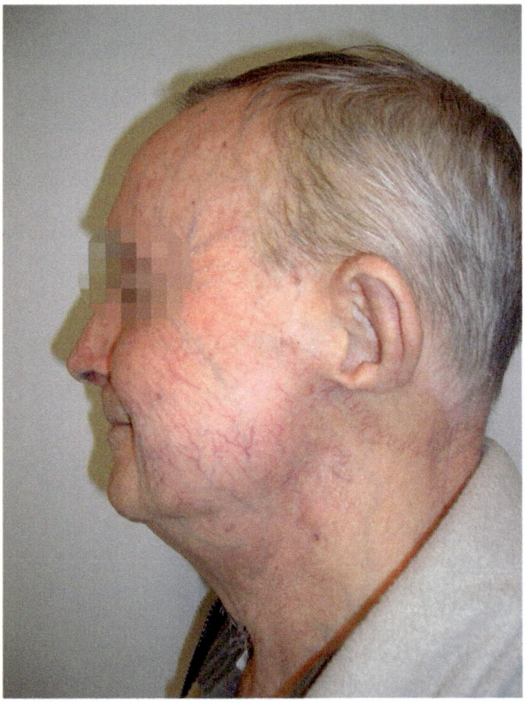

Fig. 2.112 The post XRT appearance shows no sign of recurrence, and the patient's satisfaction is reflected in their smile. In other words, the biology of success without complications and the psychology of success reflected in his physiognomy are illustrated in this clinical image: He is smiling and therefore satisfied

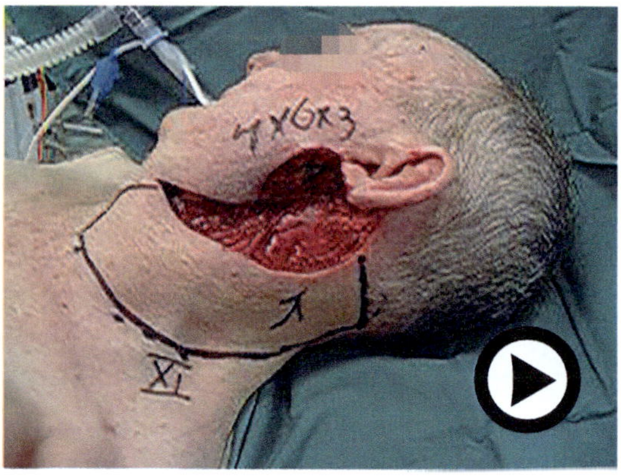

Fig. 2.113 Video 2.16 Planned operative procedure (▶ https://doi.org/10.1007/000-k6d)

The PACES characteristics were all exemplified: pain-free, aesthetic, no vascular complications, economical in terms of time and sensory recovery with the resolution of oedema.

2.1.1.11 Case 11—Malignant Development When the Patient Is Reluctant to Have Surgery, Facilitating the Ingrowth of Maggots (Figs. 2.114, 2.115, 2.116, 2.117, 2.118, 2.119, 2.120, 2.121, 2.122, 2.123, 2.124, 2.125, 2.126 and 2.127).

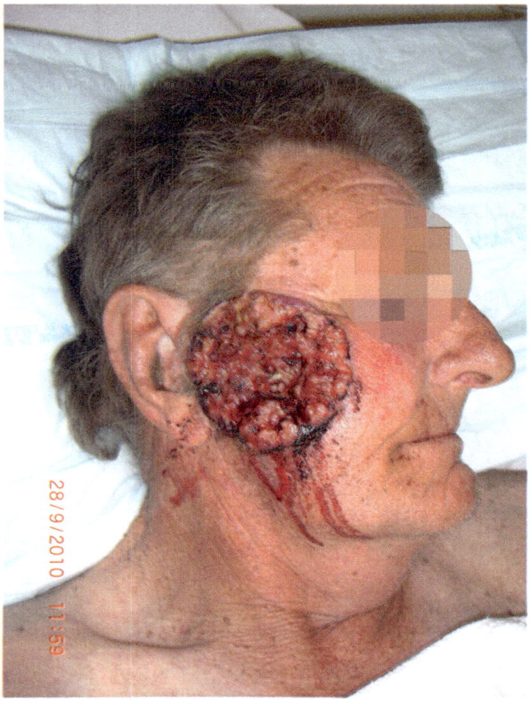

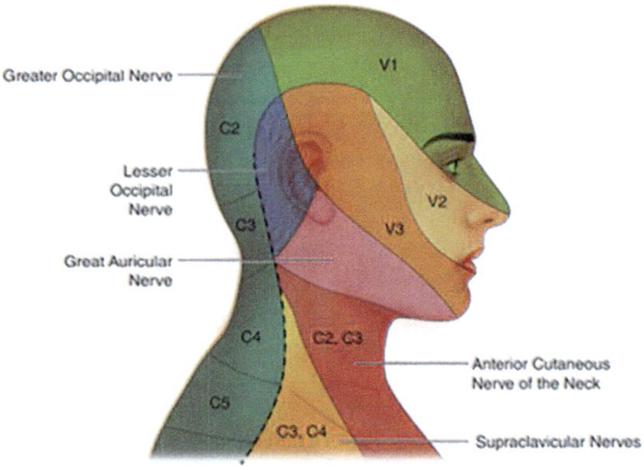

Fig. 2.114 Reluctance regarding major surgery is shown. The dermatomal mark outs become the line of incision of the dermis and epidermis, ensuring that one-third deeply is attached with only partial undermining to facilitate the closure and vascular integrity of the defect. (Reprinted with permission from Atlas, *Reconstructive Technique in Melanoma Management* (p. 19), by Felix Behan, Springer Nature 2023)

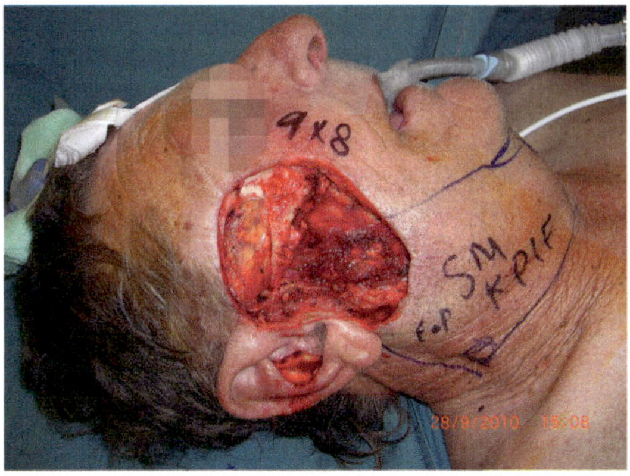

Fig. 2.115 The 9 × 8 cm surgical defect over the parotid and the mark out of the cervico-submental Keystone while leaving the medial section attached and undermined at the level of the cervical fascia

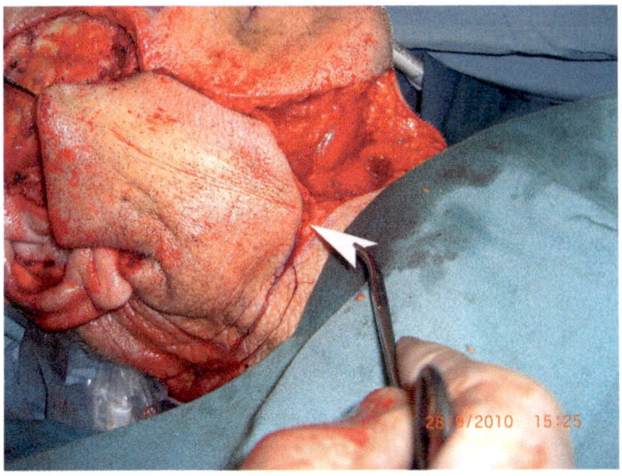

Fig. 2.118 The line of ooze from the suprafascial incision

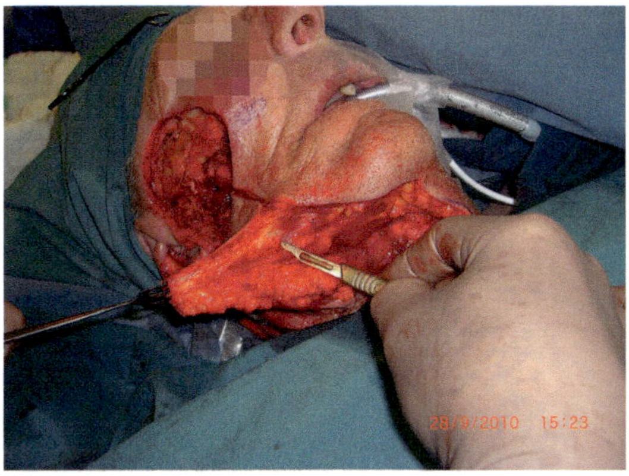

Fig. 2.116 Raising the flap at the level of the cervical fascia

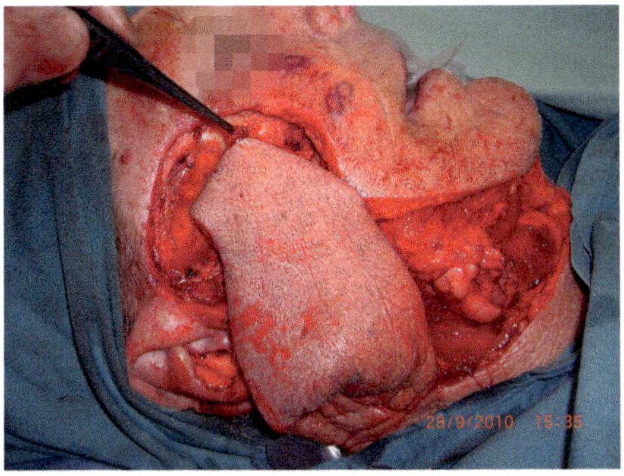

Fig. 2.119 Rotation on the sternomastoid axis is shown. Note the vascular hyperaemia from the dermal-epidermal sympathectomy. Extensive zygomatic closure is also shown

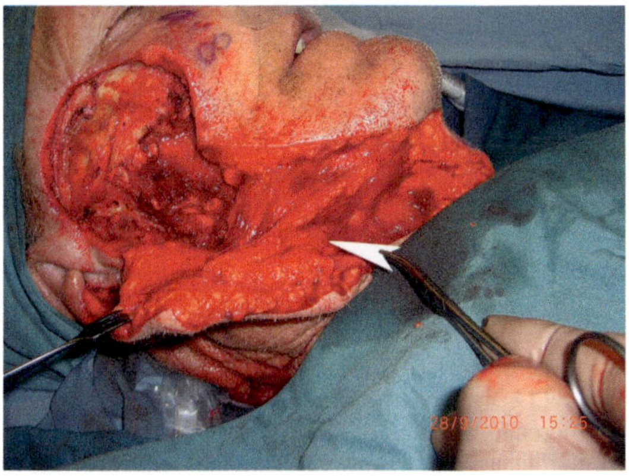

Fig. 2.117 Undermining up to the deep attachments of the sternomastoid for vascular support

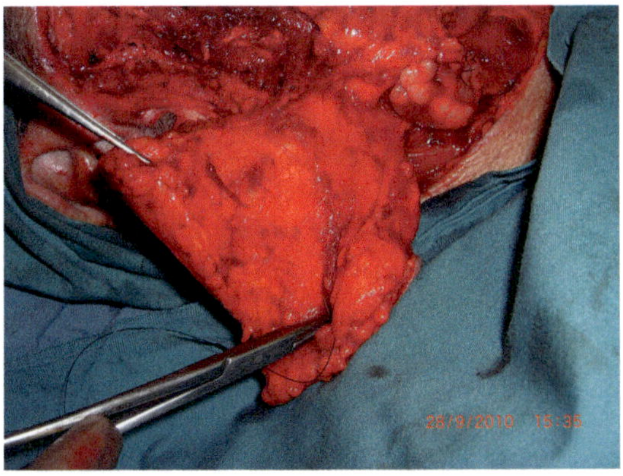

Fig. 2.120 Using Weck clips as a haemostatic technique, avoiding diathermy necrosis

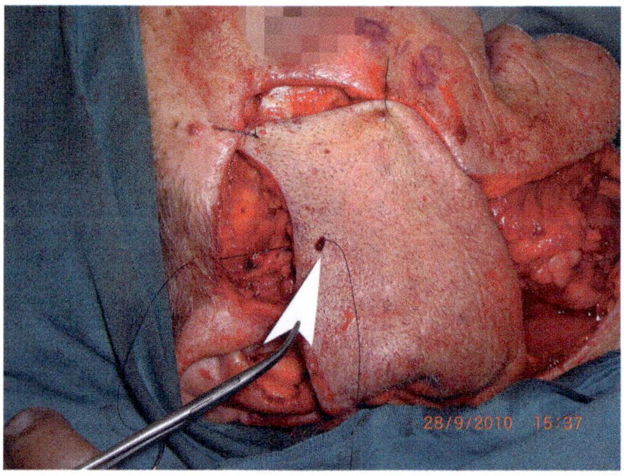

Fig. 2.121 Increased perfusion and the red dot sign (arrowed) are shown, and the white distal limit of the flaps are fully perfused after 3 min (time stamped)

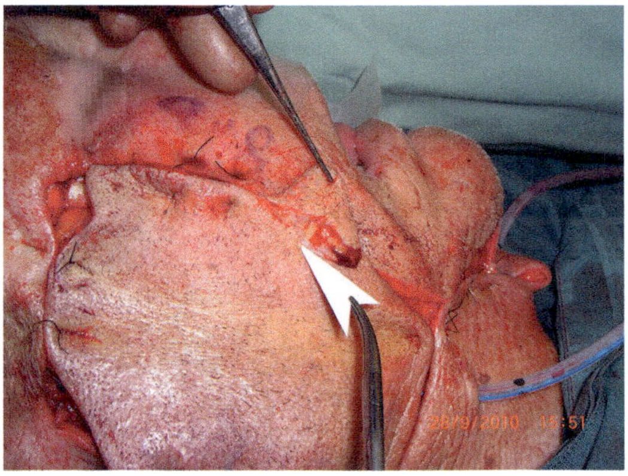

Fig. 2.123 The excess tissue is excised, allowing an aesthetic insertion of the flap

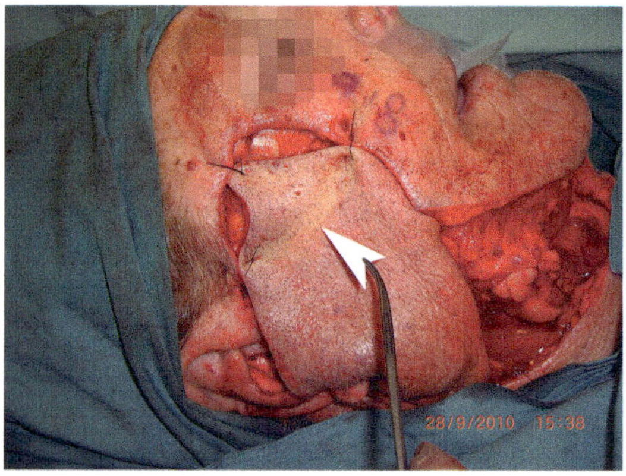

Fig. 2.122 1 min later, the white phase is being replaced by a vascular phase

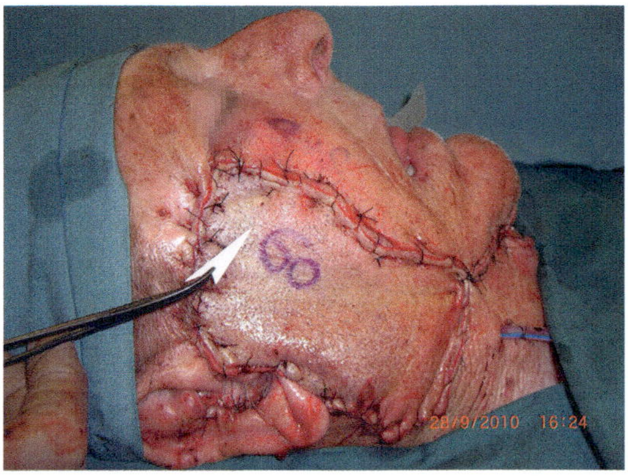

Fig. 2.124 Closure after 60 min is shown. The timeframe is noteworthy in elderly patients and exemplifies the Keystone's characteristics

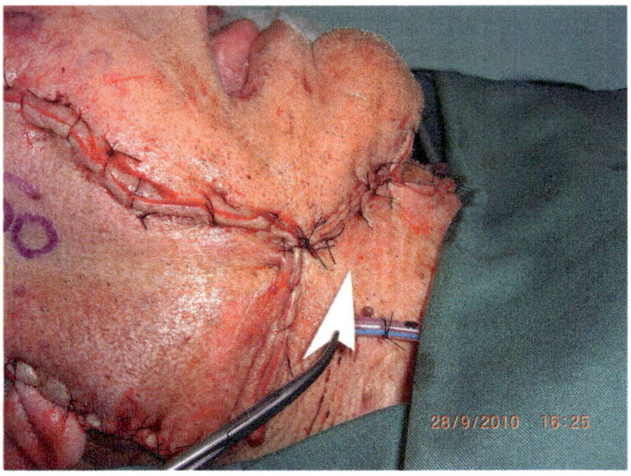

Fig. 2.125 The final closure of the neck wound and the point of maximum tension are imperative. These locking mattress sutures stay in situ for 3 weeks to avoid breakdown

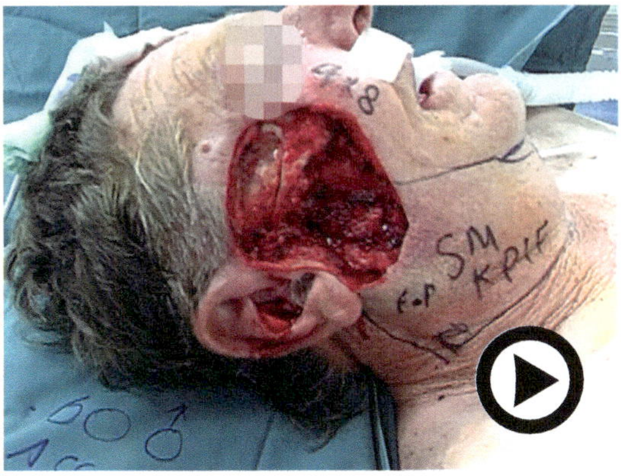

Fig. 2.127 Video 2.17 The Keystone principle of closure for a large parotid defect for the cervico-submental Keystone (▶ https://doi.org/10.1007/000-k6e)

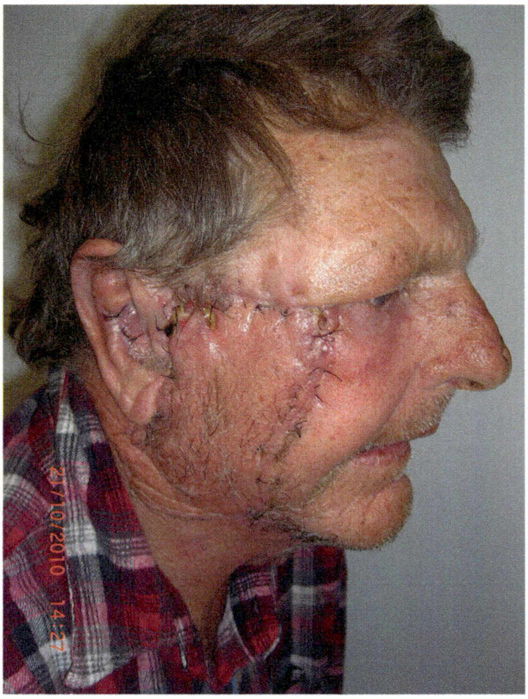

Fig. 2.126 Appearance at 24 days before XRT

The PACES characteristics were all exemplified: pain-free, aesthetic, no vascular complications, economical in terms of time and sensory recovery with the resolution of oedema.

2.1.1.12 Case 12—CA Parotid and Block Dissection Levels II, III and IV in a 68-Year-Old (Figs. 2.128, 2.129, 2.130, 2.131, 2.132 and 2.133)

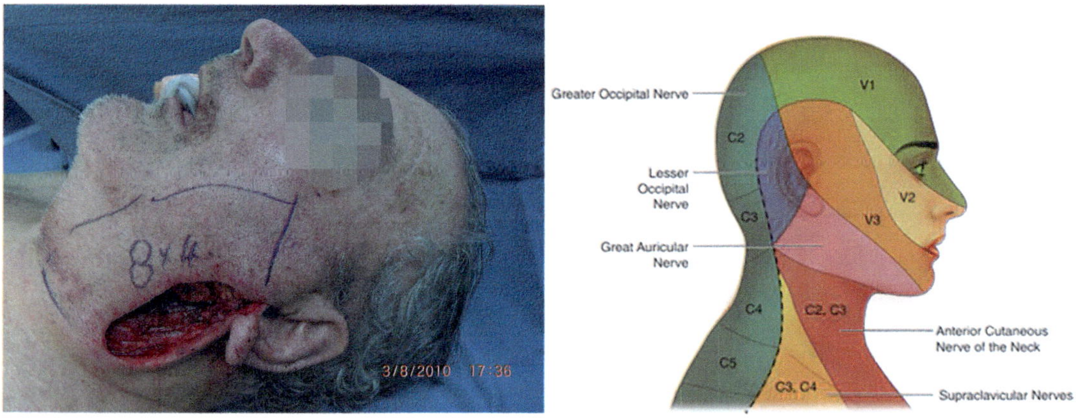

Fig. 2.128 The mark out of the Keystone reconstruction, where the skin and epidermis are excised to create a sympathectomy effect, leaves only one-third of deep attachment. This dynamic form of tightness in closure supersedes the value of facial nerve reconstruction if it is sacrificed. The dermatomal mark outs become the line of incision of the dermis and epidermis, ensuring that one-third deeply is attached with only partial undermining to facilitate the closure and vascular integrity of the defect. (Reprinted with permission from Atlas, *Reconstructive Technique in Melanoma Management* (p. 19), by Felix Behan, Springer Nature 2023)

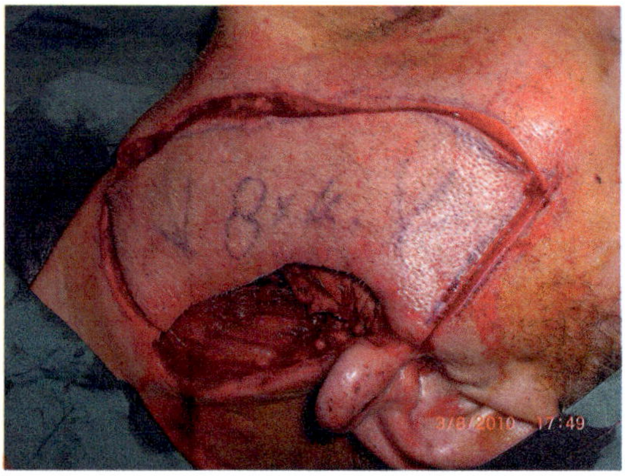

Fig. 2.129 Islanding creates the hypervascularity phase when the mark out is incised at the dermal-epidermal levels. This umbrella of tissue in the Keystone design facilitates the direct closure of the parotid defect

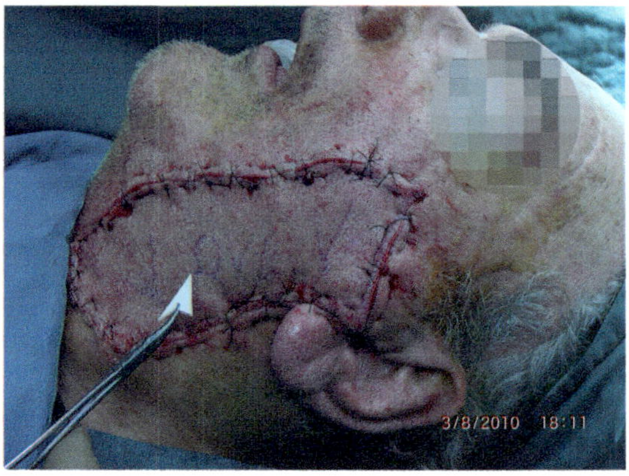

Fig. 2.130 Completion at 25 min, as timestamped

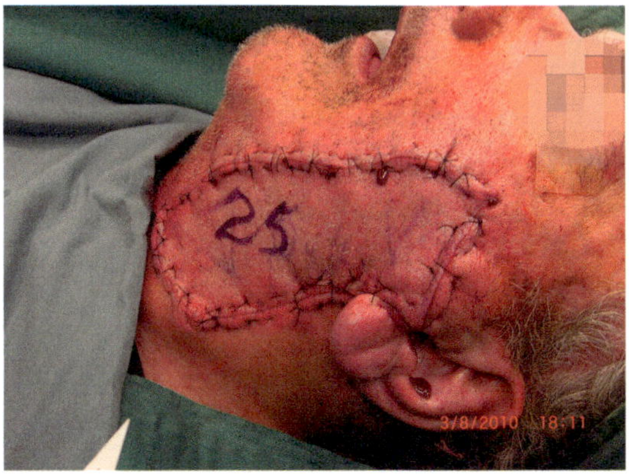

Fig. 2.131 Fully vascularised with no sites of impending necrosis

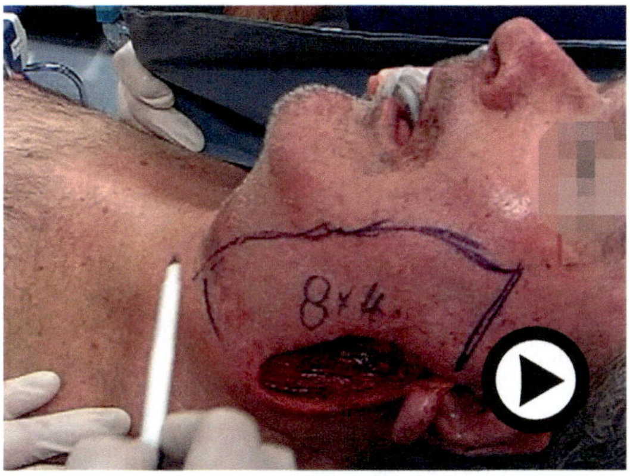

Fig. 2.132 Video 2.18 Planned operative procedure in a large parotid defect in a patient with comorbidities and blood dyscrasias (▶ https://doi.org/10.1007/000-k6f)

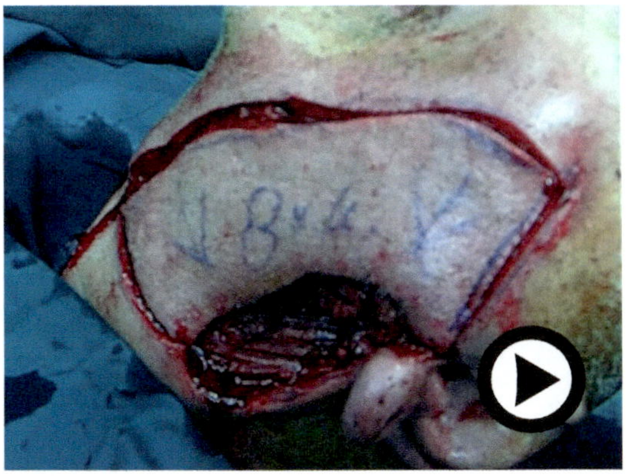

Fig. 2.133 Video 2.19 The hypervascularisation phase in a Keystone, reflecting the sympathectomy effect, as hypothesised (▶ https://doi.org/10.1007/000-k6g)

The PACES characteristics were all exemplified: pain-free, aesthetic, no vascular complications, economical in terms of time and sensory recovery with the resolution of oedema.

2.1.1.13 Case 13—CA of the External Canal Extending onto Mastoid and Parotid (Figs. 2.134, 2.135, 2.136, 2.137, 2.138, 2.139, 2.140, 2.141, 2.142, 2.143 and 2.144)

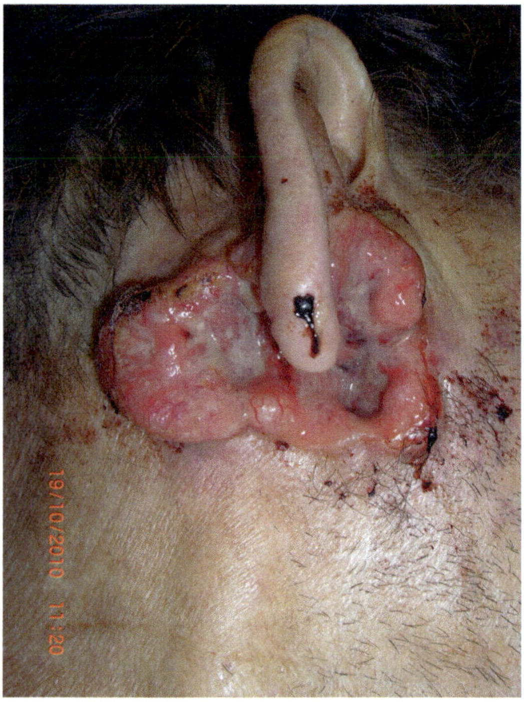

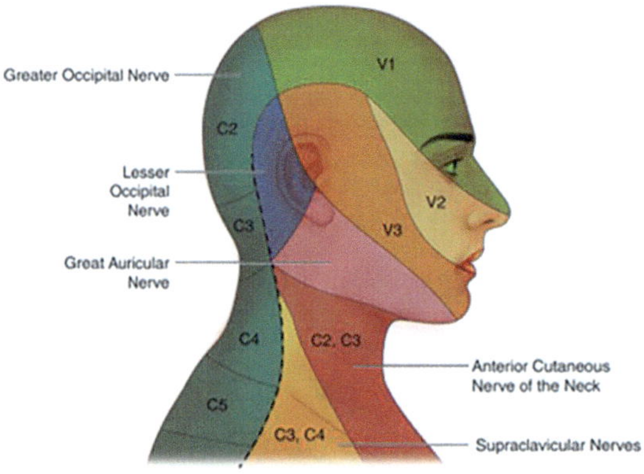

Fig. 2.134 On presentation, the biopsy confirmed SCC on this lobulated tumour mass. The dermatomal mark outs become the line of incision of the dermis and epidermis, ensuring that one-third deeply is attached with only partial undermining to facilitate the closure and vascular integrity of the defect. (Reprinted with permission from Atlas, *Reconstructive Technique in Melanoma Management* (p. 19), by Felix Behan, Springer Nature 2023)

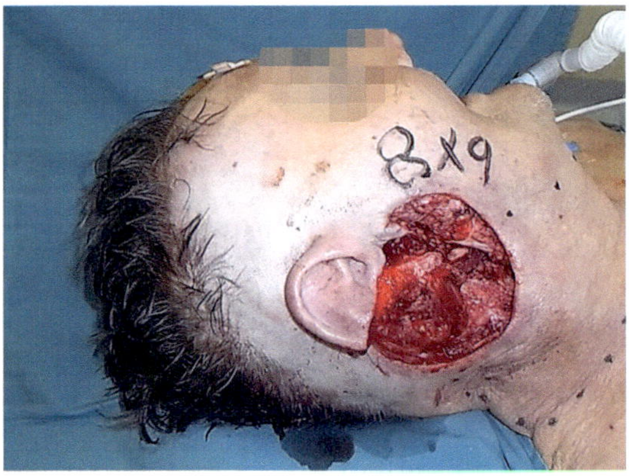

Fig. 2.135 The excision, including the external canal, mastoid and parotid

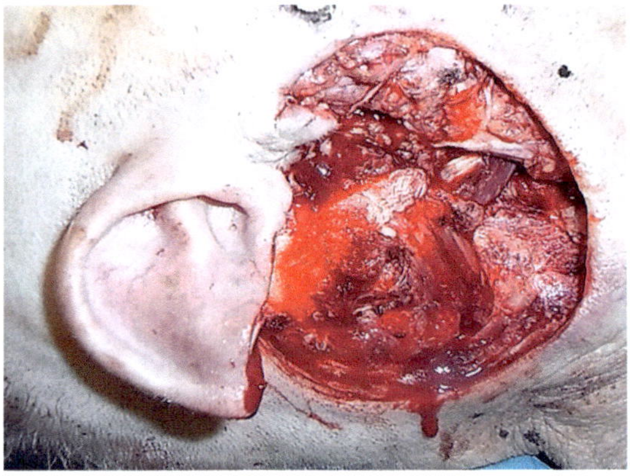

Fig. 2.136 The 8 × 9 cm surgical defect down to the temporomandibular joint (TMJ)

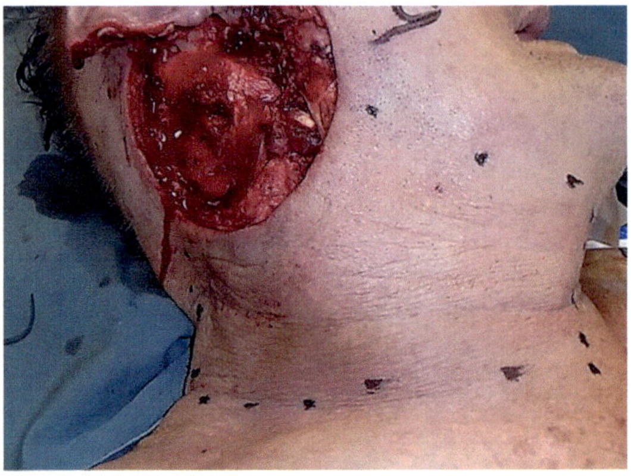

Fig. 2.137 The Keystone mark out for the cervico-submental Keystone that is to be rotated into the defect on the basis of the sternomastoid perforators

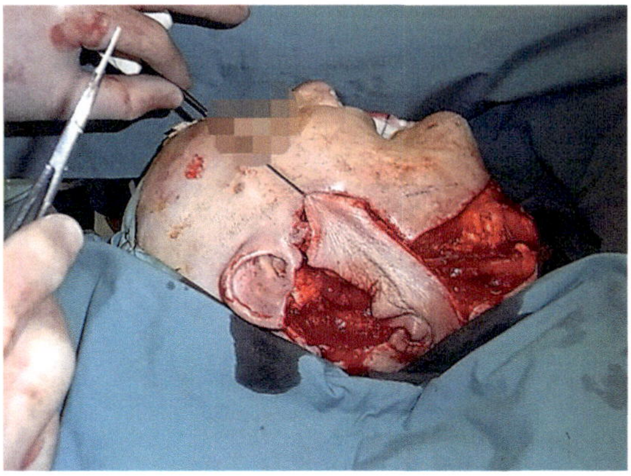

Fig. 2.138 Rotation of the flap into the defect where the anterior two-thirds has been undermined at the level of the cervical fascia

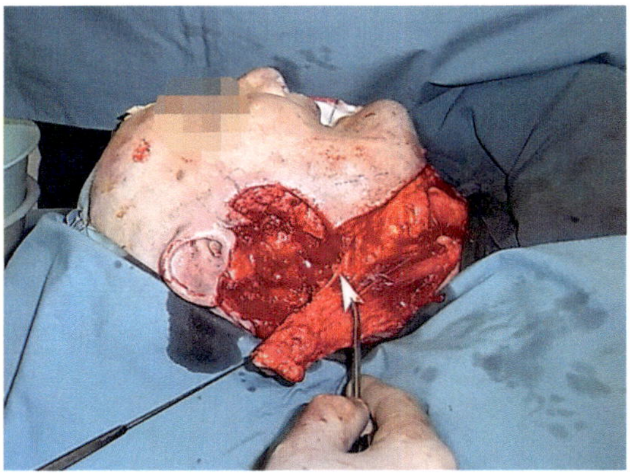

Fig. 2.139 The white arrow on the neural structures of the blocked dissection (accessory nerve)

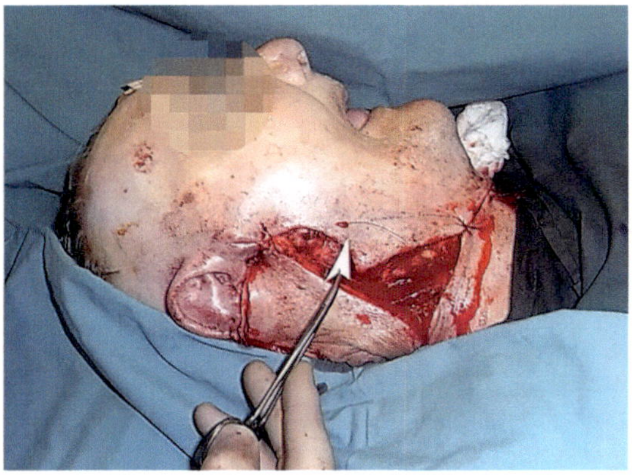

Fig. 2.140 Further staged closure of the secondary defect of the neck using our standard three-phase locking mattress suture technique

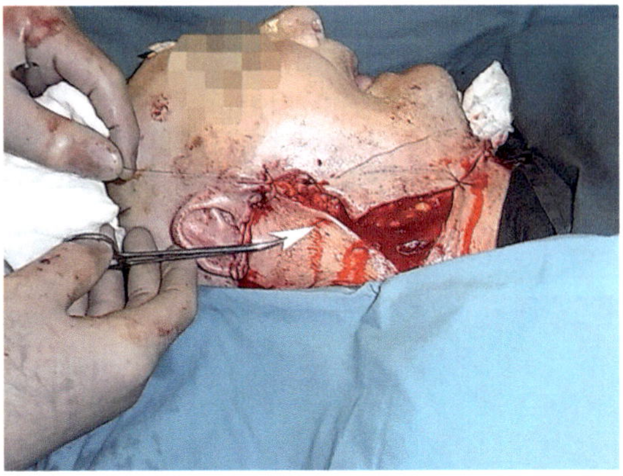

Fig. 2.141 Two red dot signs in the flap confirming its vascular reliability (white arrowed)

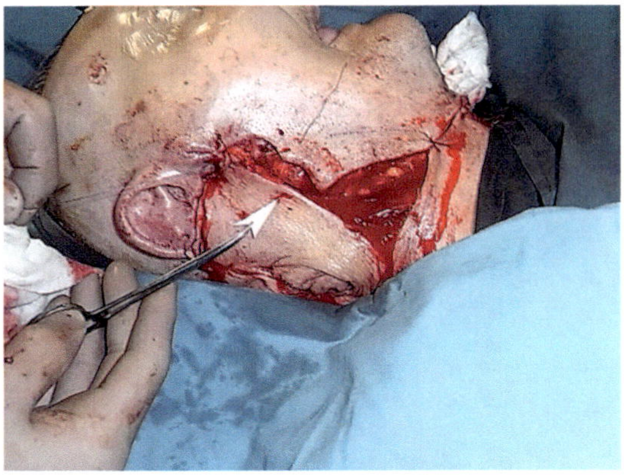

Fig. 2.142 Further progress stages in the closure

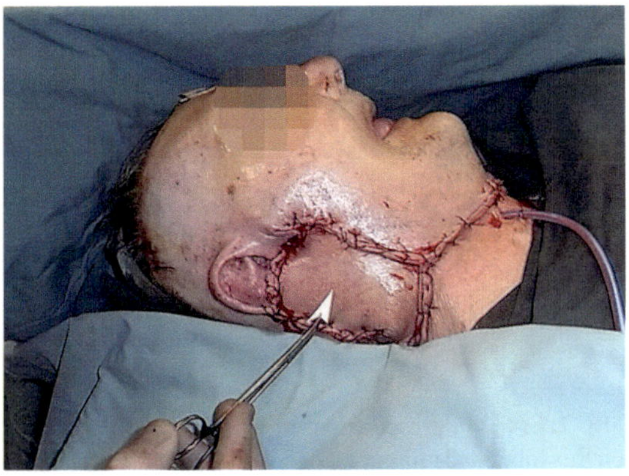

Fig. 2.143 Completion at 60 min used drainage tubes in situ. In microsurgery, drainage tubes are usually a contra-indication and a controversial issue. With the Keystone reconstructions, this is not an issue, because wounds drain

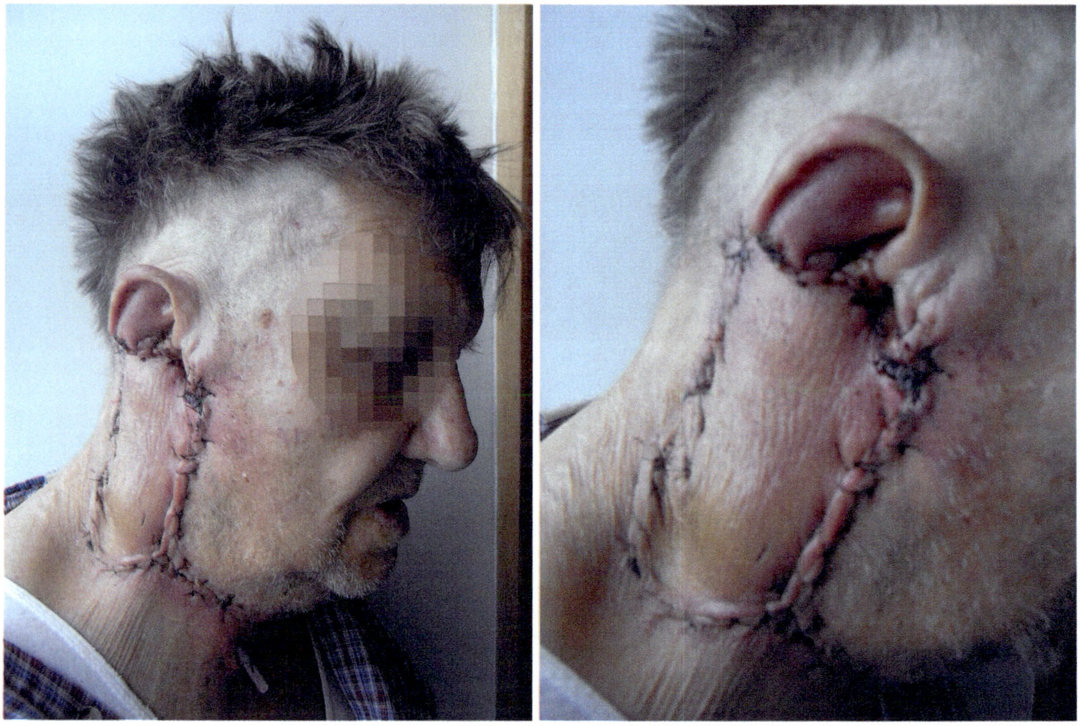

Fig. 2.144 The appearance at 8 days from our dated records exemplifies the Keystone characteristics. The standard three-phase locking mattress was used throughout, the tension suture at the neck must be left in for 3 weeks

The PACES characteristics were all exemplified: pain-free, aesthetic, no vascular complications, economical in terms of time and sensory recovery with the resolution of oedema.

2.1.1.14 Case 14—Parotid and External Canal and TMJ for an SCC (Figs. 2.145, 2.146, 2.147, 2.148, 2.149, 2.150, 2.151, 2.152, 2.153 and 2.154)

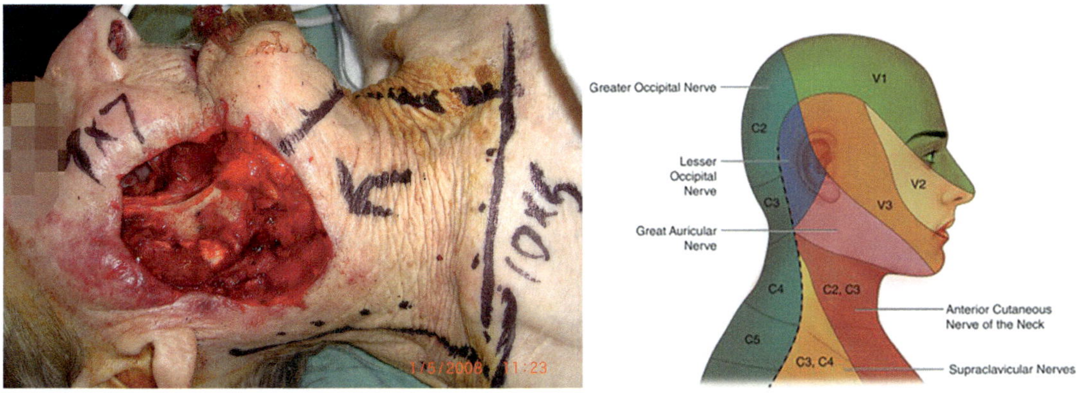

Fig. 2.145 10 × 5 cm defect and the mark out of the cervico-submental Keystone are shown, and these mark out lines are the basis for the sympathectomy effect produced as long as one-third of deeper tissues is attached. The dermatomal mark outs become the line of incision of the dermis and epidermis, ensuring that one-third deeply is attached with only partial undermining to facilitate the closure and vascular integrity of the defect. (Reprinted with permission from Atlas, *Reconstructive Technique in Melanoma Management* (p. 19), by Felix Behan, Springer Nature 2023)

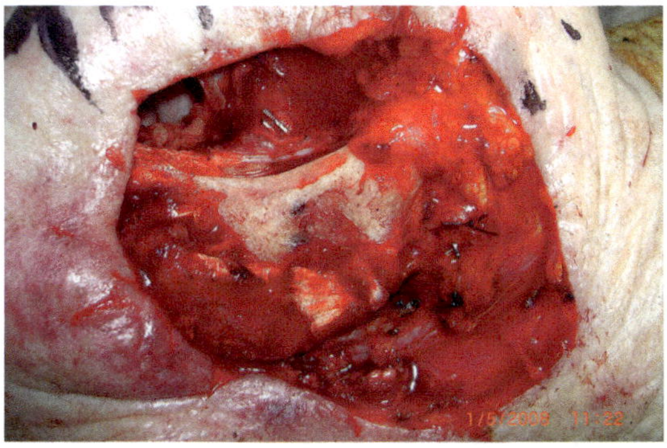

Fig. 2.146 The surgical defect and the excised ascending ramus of the mandible

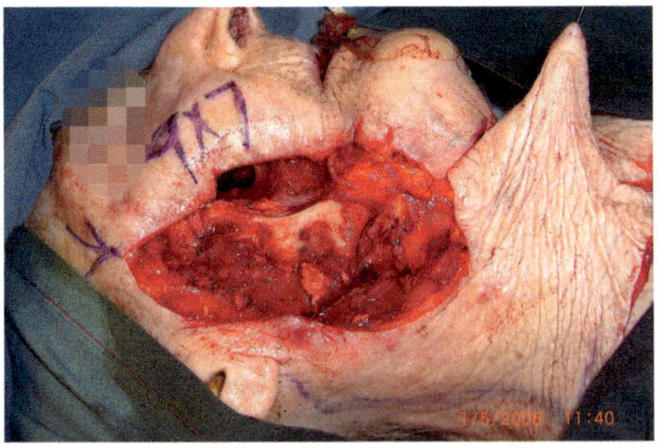

Fig. 2.147 The cervico-submental flap elevated when detached from the cervical fascia and hinged on the sternomastoid attachment

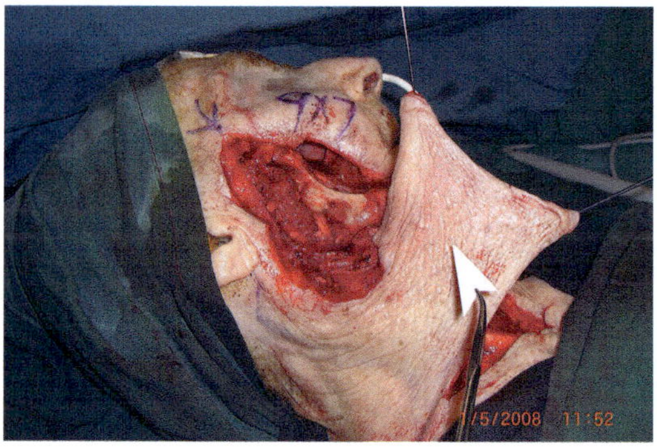

Fig. 2.148 The axis of rotation on the sternomastoid circulation

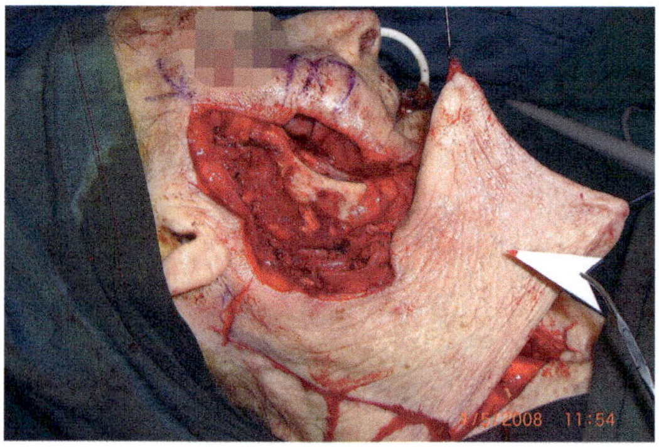

Fig. 2.149 The revascularisation phase following the sympathectomy by delineating the Keystone flap

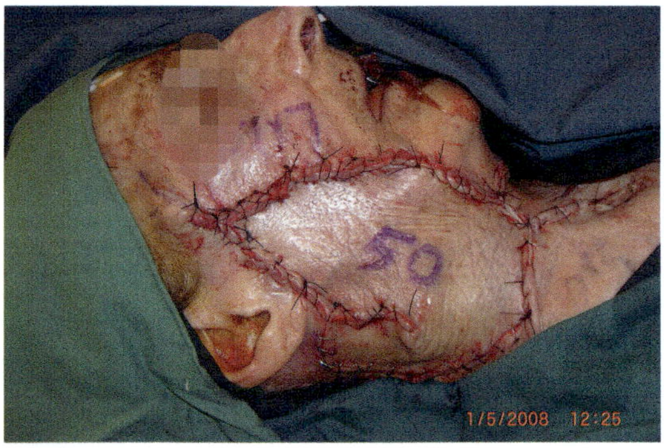

Fig. 2.150 The closure at 50 min shows no signs of impending necrosis from a vascular point of view. The standard three-phase locking mattress suture technique is applied at the key points of maximum tension but for some reason staples were used and their appearance shows the deficiency in not getting layered tissue alignment with epidermal seal

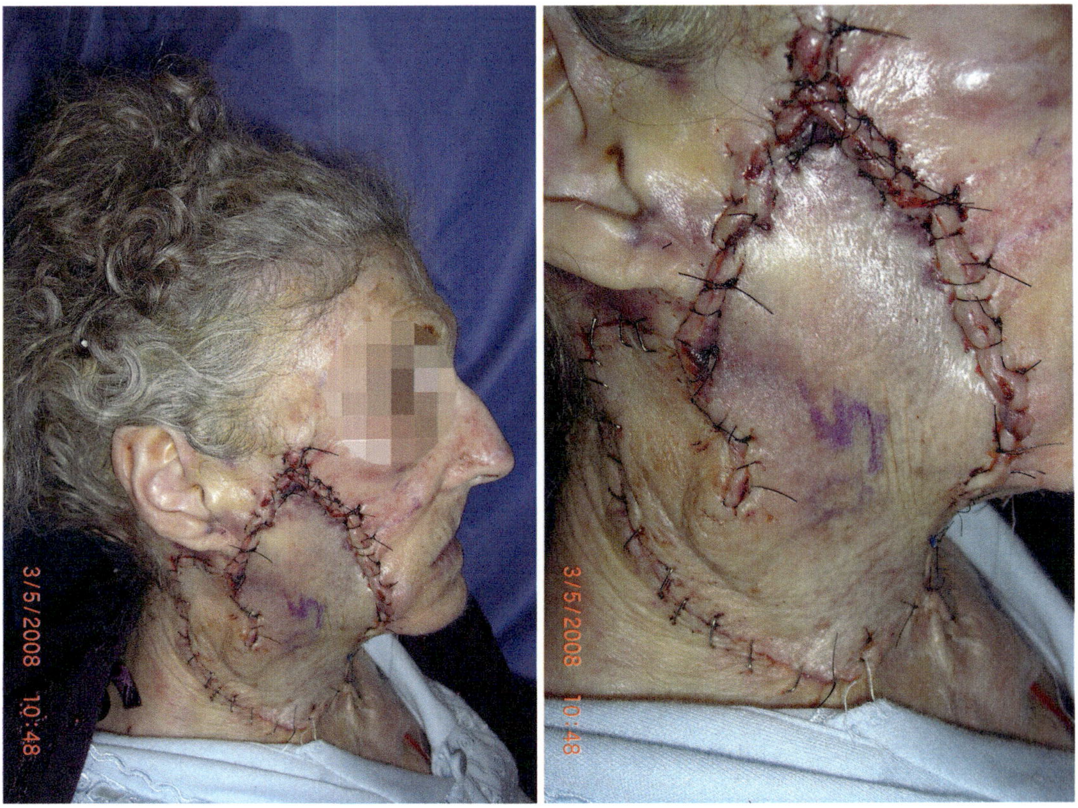

Fig. 2.151 Postoperative appearance at 2 days, with the patient exemplifying the PACES characteristics

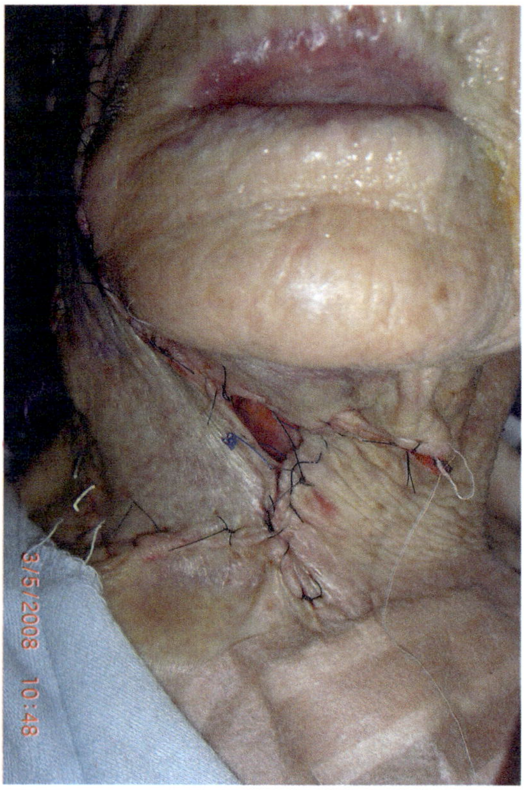

Fig. 2.152 Postoperative appearance at 2 days and the premature removal of a tension suture

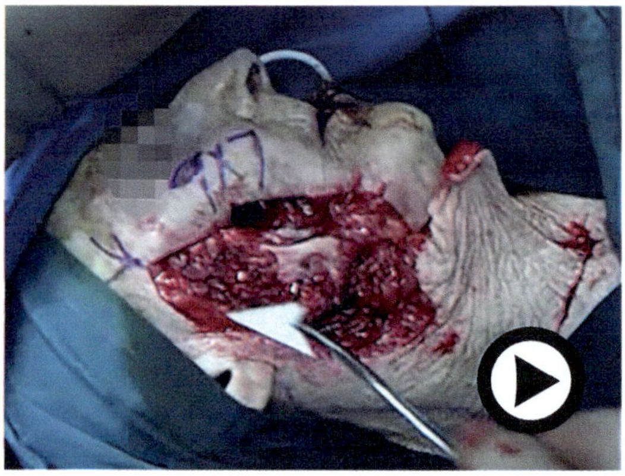

Fig. 2.153 Video 2.20 Cervico-submental flap elevation with blunt dissection and insertion into the large parotid defect (▶ https://doi.org/10.1007/000-k6h)

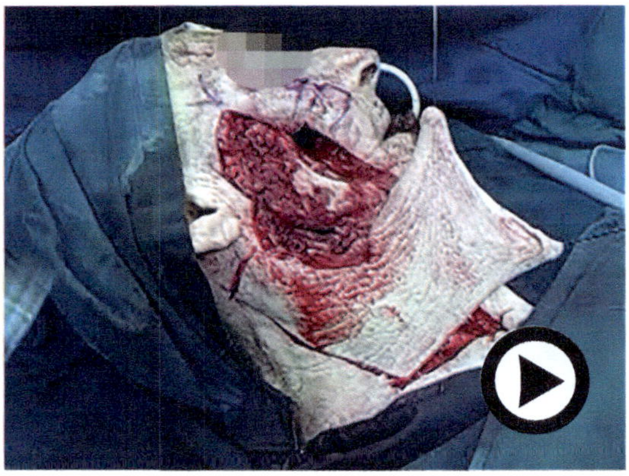

Fig. 2.154 Video 2.21 The hypervascularity of the flap initiated by the Keystone design (incision at the dermal-epidermal level only) (▶ https://doi.org/10.1007/000-k6j)

The PACES characteristics were all exemplified: pain-free, aesthetic, no vascular complications, economical in terms of time and sensory recovery with the resolution of oedema.

2.1.1.15 Case 15—Parotid SCC Neck Clearance with Failed XRT (Figs. 2.155, 2.156, 2.157, 2.158, 2.159, 2.160, 2.161 and 2.162)

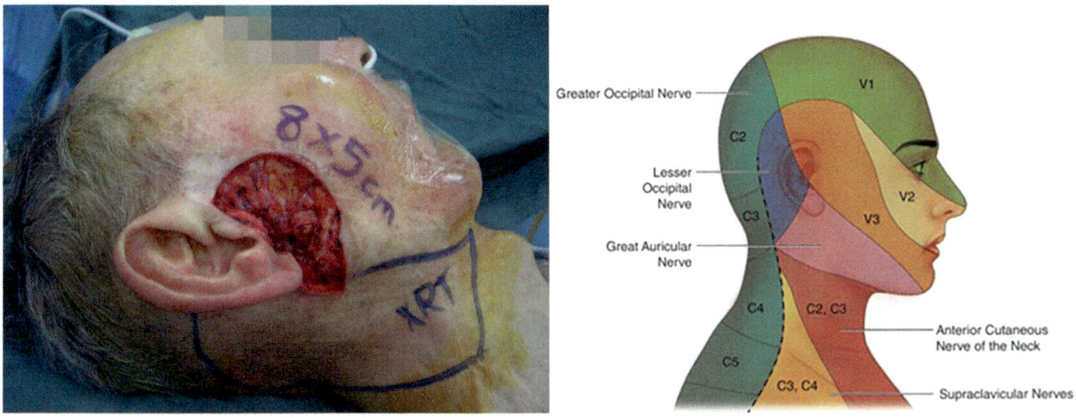

Fig. 2.155 The 8 × 5 cm surgical defect over the parotid following failed XRT and the cervico-submental Keystone mark out of the dermis epidermis can stimulate hypervascularisation as long as one-third of deep attachment is retained. The dermatomal mark outs become the line of incision of the dermis and epidermis, ensuring that one-third deeply is attached with only partial undermining to facilitate the closure and vascular integrity of the defect. (Reprinted with permission from Atlas, *Reconstructive Technique in Melanoma Management* (p. 19), by Felix Behan, Springer Nature 2023)

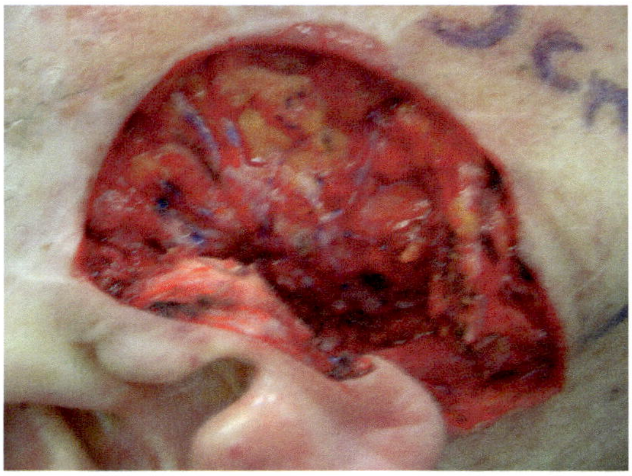

Fig. 2.156 A dissected facial nerve

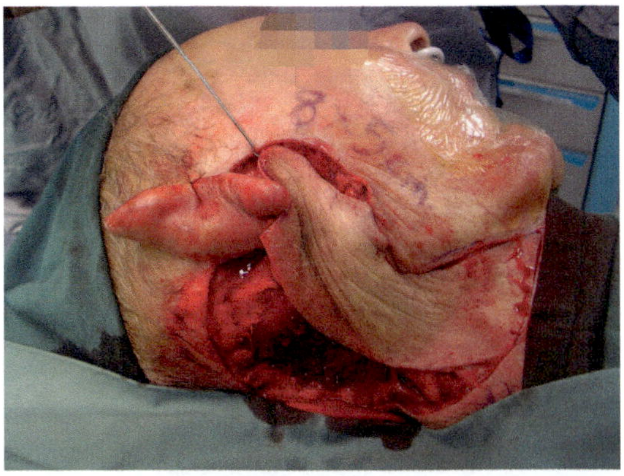

Fig. 2.157 Staged surgical closure with advancement, rotation and transposition before closing under tension, facilitated by the hypervascularisation

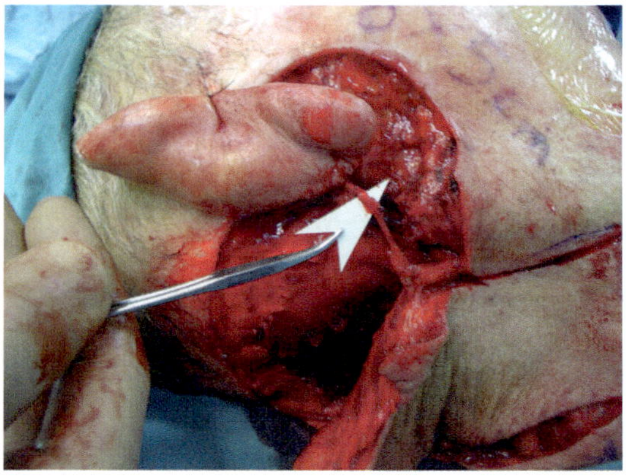

Fig. 2.158 A white arrow indicating part of the block dissection and the preservation of the accessory nerve

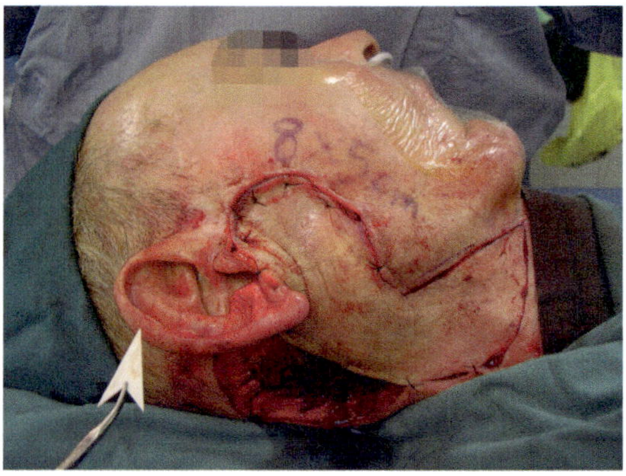

Fig. 2.159 Before closing over the mastoid defect via direct apposition

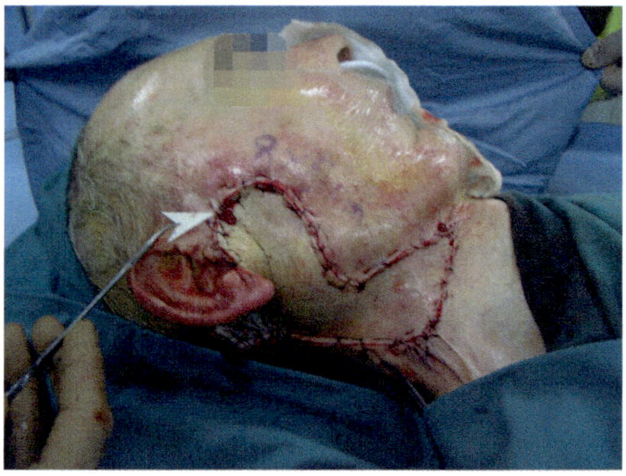

Fig. 2.160 No sign of necrosis in spite of closing under tension

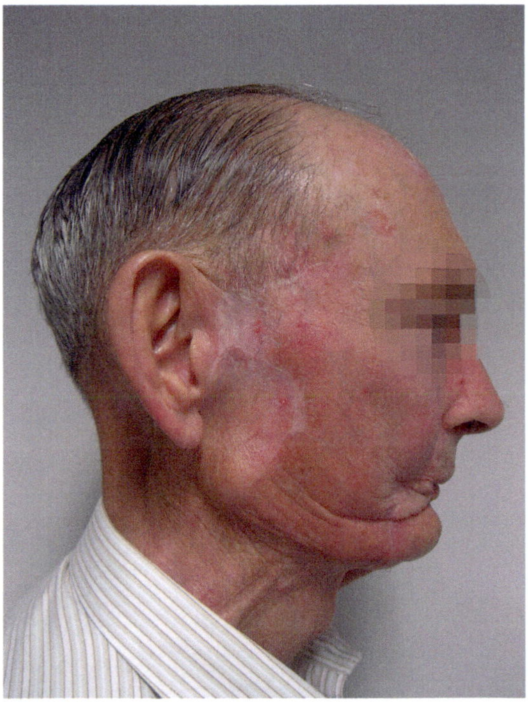

Fig. 2.161 Postoperative appearance at 1 year and no complications from the microsurgical jaw replacement

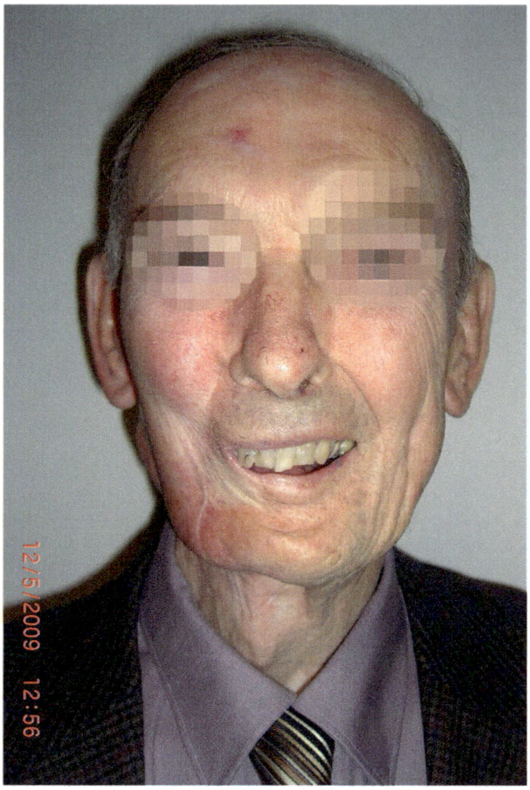

Fig. 2.162 Postoperative appearance 3 years tumour-free is shown, and the patient's happy appearance reflects his satisfaction with being asymptomatic

The PACES characteristics were all exemplified: pain-free, aesthetic, no vascular complications, economical in terms of time and sensory recovery with the resolution of oedema.

2.1.1.16 Case 16—Melanoma of the Conchal Fossa (Figs. 2.163, 2.164, 2.165, 2.166, 2.167, 2.168 and 2.169)

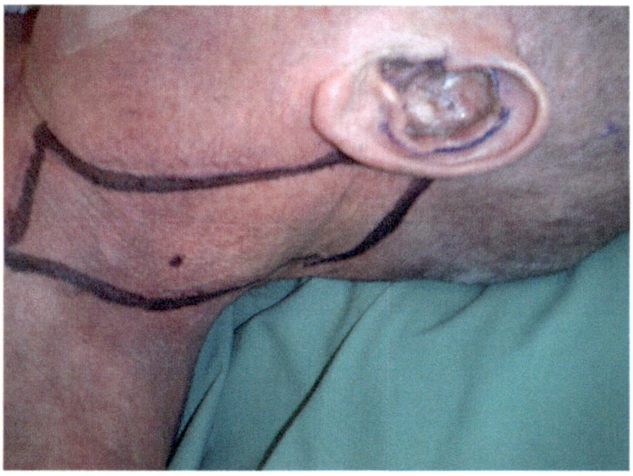

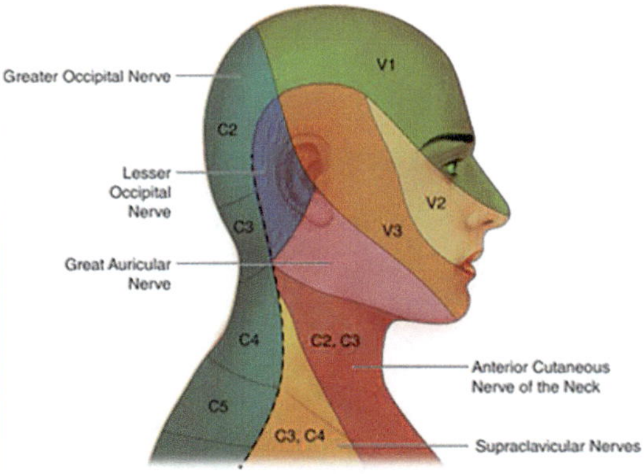

Fig. 2.163 The dermal mark out of the Keystone to be inserted into the conchal fossa, with a bridge delineated and de-epithelialised to allow the reapposition of the helix, another confirmation of the vascular reliability of the Keystone concept. The dermatomal mark outs become the line of incision of the dermis and epidermis, ensuring that one-third deeply is attached with only partial undermining to facilitate the closure and vascular integrity of the defect. (Reprinted with permission from Atlas, *Reconstructive Technique in Melanoma Management* (p. 19), by Felix Behan, Springer Nature 2023)

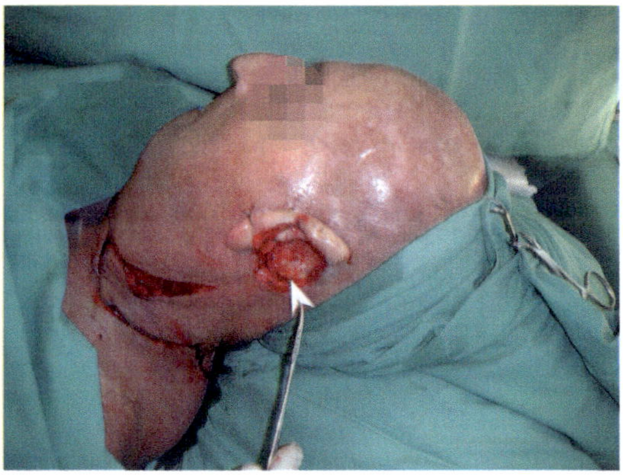

Fig. 2.164 The size of the surgical defect

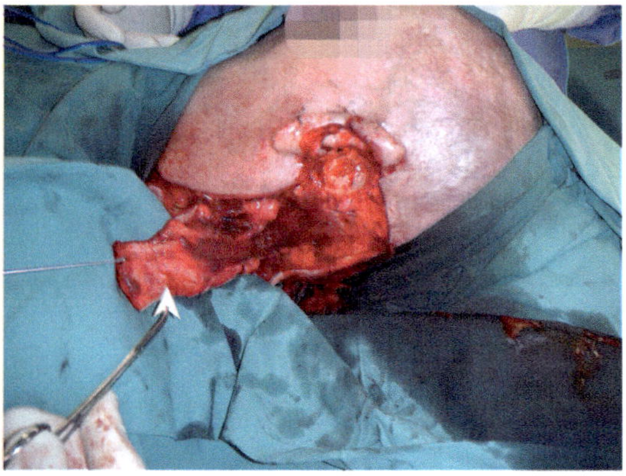

Fig. 2.165 The flap being rotated and raised at the fascial level to be inserted into the defect, allowing the helix to fall back into alignment

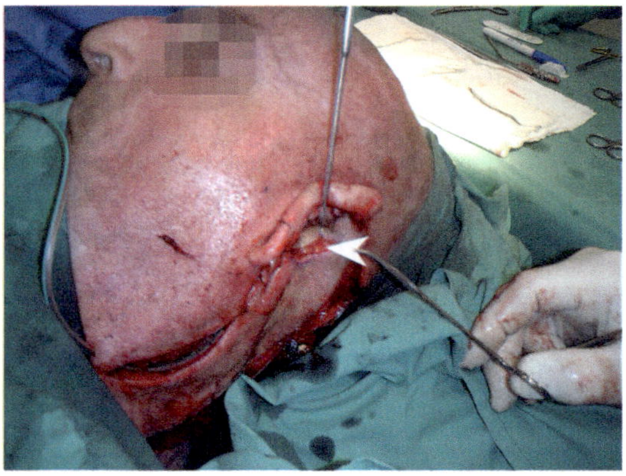

Fig. 2.166 Creating the de-epithelialised bridge, allowing the helix to be surgically inserted

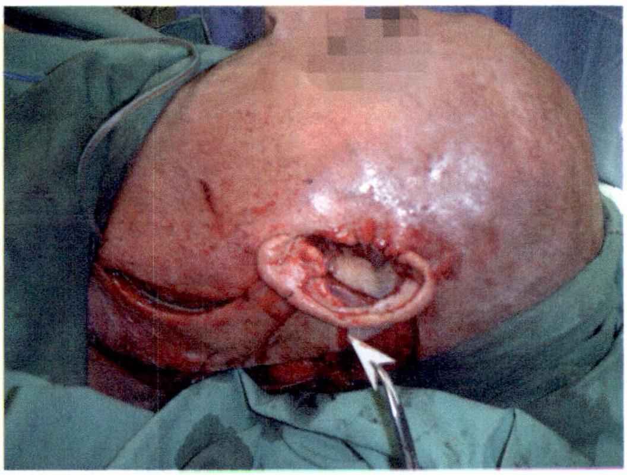

Fig. 2.167 The vascular integrity of the conchal reconstruction with the helix realigned is shown. This is another indication of the hypervascularity created to ensure such a reconstructive manoeuvre

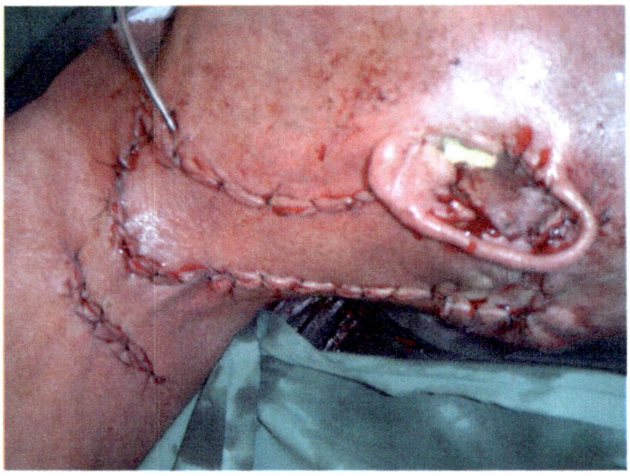

Fig. 2.168 Completion with drainage

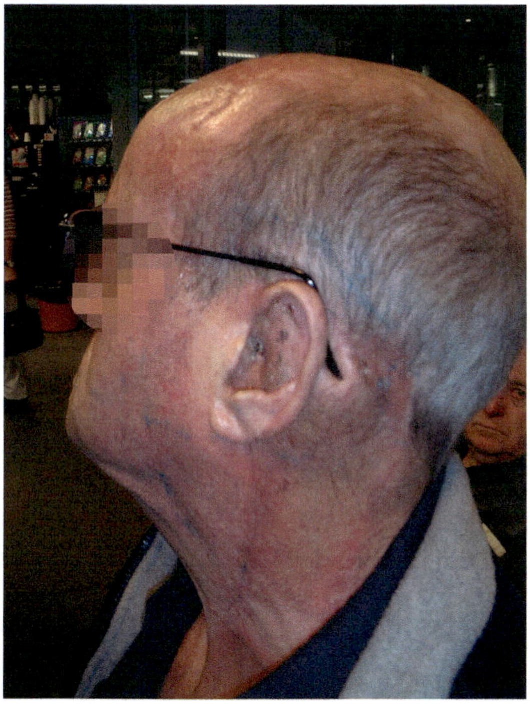

Fig. 2.169 The value of the helix repair to support spectacles and appearance at 4 weeks

The PACES characteristics were all exemplified: pain-free, aesthetic, no vascular complications, economical in terms of time and sensory recovery with the resolution of oedema.

2.1.1.17 Case 17—Facial Nerve Dissection with the Removal of the Parotid Tumour and the Keystone Closure (Figs. 2.170, 2.171, 2.172, 2.173, and 2.174)

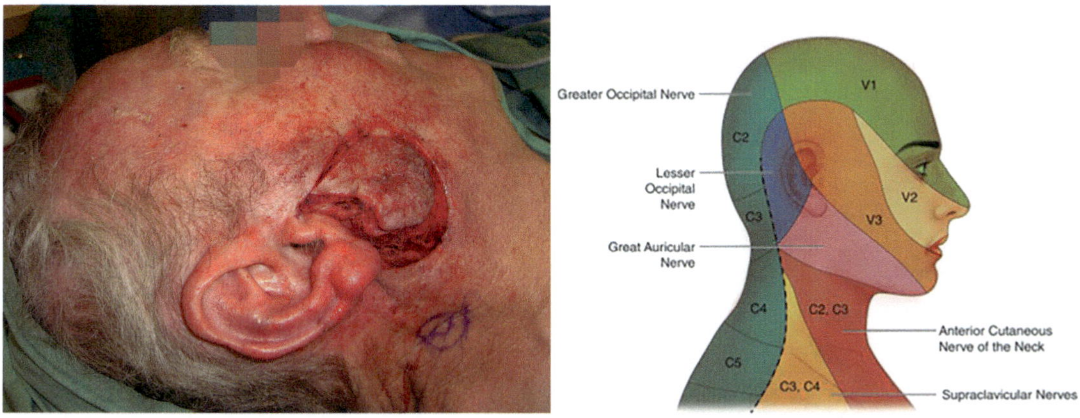

Fig. 2.170 SCC over the parotid and cervico-submental Keystone is shown. The dermatomal mark outs become the line of incision of the dermis and epidermis, ensuring that one-third deeply is attached with only partial undermining to facilitate the closure and vascular integrity of the defect. (Reprinted with permission from Atlas, *Reconstructive Technique in Melanoma Management* (p. 19), by Felix Behan, Springer Nature 2023)

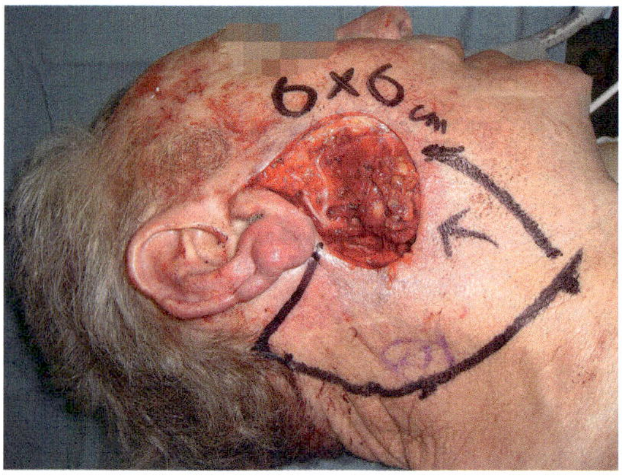

Fig. 2.171 The 6 × 6 cm surgical defect showing the dissected facial nerve in depth and the mark out and design of the cervico-submental Keystone

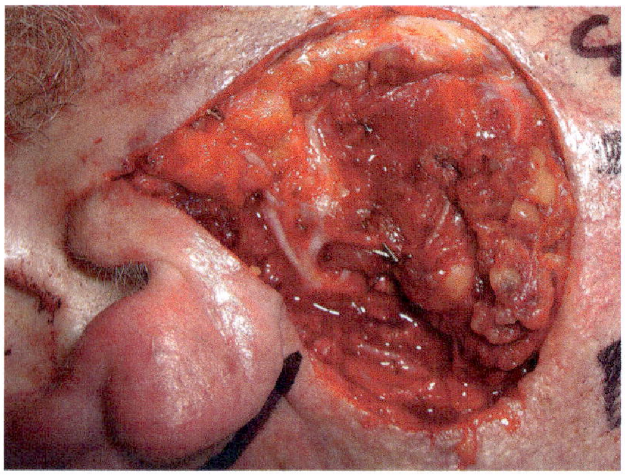

Fig. 2.172 The 6 × 6 cm surgical defect showing the dissected facial nerve in depth

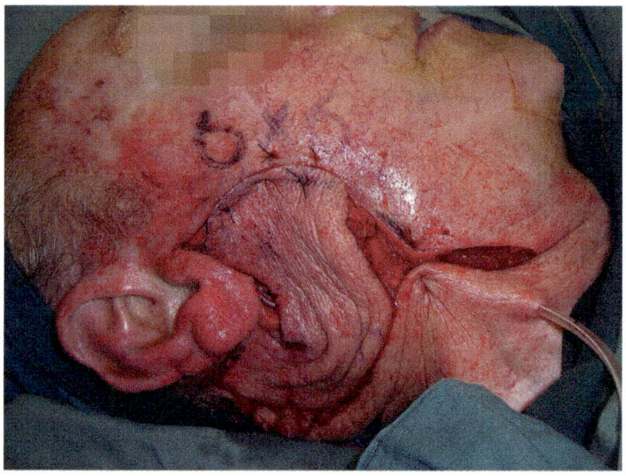

Fig. 2.173 The standard three-phase locking mattress suture technique and the closure of the neck defect via direct apposition, evident under tension (a 3-week suture insert)

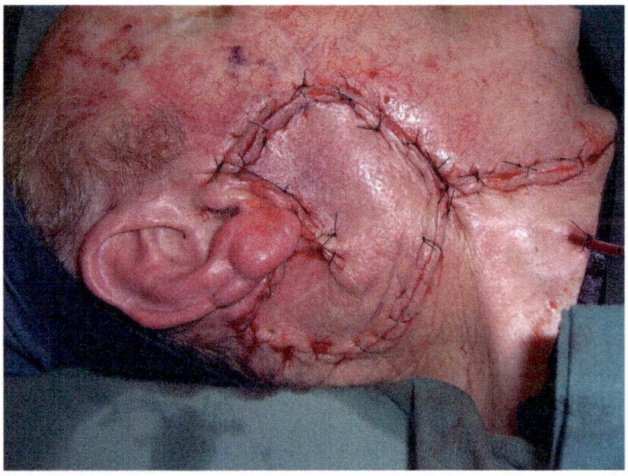

Fig. 2.174 The hypervascularity is noted on the wound closure, completed in 45 min

The PACES characteristics were all exemplified: pain-free, aesthetic, no vascular complications, economical in terms of time and sensory recovery with the resolution of oedema.

2.1.1.18 Case 18—SCC Secondary over the Mastoid, Postauricular Defect + Parotid (Figs. 2.175, 2.176, 2.177, 2.178, 2.179, 2.180, 2.181, 2.182, 2.183, 2.184, 2.185, 2.186, 2.187 and 2.188)

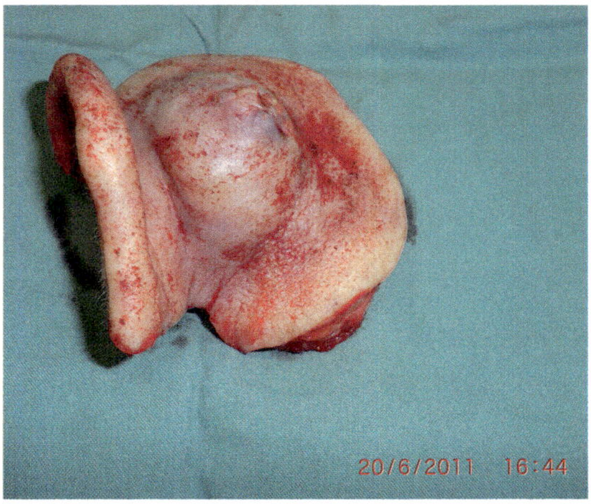

Fig. 2.175 Tumour specimen of the mastoid

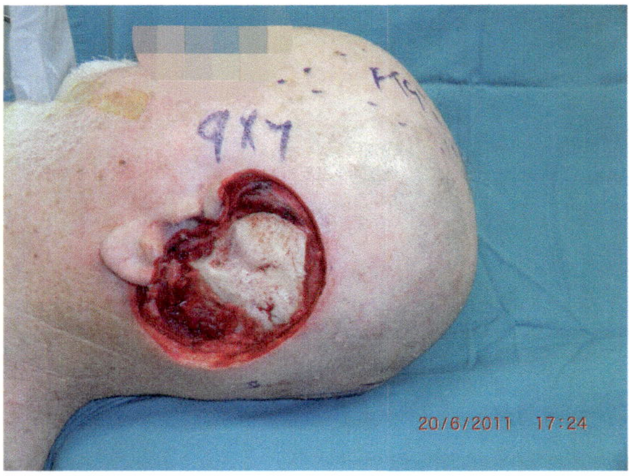

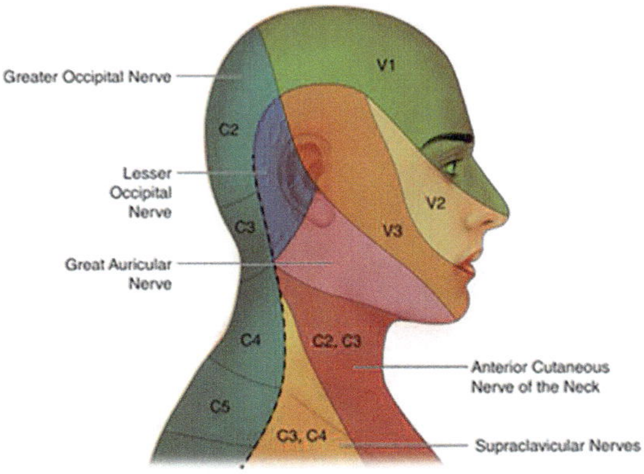

Fig. 2.176 A 9 × 7 cm surgical defect is shown. The dermatomal mark outs become the line of incision of the dermis and epidermis, ensuring that one-third deeply is attached with only partial undermining to facilitate the closure and vascular integrity of the defect. (Reprinted with permission from Atlas, *Reconstructive Technique in Melanoma Management* (p. 19), by Felix Behan, Springer Nature 2023)

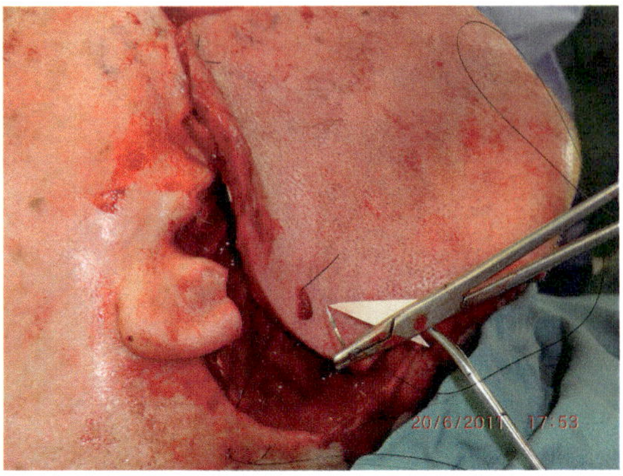

Fig. 2.177 The hypervascularity sign in the flap producing the red dot sign at the suture point (white arrowed), reflecting hypervascularity in the flap

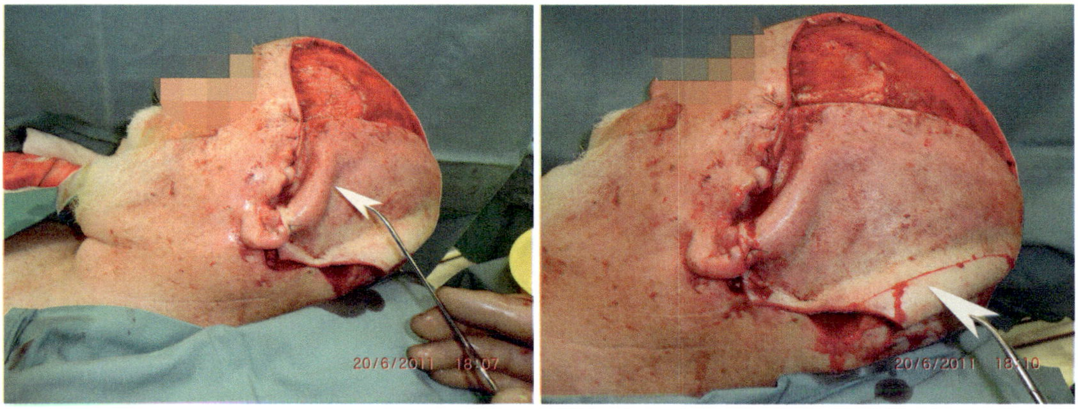

Fig. 2.178 Staged closure and reconstructing a helix with tissue folds

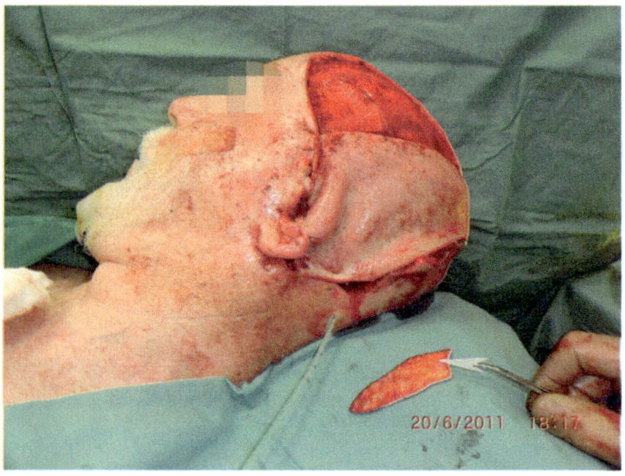

Fig. 2.179 The full-thickness graft for the tight occipital closure

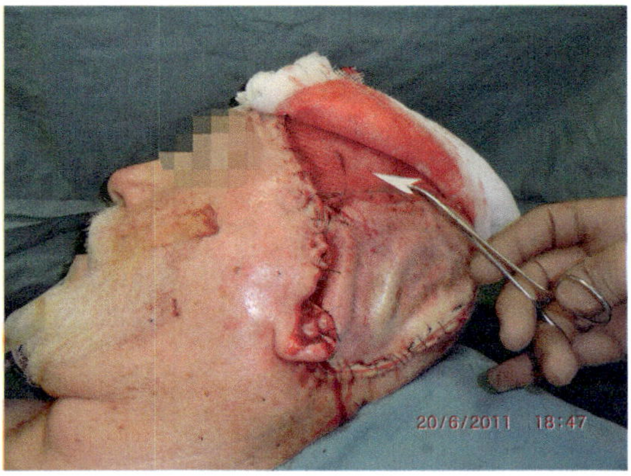

Fig. 2.181 The mesh graft for the pericranial defect

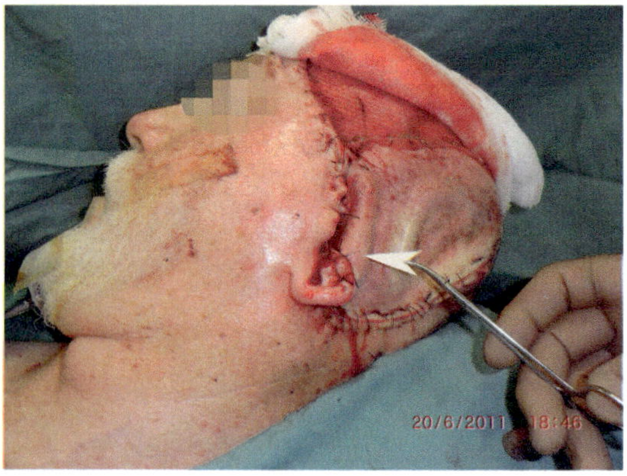

Fig. 2.180 The folds of tissue used to create the helix

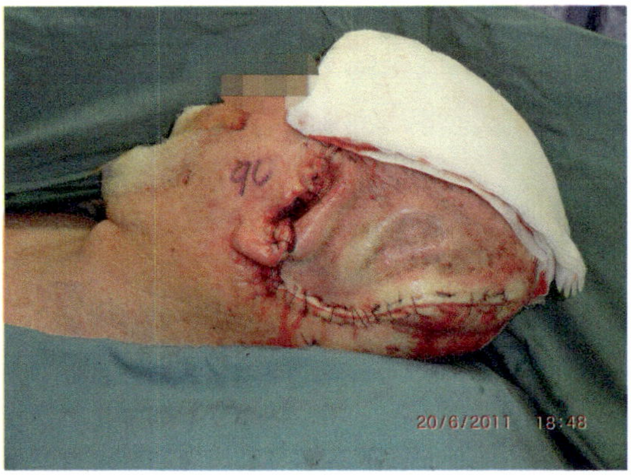

Fig. 2.182 The graft has been inserted, and the whiteness around the suture line indicates the need for a graft rather than further closure under tension—which is just a cautionary manoeuvre that can be completed in 90 min

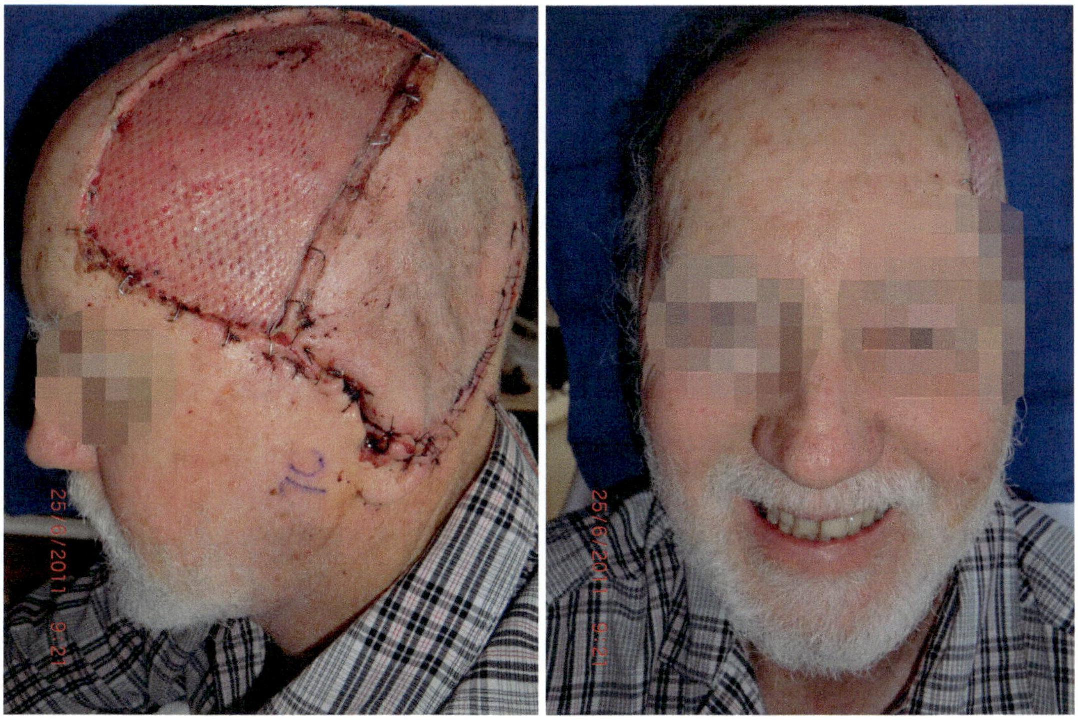

Fig. 2.183 The appearance at 5 days reflects the patient's satisfaction, and all the characteristics of the Keystone have been exemplified

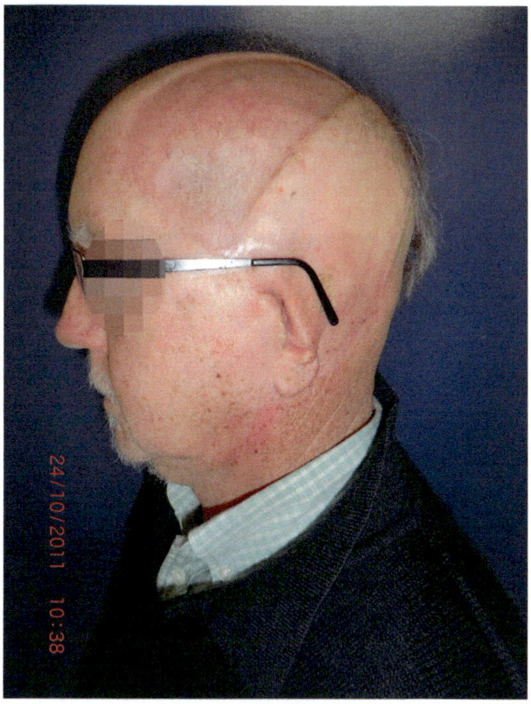

Fig. 2.184 Postoperative appearance at 4 months, with the patient wearing spectacles

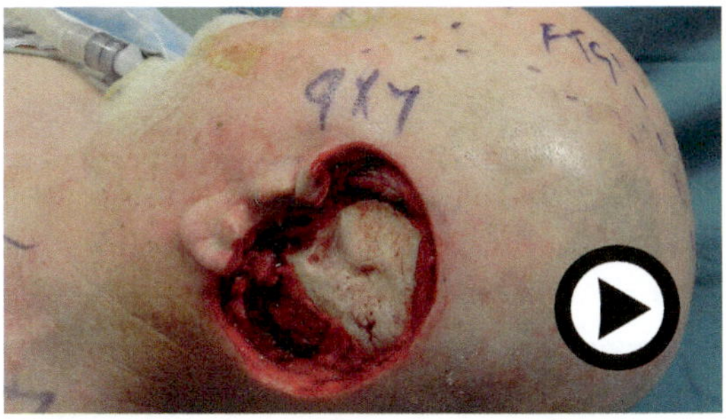

Fig. 2.185 Video 2.22 The planned operative procedure (▶ https://doi.org/10.1007/000-k6k)

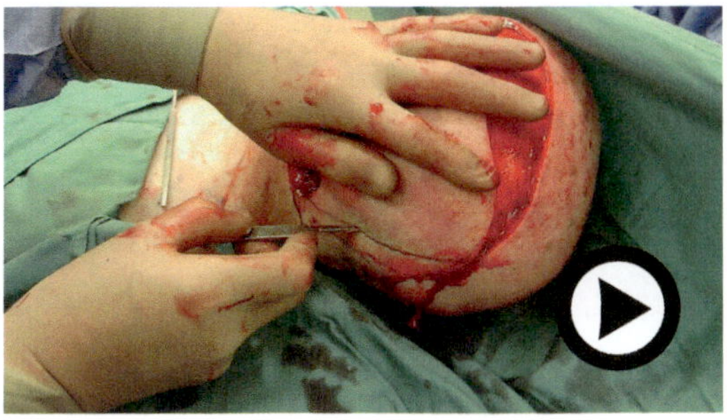

Fig. 2.186 Video 2.23 The use of a scalp flap for a parotid defect using Keystone principles—blunt dissection without skeletonising the perforators (▶ https://doi.org/10.1007/000-k6m)

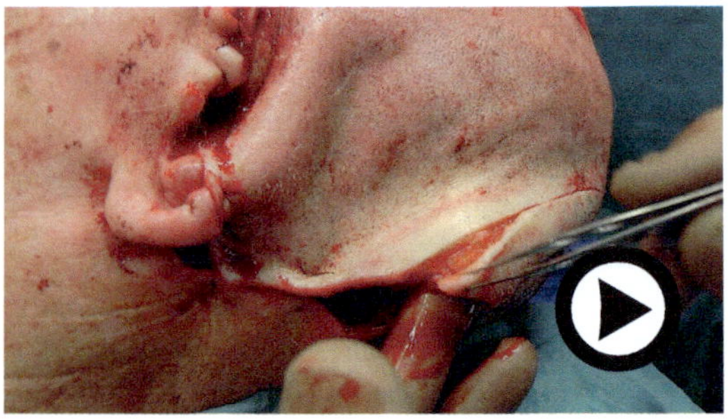

Fig. 2.187 Video 2.24 More characteristics of the Keystone when applied to a scalp rotation flap (▶ https://doi.org/10.1007/000-k6n)

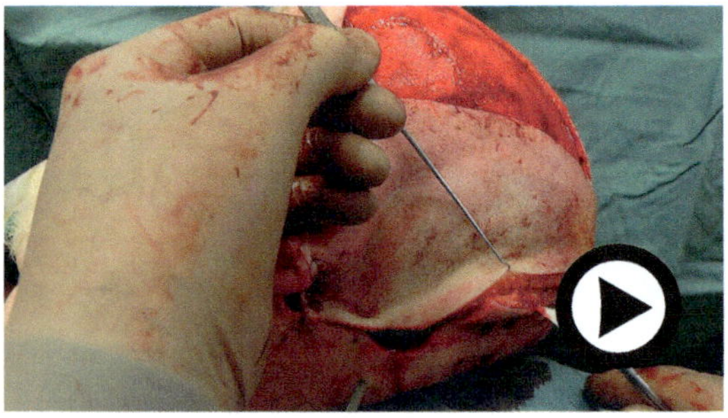

Fig. 2.188 Video 2.25 Keystone characteristics of the suprafascial circulation, allowing one to excise dog ears in transit (▶ https://doi.org/10.1007/000-k6p)

The PACES characteristics were all exemplified: pain-free, aesthetic, no vascular complications, economical in terms of time and sensory recovery with the resolution of oedema.

2.1.1.19 Case 19—A Facial Keystone for an SCC of the External Canal After a Parotidectomy (Figs. 2.189, 2.190, 2.191, and 2.192)

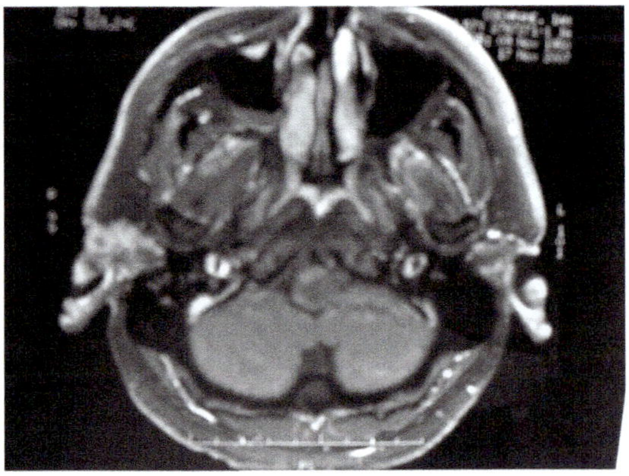

Fig. 2.189 An X-ray of the external canal showing the dimensions of the SCC

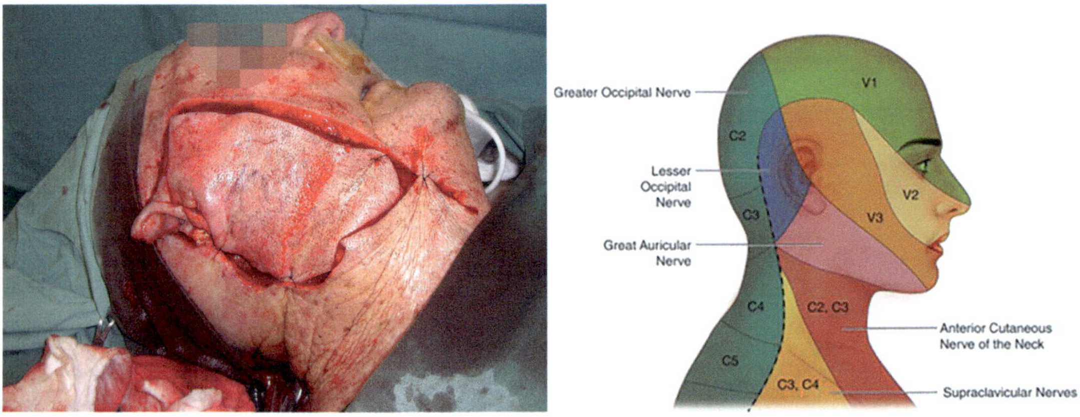

Fig. 2.190 An outline of the facial Keystone in the V2 distribution is shown. The skin and epidermis are divided to create a flap that is hypervascularised with one-third deep attachment. A red dot sign is evident as well, confirming the nature of this hypervascularised tissue, which ensures healing. The dermatomal mark outs become the line of incision of the dermis and epidermis, ensuring that one-third deeply is attached with only partial undermining to facilitate the closure and vascular integrity of the defect. (Reprinted with permission from Atlas, *Reconstructive Technique in Melanoma Management* (p. 19), by Felix Behan, Springer Nature 2023)

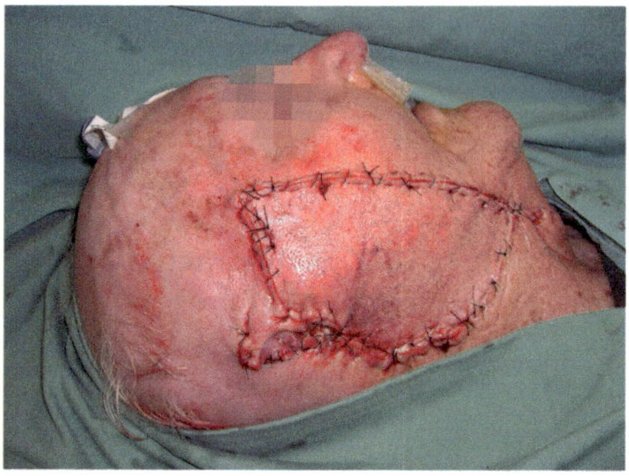

Fig. 2.191 Fully closed in 35 min

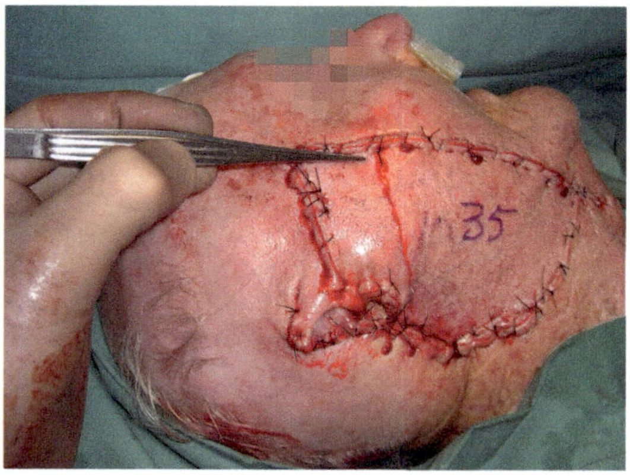

Fig. 2.192 Notice the number of red dot signs in this flap even when closed under tension, used to give an excellent aesthetic outcome in 35 min

The PACES characteristics were all exemplified: pain-free, aesthetic, no vascular complications, economical in terms of time and sensory recovery with the resolution of oedema.

2.1.1.20 Case 20—Recurrent SCC over the R Parotid Sequential Keystone Scars Is not an Impedance (Figs. 2.193, 2.194, 2.195, 2.196, 2.197, 2.198 and 2.199)

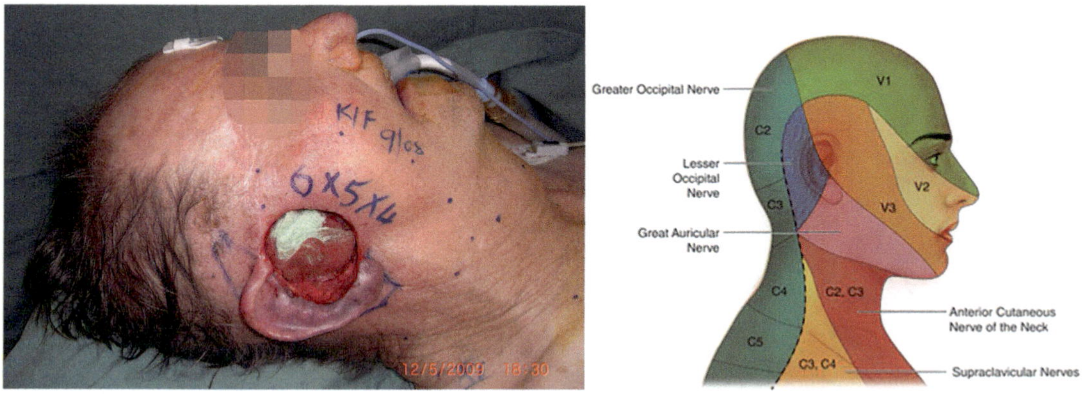

Fig. 2.193 Recurrent SCC R parotid over the external canal produces a necrotic ear recurrence, and the surgical excision is 6 × 5 × 4 cm, revealing the R external canal (6.30 pm). The dermatomal mark outs become the line of incision of the dermis and epidermis, ensuring that one-third deeply is attached with only partial undermining to facilitate the closure and vascular integrity of the defect. (Reprinted with permission from Atlas, *Reconstructive Technique in Melanoma Management* (p. 19), by Felix Behan, Springer Nature 2023)

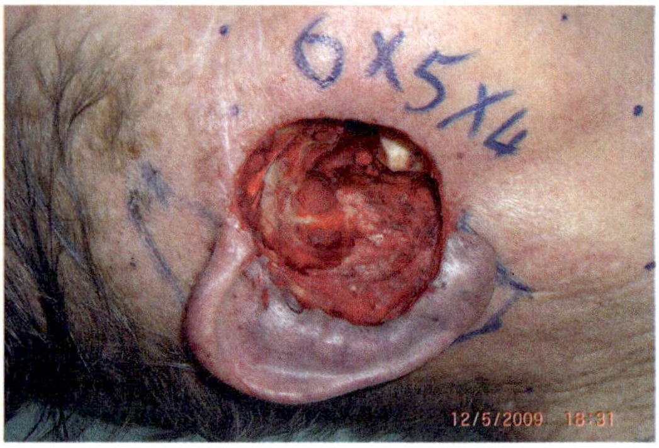

Fig. 2.194 The cervico-submental design is used to close the defect. Note the cyanotic appearance of the ear, helix and lobule, which are islanded to create increased blood flow to the anatomical site

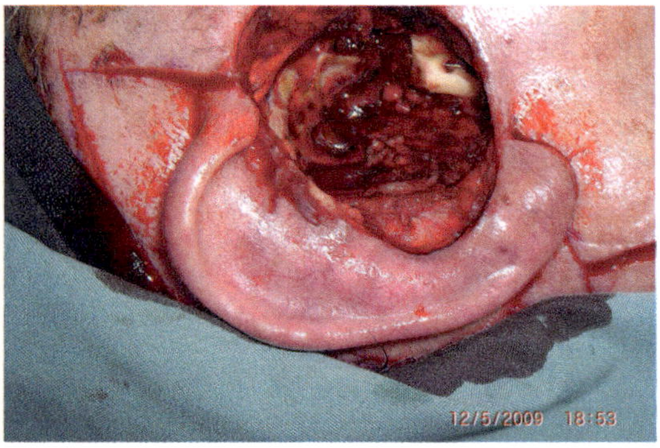

Fig. 2.195 Note that the island outlined around the ear through the skin and epidermis becomes hypervascularised, and the cyanotic appearance disappears in 20 min, as timestamped on the image (6.53 pm)

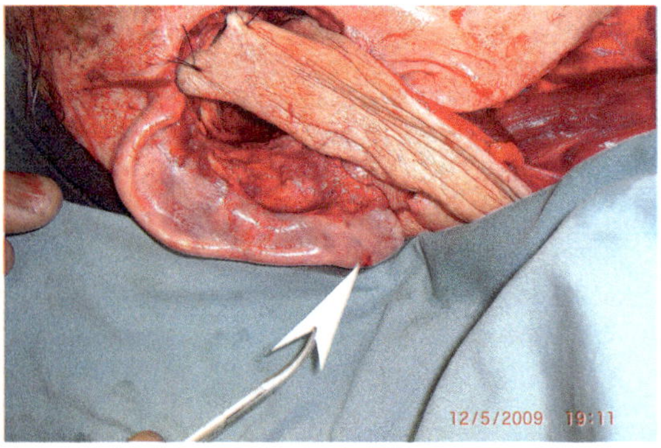

Fig. 2.196 Notice that the arrow points to the red dot sign in the hypervascularised lobule of the ear, consistent with a salvage manoeuvre, while the cervico-submental Keystone closes the defect (7.12 pm)

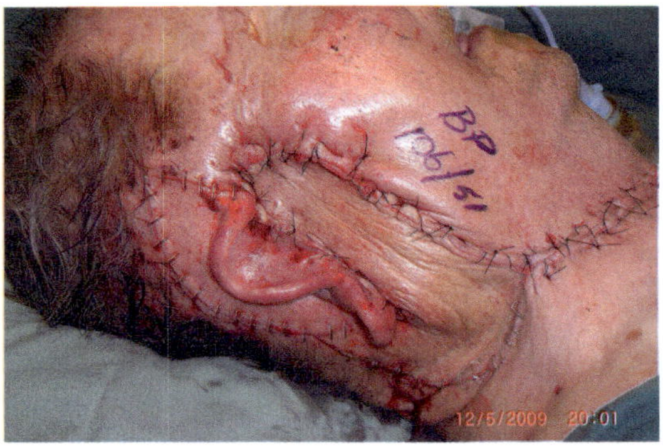

Fig. 2.197 Closure under tension, with the ear back to normal (8.01 pm). Some technicians prefer staples who adopt this technique until they see the value of the standard three-phase locking mattress suture technique using nylon (speed and aesthetcis)

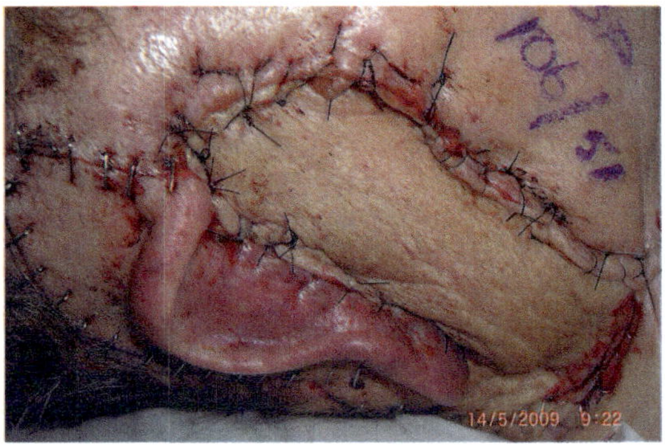

Fig. 2.198 Appearance at 2 days—no flap necrosis and a normal ear

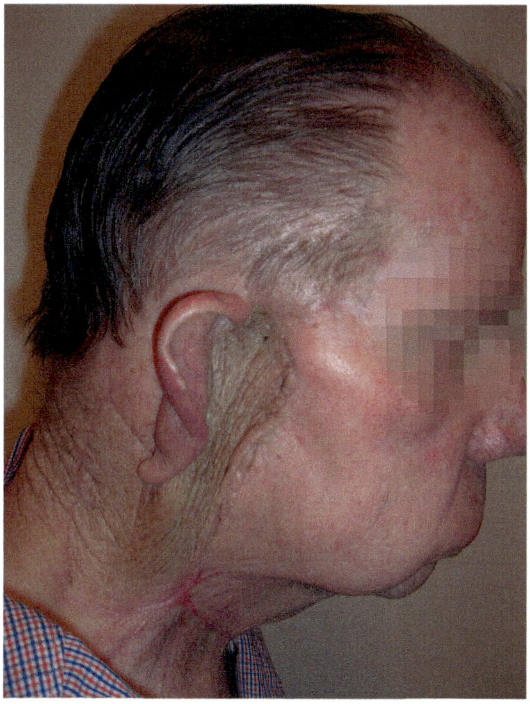

Fig. 2.199 The appearance at 2 months shows that the closure under tension eliminates any need for facial nerve reconstruction

The PACES characteristics were all exemplified: pain-free, aesthetic, no vascular complications, economical in terms of time and sensory recovery with the resolution of oedema.

2.1.1.21 Case 21—Dermatofibrosarcoma in a 75-Year-Old, Creating a 5 × 2 cm Defect (Figs. 2.200, 2.201, 2.202, 2.203, 2.204, 2.205 and 2.206)

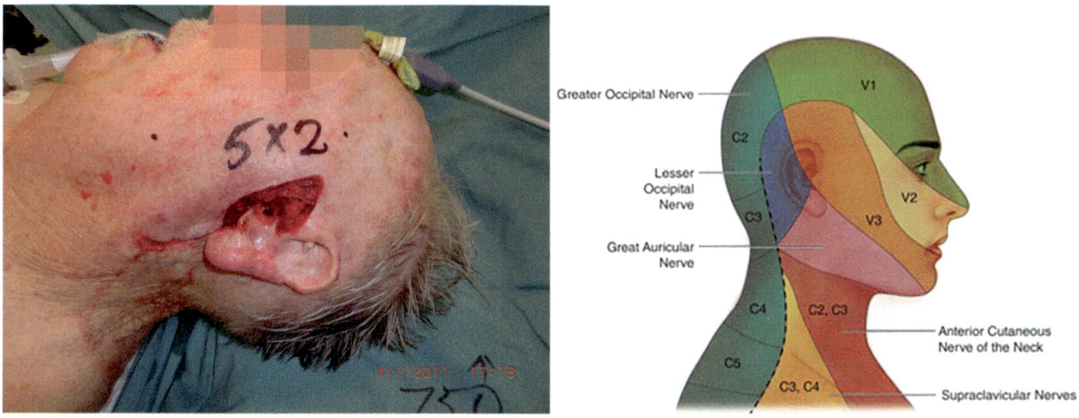

Fig. 2.200 Closure with a preauricular Keystone was carried out with closure under tension. The dermatomal mark outs become the line of incision of the dermis and epidermis, ensuring that one-third deeply is attached with only partial undermining to facilitate the closure and vascular integrity of the defect. (Reprinted with permission from Atlas, *Reconstructive Technique in Melanoma Management* (p. 19), by Felix Behan, Springer Nature 2023)

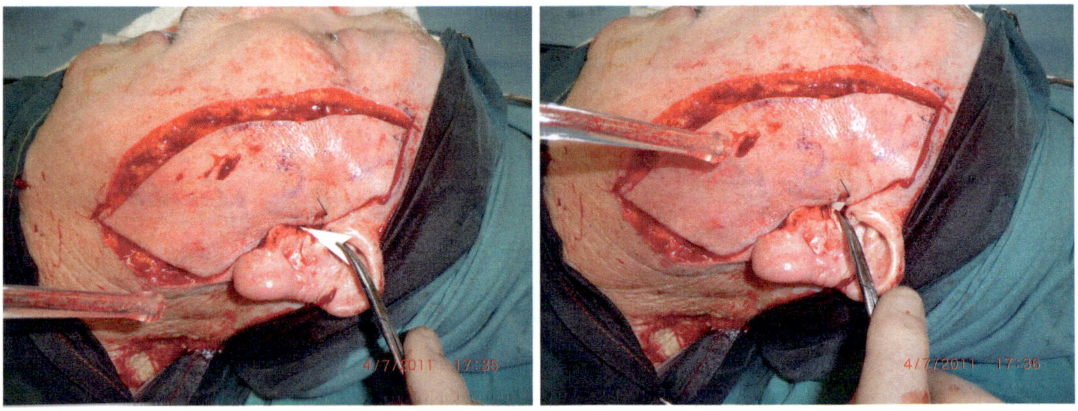

Fig. 2.201 All the Keystone characteristics are evident with hypervascularisation and the red dot sign—a guarantee of vascular integrity that ensures a safe closure. The dermal-epidermal outline of the Keystone allows closure under tension, with hypervascularisation and red dot sign indicators present

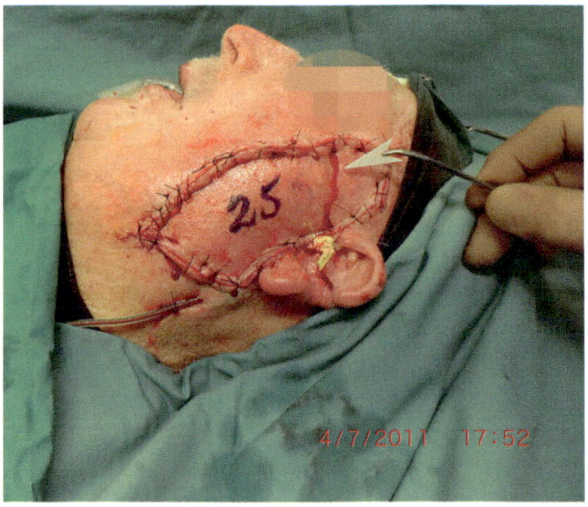

Fig. 2.202 Closure in 25 min (timestamped) and fully vascularised

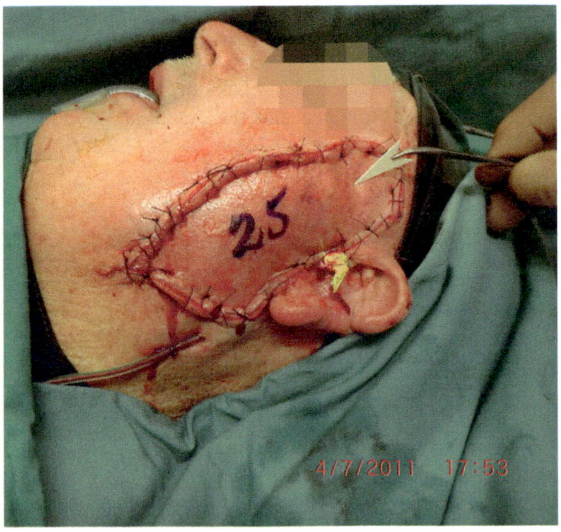

Fig. 2.203 No sign of any vascular impedance is shown. A normal vascular appearance has been achieved with the Keystone without lines of tension

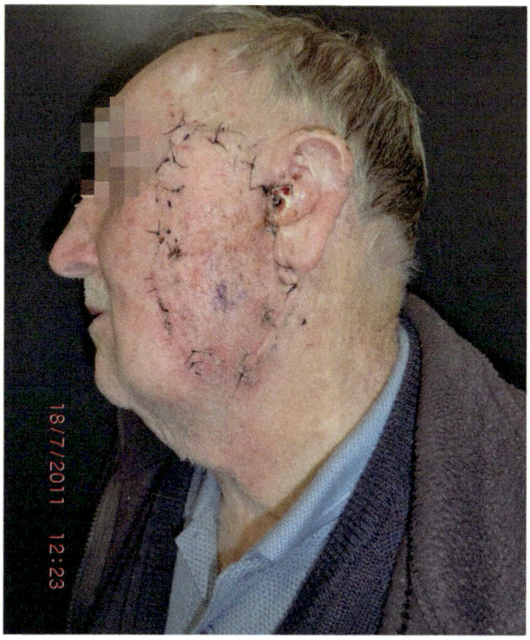

Fig. 2.204 Appearance at 2 weeks in the middle of the wound-dressing sequence and the standard three-phase suture removal technique (12.23 pm)

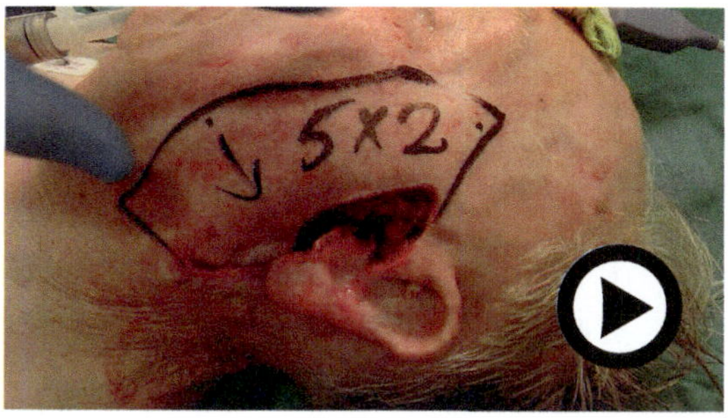

Fig. 2.205 Video 2.26 The operative details of raising a preauricular Keystone randomly based on the superficial muscular aponeurotic system (SMAS) fascia (▶ https://doi.org/10.1007/000-k6q)

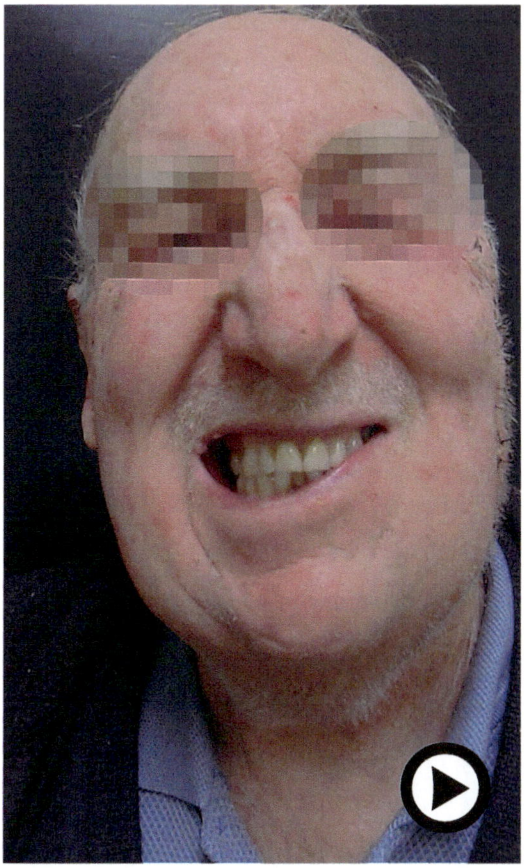

Fig. 2.206 Video 2.27 Patient response showing all the characteristics of the Keystone (PACES), with the patient's acknowledgement (▶ https://doi.org/10.1007/000-k6r)

The PACES characteristics were all exemplified: pain-free, aesthetic, no vascular complications, economical in terms of time and sensory recovery with the resolution of oedema.

2.1.1.22 Case 22—Submental Keystone for the Closure of a Submental Defect (Figs. 2.207, 2.208, 2.209, 2.210, 2.211, 2.212, 2.213, 2.214, 2.215, 2.216, 2.217, 2.218, 2.219, 2.220 and 2.221).

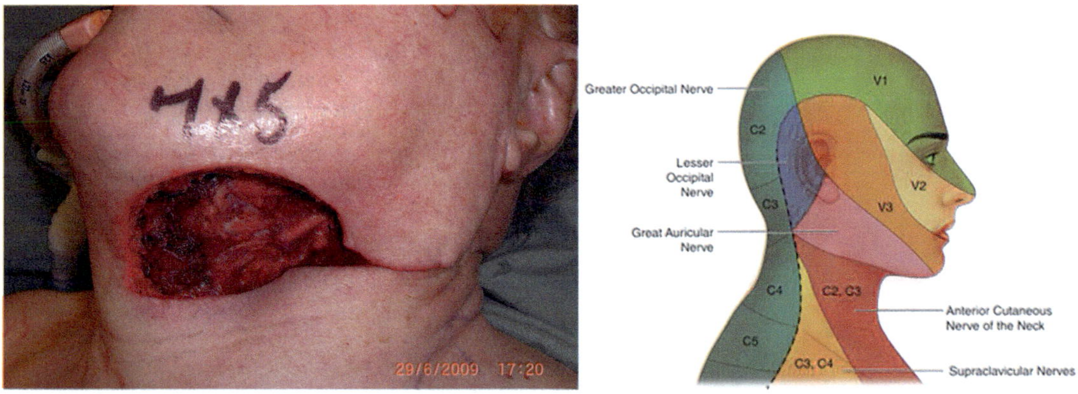

Fig. 2.207 A submental gland and mandibular trim for an SCC recurrence is shown. The dermatomal mark outs become the line of incision of the dermis and epidermis, ensuring that one-third deeply is attached with only partial undermining to facilitate the closure and vascular integrity of the defect. (Reprinted with permission from Atlas, *Reconstructive Technique in Melanoma Management* (p. 19), by Felix Behan, Springer Nature 2023)

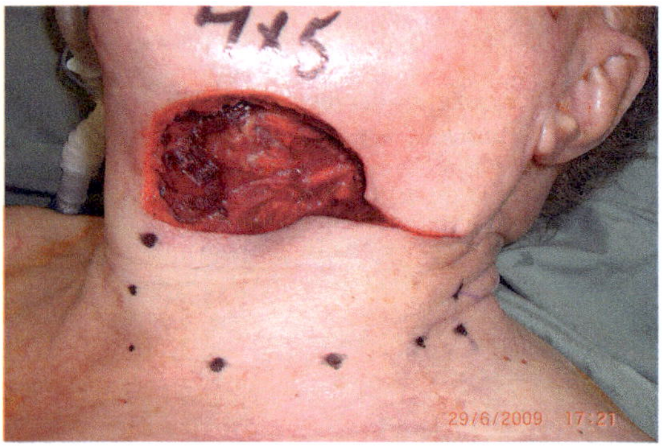

Fig. 2.208 The mark out of the cervical Keystone has been part of the nodal clearance. Note that this is a Keystone raised on undermined tissue, which is normally contraindicated, but the hypervascularity that is produced guarantees intact healing without necrosis

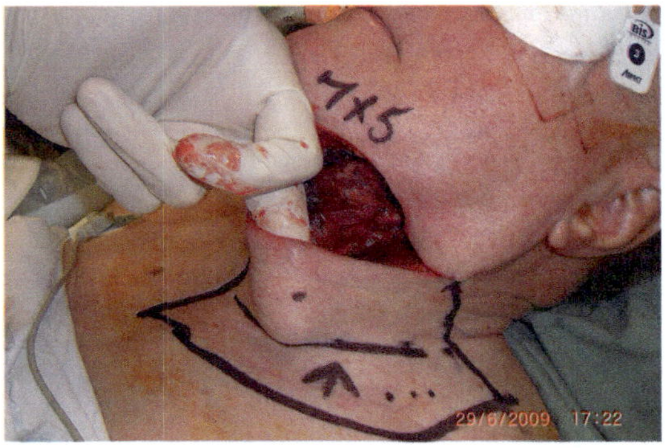

Fig. 2.209 Undermining is not a contraindication for Keystone application. By islanding around the mark out the flaps become hypervascularised when delineated around the dermatomal mark out, ensuring a good clinical closure. It is based on random supraclavicular perforators (which are dotted, and the arrow indicates the line of direct closure with supply from the subdermal plexus)

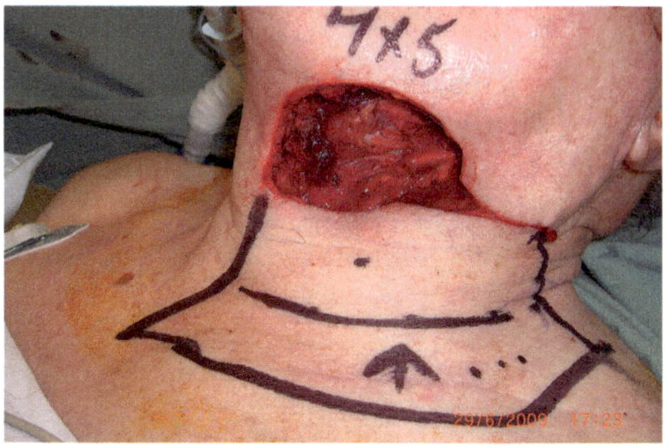

Fig. 2.210 Undermined neck tissue closed with a Keystone mark out following a nodal clearance

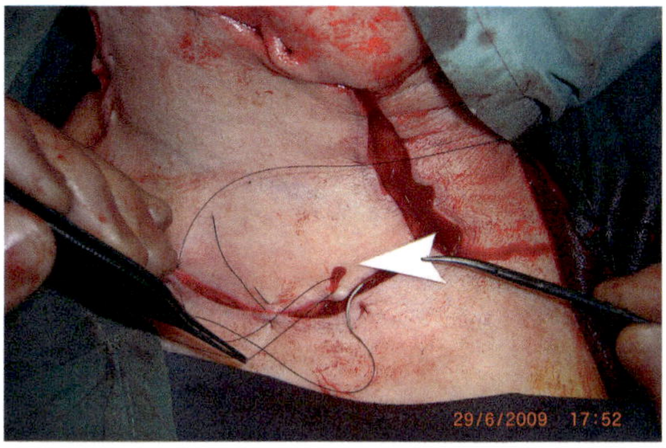

Fig. 2.211 The vascular characteristics of hypervascularisation and the red dot sign are evident at the suture exit point

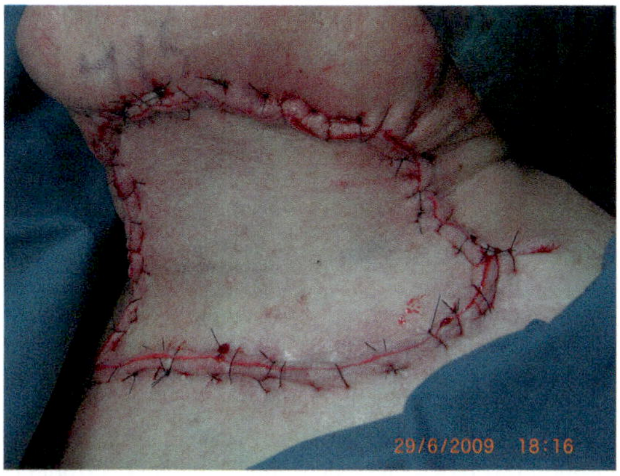

Fig. 2.212 The wound closure under tension after 60 min

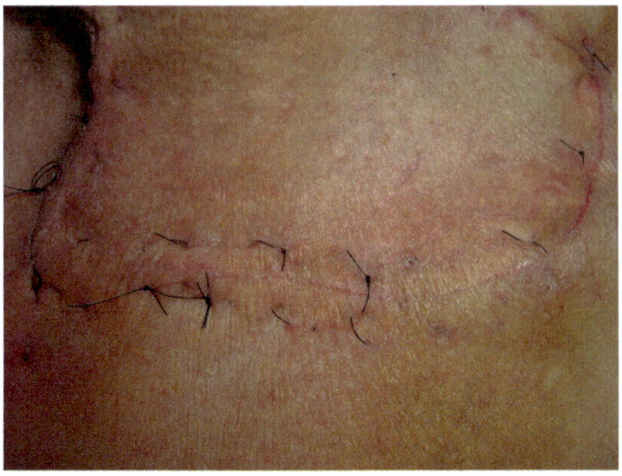

Fig. 2.213 Appearance at 2 weeks with a staged removal of the locking mattress sutures and the continuous nylon epidermal closure

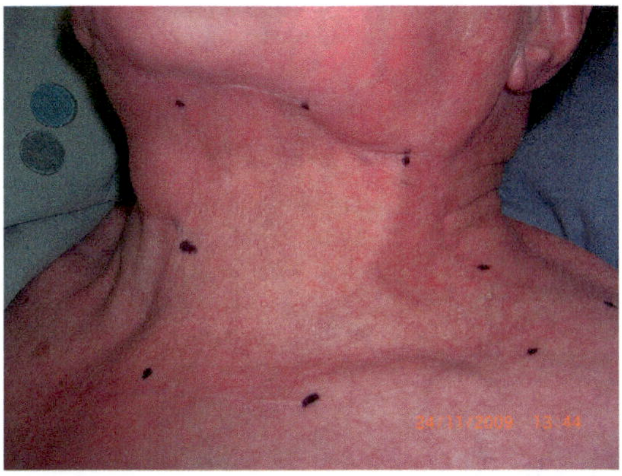

Fig. 2.214 A preauricular recurrence is shown 5 months later, and the previous Keystone closure has been dotted in outline to show excellent wound closure and healing

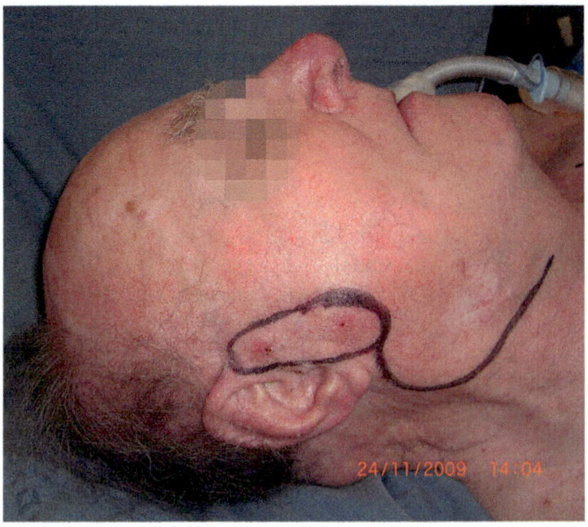

Fig. 2.215 Two foci of preauricular recurrence, with the Keystone design outlined

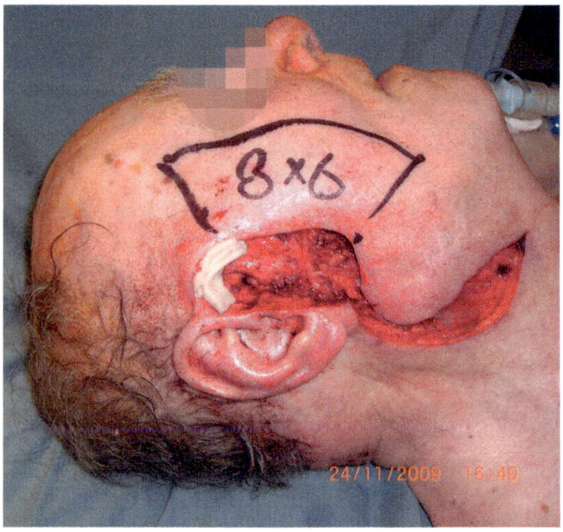

Fig. 2.216 No encroaching on the previous reconstructive site, as scarring does not embarrass revascularisation in the Keystone

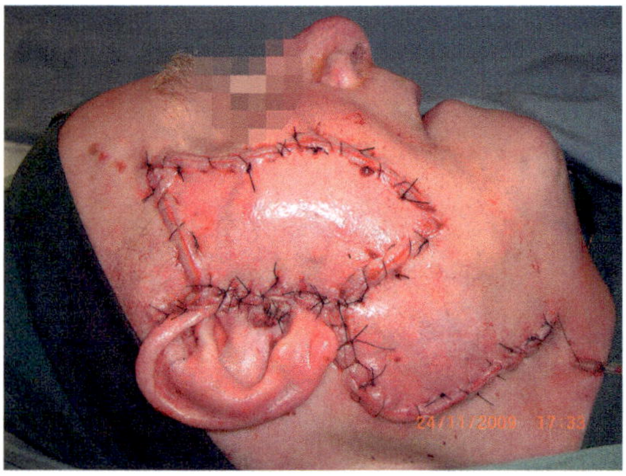

Fig. 2.217 The hypervascularisation features are based on parotid perforators of the carotid

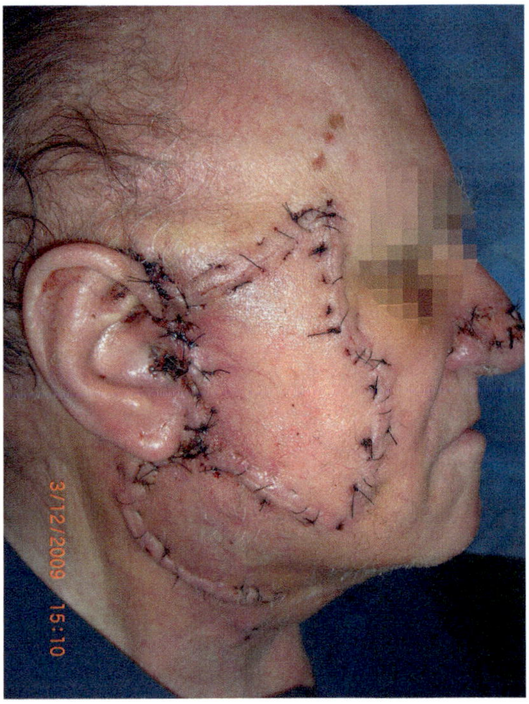

Fig. 2.218 The appearance of the wound after 10 days is shown, and the flap closure shows no indication of necrosis, consistent with the hypervascularisation of the Keystone principle

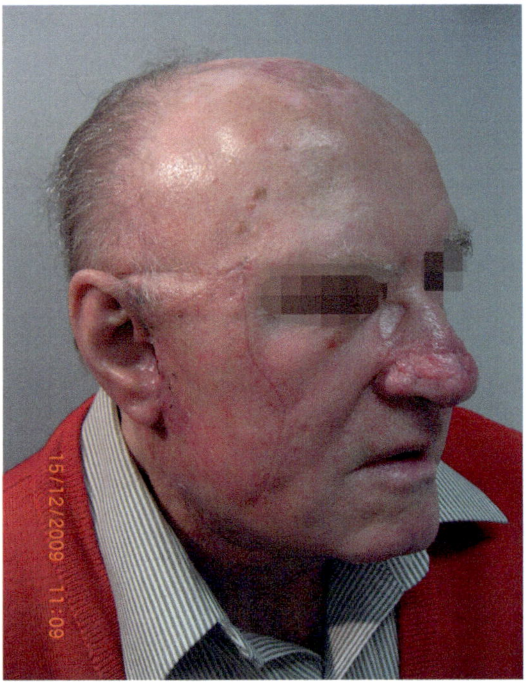

Fig. 2.219 Appearance at 3 weeks—acceptable aesthetic outcome, with a pleased patient

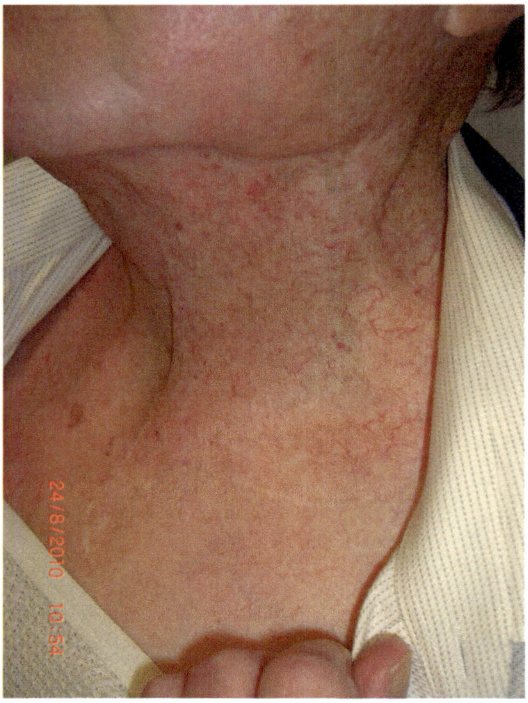

Fig. 2.220 Appearance of the submental closure at 8 months (Fig. 2.197 series above)

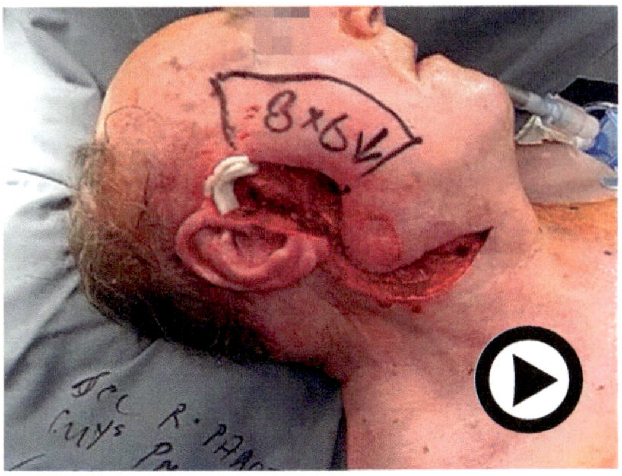

Fig. 2.221 Video 2.28 The delineation of the Keystone in the preauricular plane, which facilitates direct closure (▶ https://doi.org/10.1007/000-k6s)

The PACES characteristics were all exemplified: pain-free, aesthetic, no vascular complications, economical in terms of time and sensory recovery with the resolution of oedema.

2.1.1.23 Case 23—Preauricular Mass Parotid Clearence in a Patient with Chronic Lymphocytic Leukaemia (CLL) on Immunotherapy (Figs. 2.222, 2.223, 2.224, 2.225, 2.226, 2.227, 2.228, 2.229, 2.230, 2.231, 2.232, 2.233, 2.234, 2.235 and 2.236)

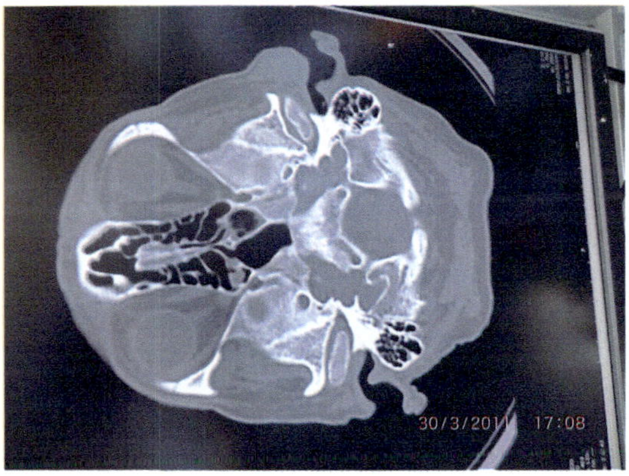

Fig. 2.223 CT verification of the mass, including the involvement of the external canal done—with Professor Sizeland as part of the oncology duet

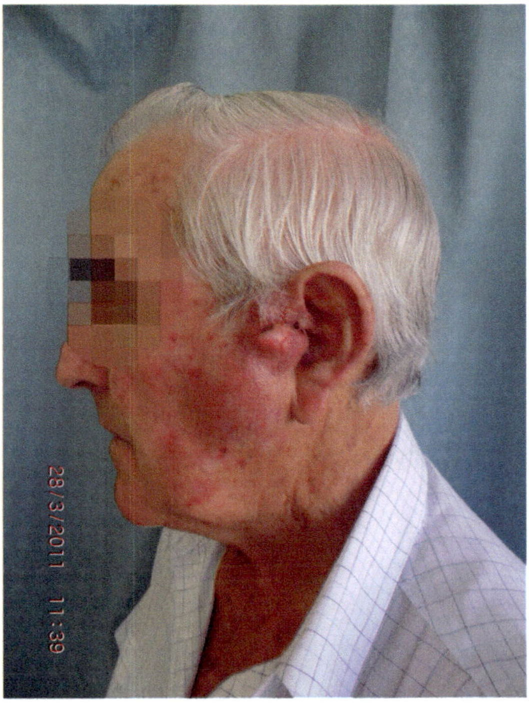

Fig. 2.222 The flap is hypervascularised by creating an island delineating the V2 dermatome; the cyanotic changes disappear; it is based on sternomastoid perforators, but the hypervascularisation from the suprafascial and infrafascial input allows this to trim off the dog ear at the intraoperative phase, avoiding any delayed procedure. The dermatomal mark outs become the line of incision of the dermis and epidermis, ensuring that one-third deeply is attached with only partial undermining to facilitate the closure and vascular integrity of the defect. (Reprinted with permission from Atlas, *Reconstructive Technique in Melanoma Management* (p. 19), by Felix Behan, Springer Nature 2023)

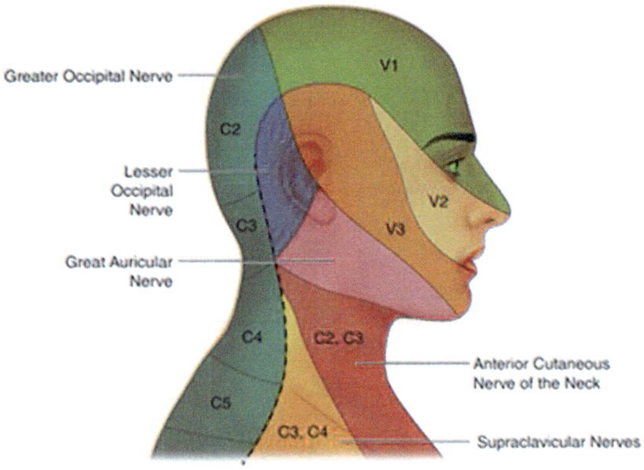

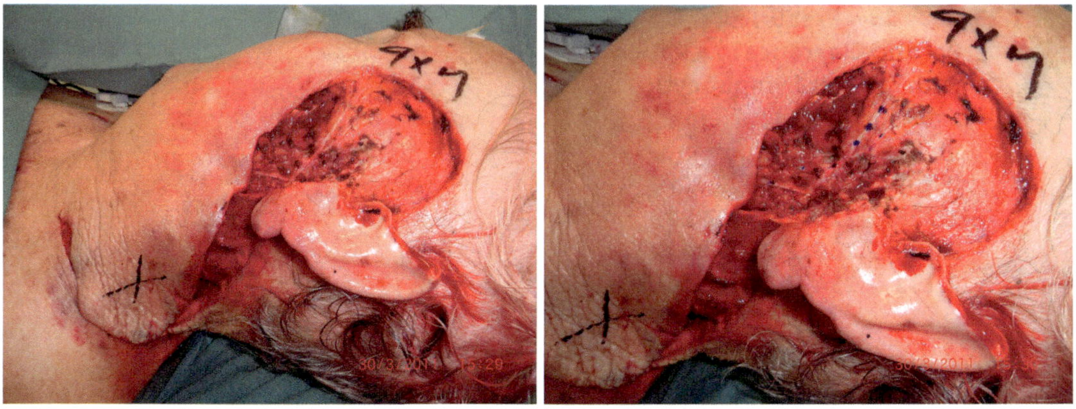

Fig. 2.224 Closing that flap directly would have caused necrosis of the tissue indicated with the X cross, and to avoid that we have hypervascularised the V2 area of the dermatome to facilitate closure under tension. The seventh nerve is dotted as a precaution to avoid sutures

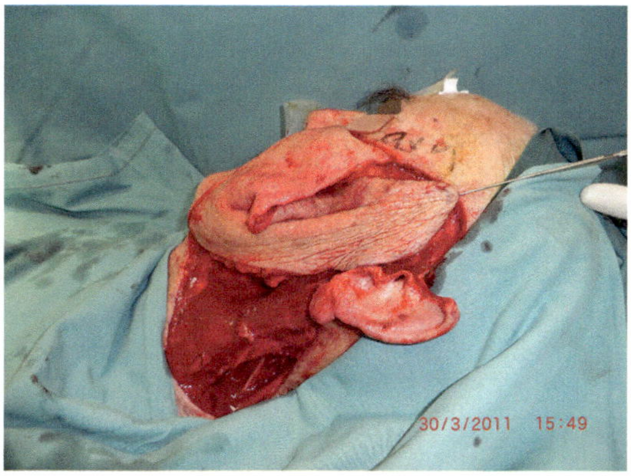

Fig. 2.225 Staged closure before definitive insertion

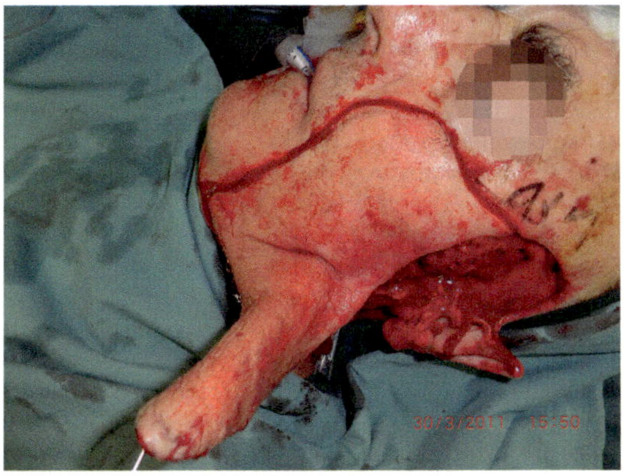

Fig. 2.227 The flap is hypervascularised when the islanding is completed at the dermal-epidermal level

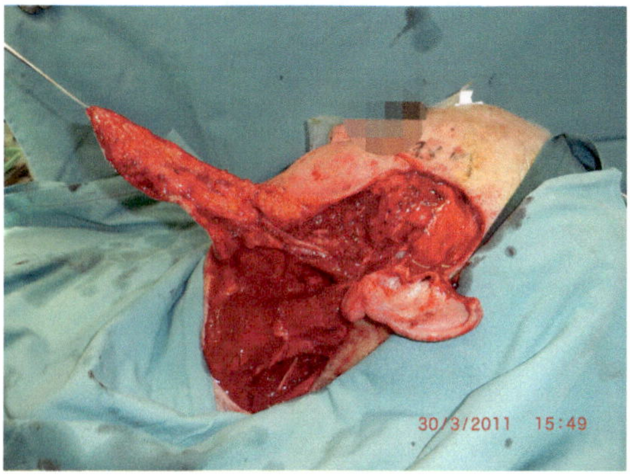

Fig. 2.226 The retracted flap at the base down to the sternomastoid microperforators without any delineation

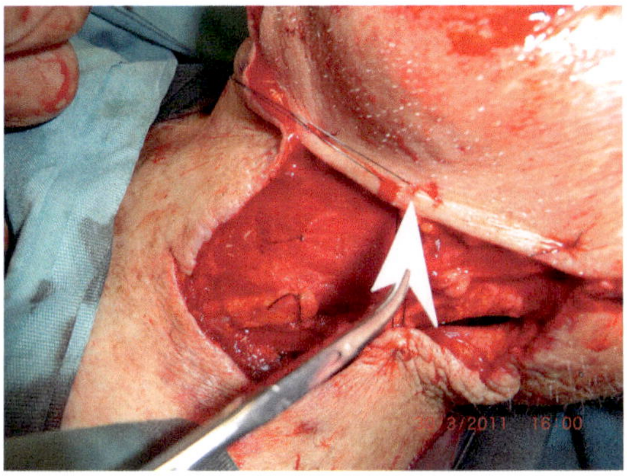

Fig. 2.228 The red dot signs (arrowed) are confirmation of the hypervascularity phase

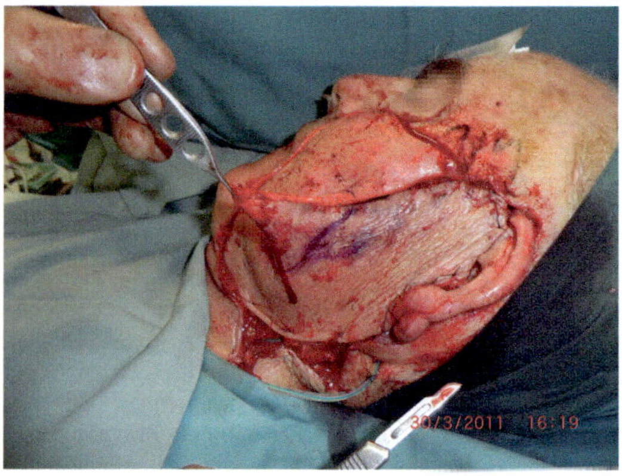

Fig. 2.229 The dog ear has been excised without imperilling distal perfusion

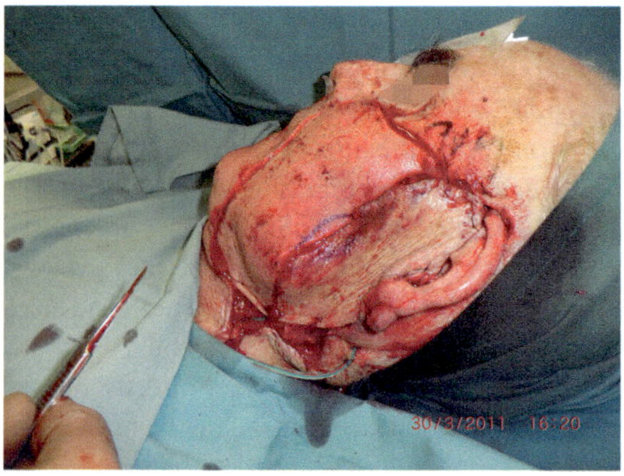

Fig. 2.230 The final closure

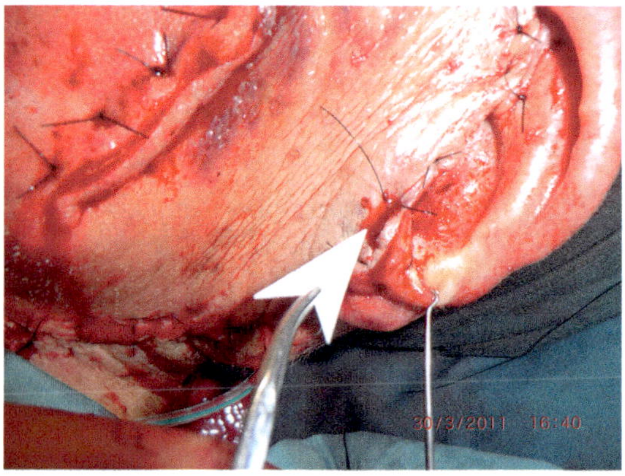

Fig. 2.231 The red dot sign at the suture point

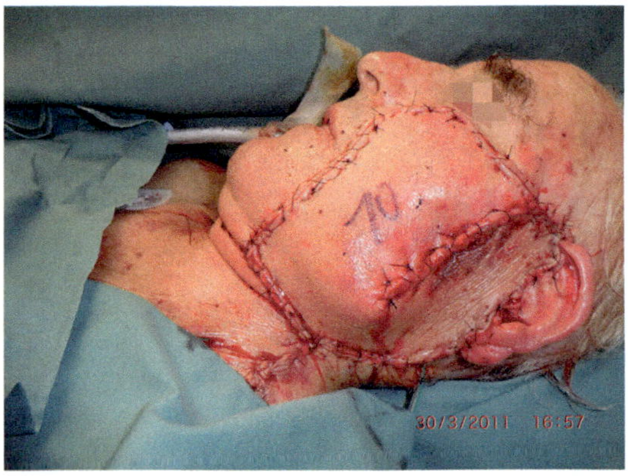

Fig. 2.232 The final closure with a 70 min timeframe compares favourably with alternative methods of reconstruction, and the PACES characteristics are all exemplified

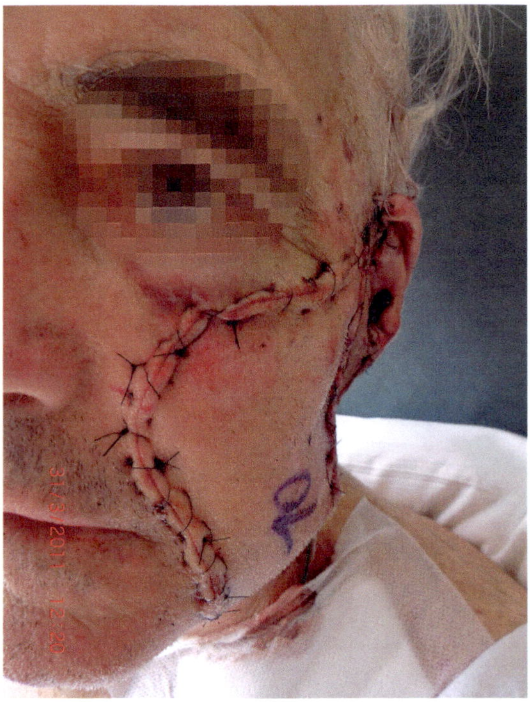

Fig. 2.233 Another view of Fig. 2.232 without any evidence of marginated necrosis

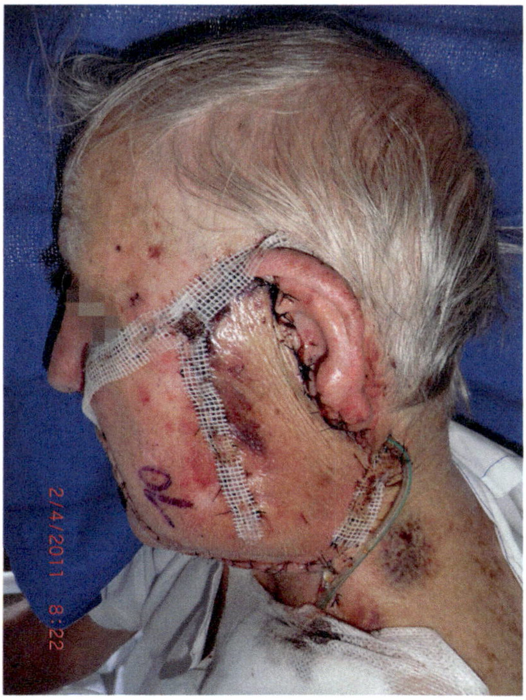

Fig. 2.234 Appearance at 3 days is shown. The ear helix has been islanded above and below during the procedure, to remove any cyanotic phase. No necrosis developed, indicating the reliability of the hypervascularisation, which avoids a secondary procedure regarding scar revision

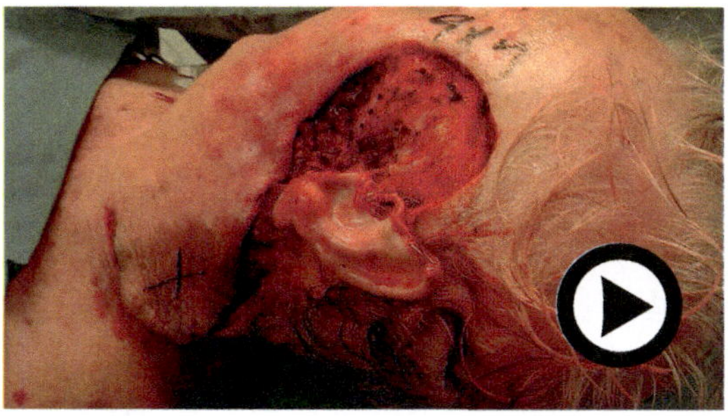

Fig. 2.235 Video 2.29 The clinical background, and the technique of the Keystone closure is detailed in this application (▶ https://doi.org/10.1007/000-k6t)

The PACES characteristics were all exemplified: pain-free, aesthetic, no vascular complications, economical in terms of time and sensory recovery with the resolution of oedema.

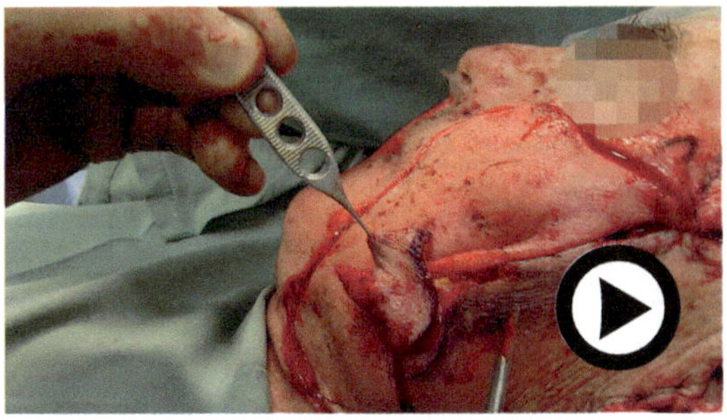

Fig. 2.236 Video 2.30 The dog ear excision, showing the reliability of the hypervascularisation resulting from the Keystone design in the dermatomes (▶ https://doi.org/10.1007/000-k6v)

2.1.1.24 Case 24—3 × 3 cm Defect Conchal Fossa Involving the Mastoid Bone

A mitotic lesion of the conchal fossa shows the excision and closure technique using the Keystone principle along the C2 and C3 dermatomes with an incontinuity neck dissection. The helical rim closure fits into the de-epithelialised section in the distal third of the cervical Keystone, and the closure has been completed. The neck wounds, following levels II, III and IV for the neck dissection, have also been directly closed, including the helical bridge. This technique has universal applications for conchal fossa and helical reconstructions reflecting the double islanding technique of the Keystone and the conchal fossa defect (Figs. 2.237, 2.238, 2.239, 2.240, 2.241, 2.242 and 2.243).

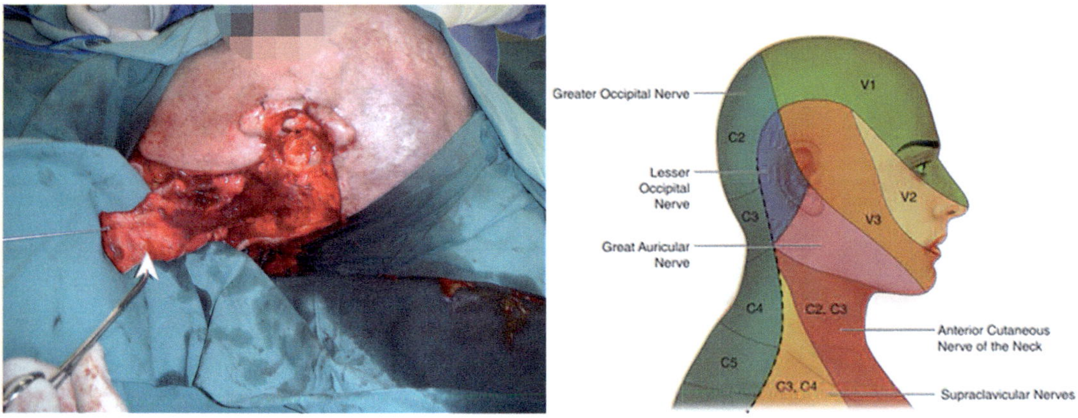

Fig. 2.237 This excision of a mitotic lesion of the L conchal fossa mastoid tip includes levels II, III and IV neck dissection. The dermatomal mark outs become the line of incision of the dermis and epidermis, ensuring that one-third deeply is attached with only partial undermining to facilitate the closure and vascular integrity of the defect. (Reprinted with permission from Atlas, *Reconstructive Technique in Melanoma Management* (p. 19), by Felix Behan, Springer Nature 2023)

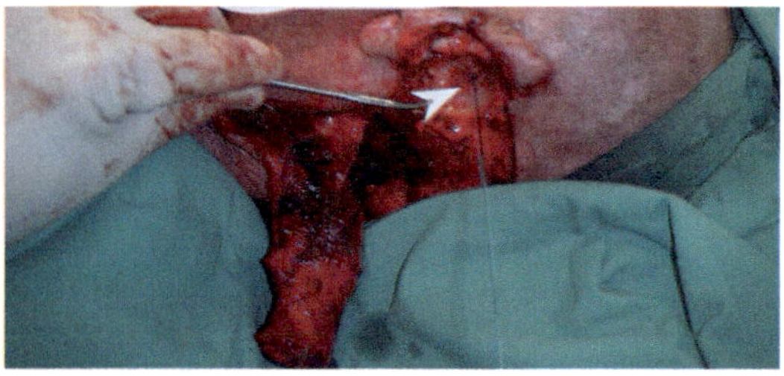

Fig. 2.238 The size of the mitotic defect, including the 3 × 3 cm mastoid bone

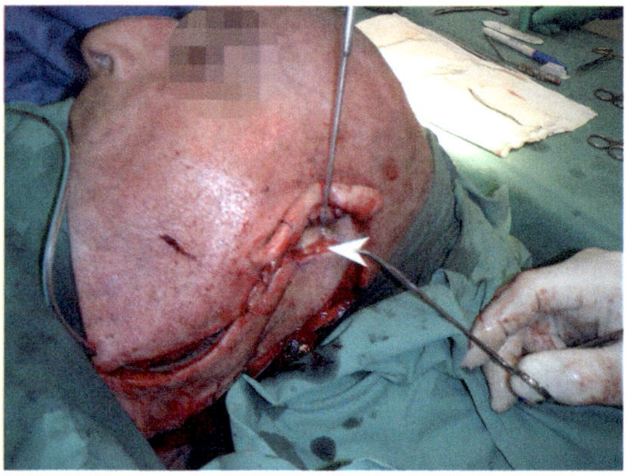

Fig. 2.239 The C2 and C3 cervical Keystone closes the defect, but for the helix of the ear to be inserted, a de-epithelialised section allows this to be sutured in situ. This completes the ear reconstruction, and the hypervascularity phase allows one to reattach the helix along a de-epithelialised bridge

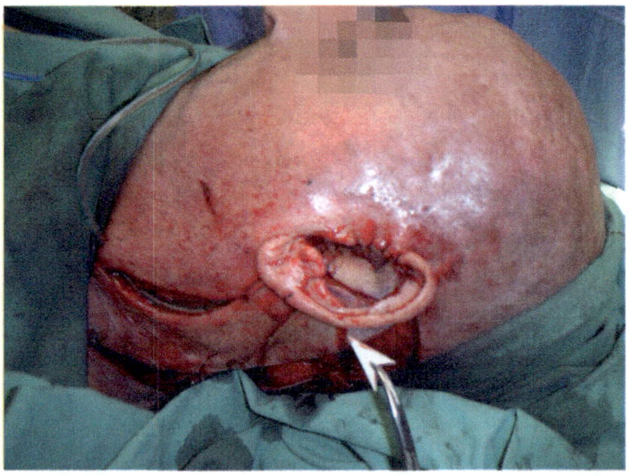

Fig. 2.240 The wound closure of the conchal fossa, including the cervical Keystone flap, is shown. Note that the Keystone is in the hyperaemic phase despite having a de-epitherialised section along which the helical rim is inserted. This is another indication that the hypervascularity phase and the reliability of the Keystone improve circulation. In other words it is a double islanding technique based on the vascular reliability of filamentous perforators

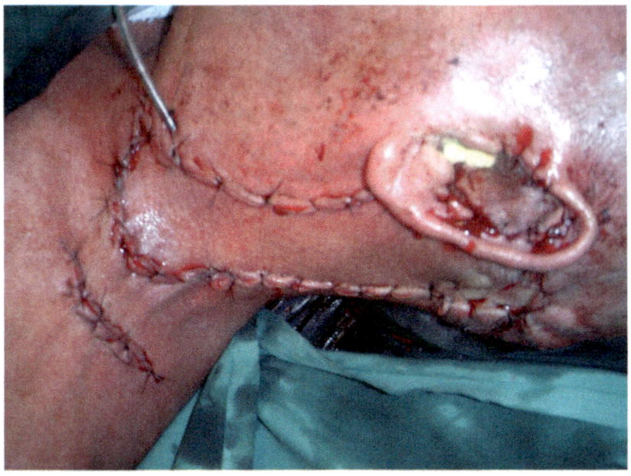

Fig. 2.241 The completion of the standard three-phase suture technique, with the viable flap in the conchal fossa and the neck wound closed completely under Redivac seal

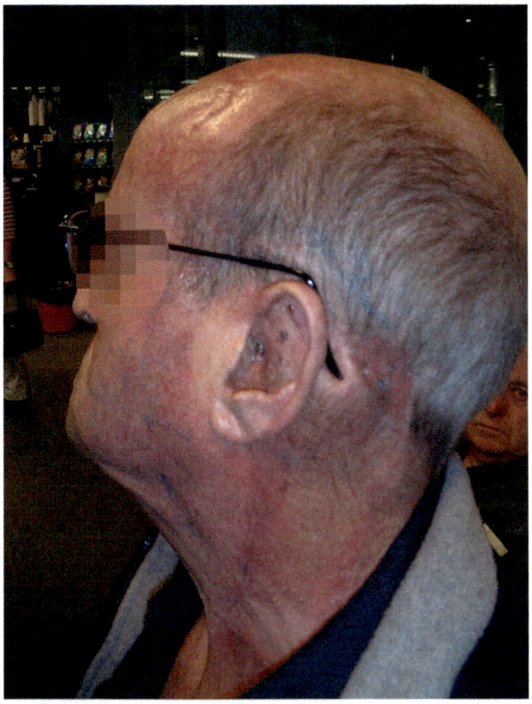

Fig. 2.242 Complete healing, no evidence of vascular impedance and postoperative appearance at 6 months showing no evidence of recurrence

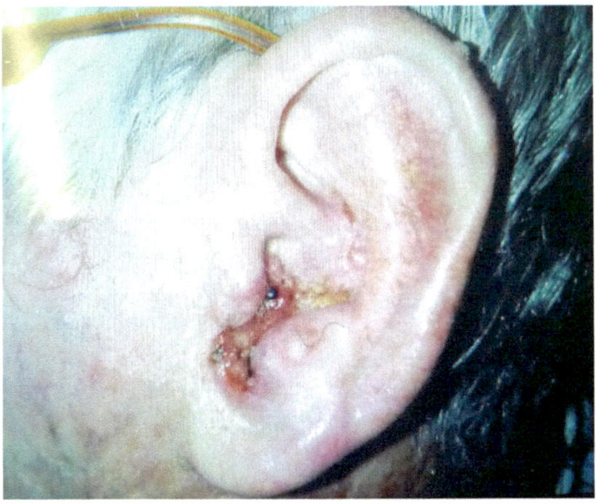

Fig. 2.243 The malignancy of the conchal fossa of the L ear involving the external auditory bony canal

The PACES characteristics were all exemplified: pain-free, aesthetic, no vascular complications, economical in terms of time and sensory recovery with the resolution of oedema.

2.1.1.25 Case 25—Partial Ear Amputation for Conchal Fossa Defect Closed with an Omega (u) Variant of the Keystone (U) variant of the Keystone (Figs. 2.243, 2.244, 2.245, 2.246, 2.247, 2.248, 2.249, 2.250, 2.251 and 2.252)

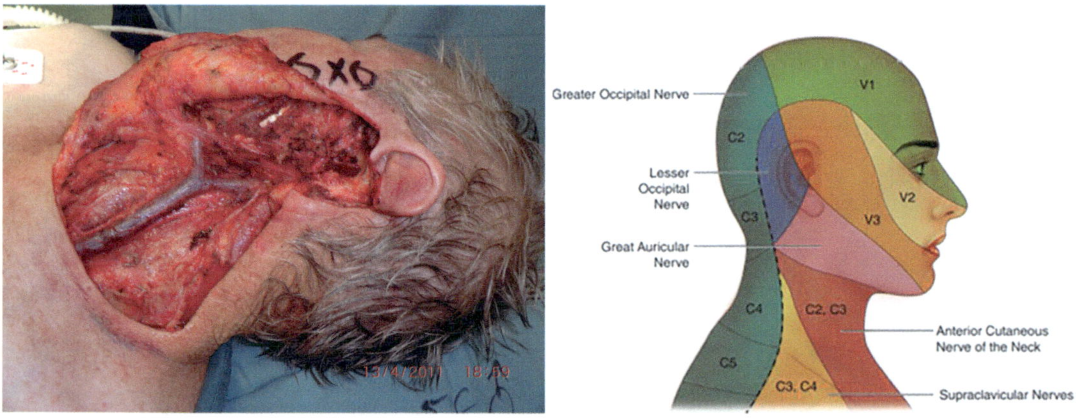

Fig. 2.244 This illustrates the importance of retaining all vascular drainage points. The oncological defect is 6 × 6 cm, involving a partial amputation of the ear, leaving the upper helix as the only remnant. The oncological clearance (DUET procedure by Sizeland) of neck glands levels II, III and IV is shown, and the external jugular vein is retained to optimise venous drainage should venous necrosis occur. The dermatomal mark outs become the line of incision of the dermis and epidermis leaving one-third deeply attached with only partial undermining to facilitate closure of the defect. (Reprinted with permission from Atlas, *Reconstructive Technique in Melanoma Management* (p. 19), by Felix Behan, Springer Nature 2023)

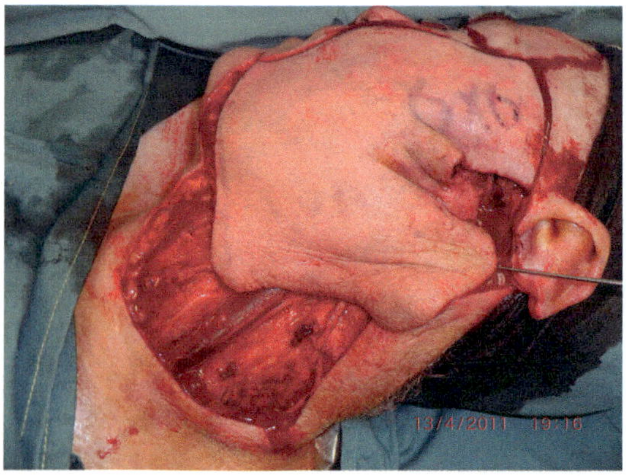

Fig. 2.245 The lower cervical tissues are parts of the neck flap rotated into the defect, creating the omega variant of the Keystone. Islanding is an essential requirement of the technique. It is designed along the nasolabial line, part of its hypervascularisation technique, to prevent flap necrosis when closed under tension. The red dot sign is consistently evident

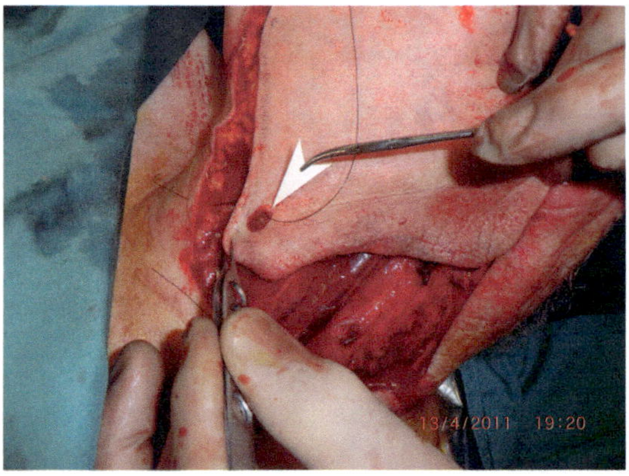

Fig. 2.246 The arrow shows the hyperaemic phase at the apex of the flap, the red dot sign at the suture point bleeding more on the flap side than on the receiving site. The site of potential necrosis at the apex is overcome by this hypervascularisation technique of islanding at the dermal-epidermal level without excessive undermining

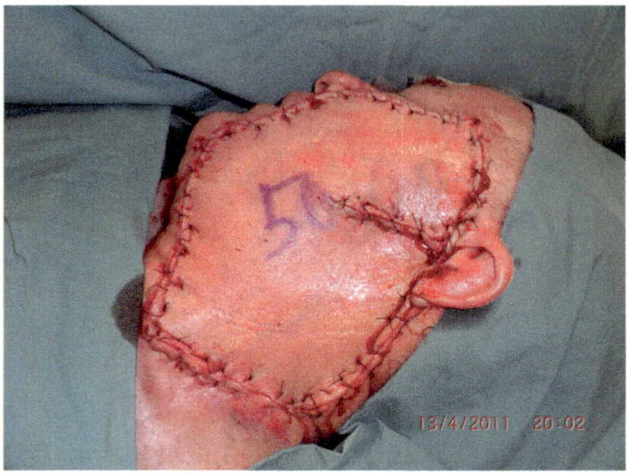

Fig. 2.247 Finally, the U-shaped omega-variant Keystone allows direct closure using the standard three-phase suture technique. Such is the reliabilty of the hyperaemia. Any dog ears of redundent tissue can be trimmed

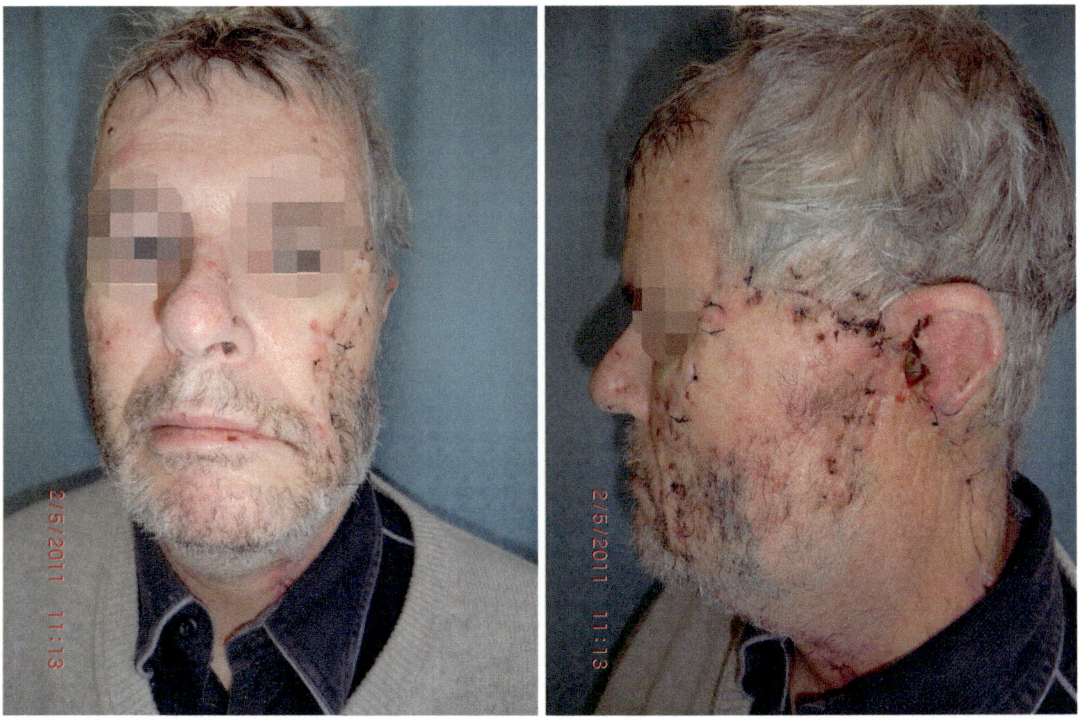

Fig. 2.248 Postoperative appearance at 2 weeks with a sequential staged removal of sutures to avoid any rupture in this single-layer suture technique

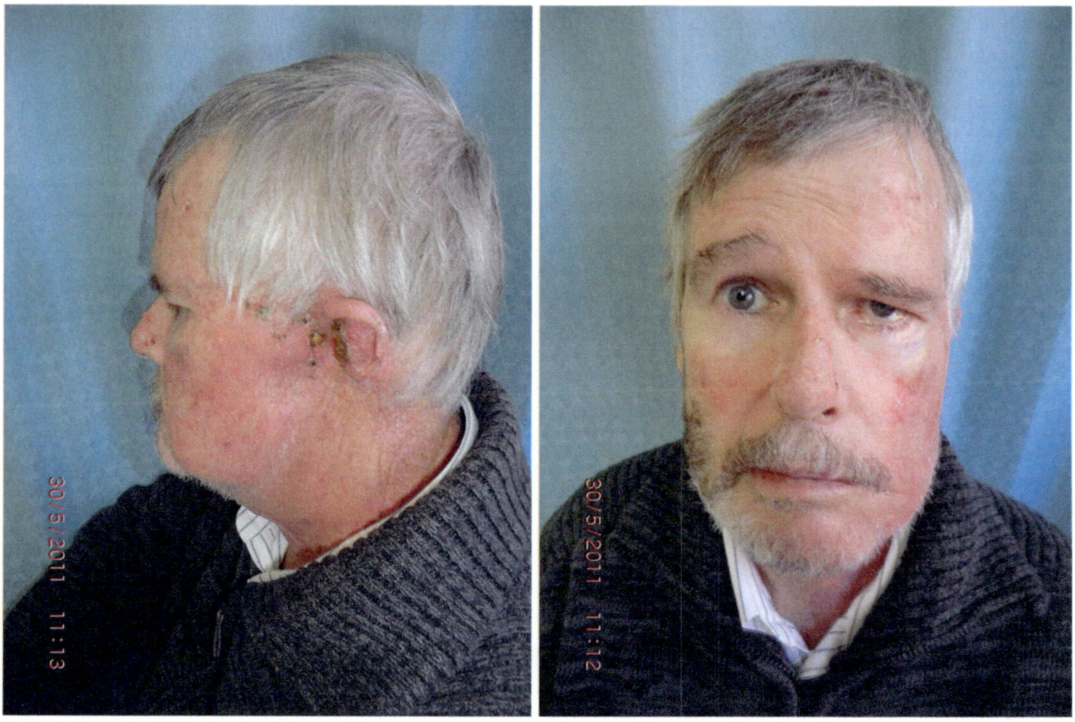

Fig. 2.249 Postoperative appearance at 6 weeks shows the removal of sutures. Note how the islanding of the neck flaps eliminates necrosis

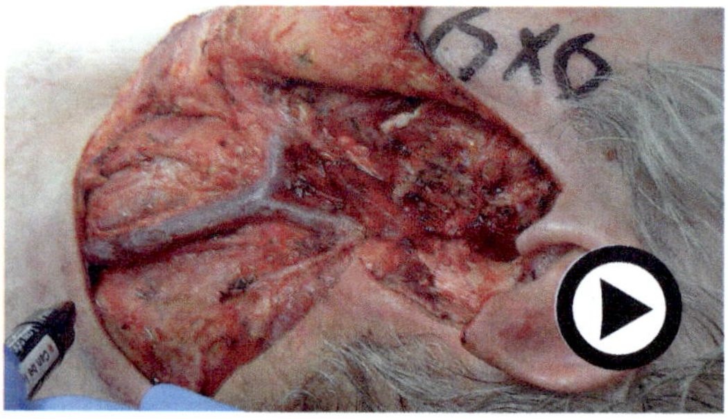

Fig. 2.250 Video 2.31 A diagram of the design of the Keystone used to hypervascularise the flap with closure under tension, thus avoiding facial nerve reconstruction (▶ https://doi.org/10.1007/000-k6w)

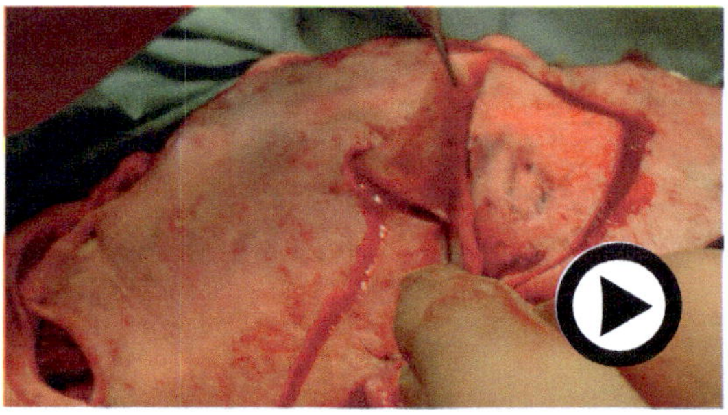

Fig. 2.251 Video 2.32 The reconstruction and the value of excising the dog ear pleat to eliminate a second stage because of the hypervascularisation (▶ https://doi.org/10.1007/000-k6x)

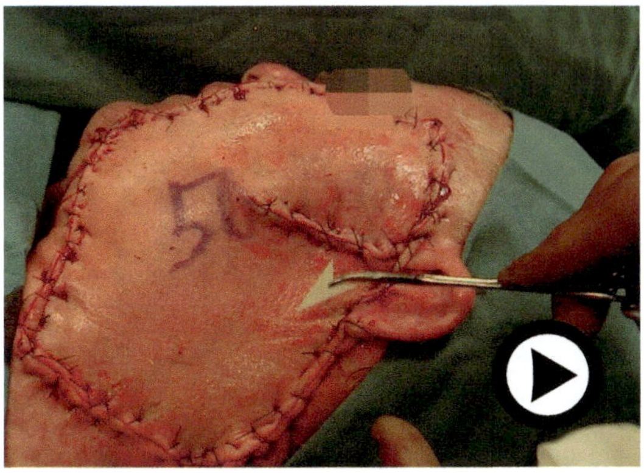

Fig. 2.252 Video 2.33 The postoperative appearance, confirming the absence of any necrosis with closure under tension as a solution for facial nerve deficiency. Note the absence of any necrosis or vascular impendence (▶ https://doi.org/10.1007/000-k6y)

The PACES characteristics were all exemplified: pain-free, aesthetic, no vascular complications, economical in terms of time and sensory recovery with the resolution of oedema.

2.1.1.26 Case 26—Major 8 × 6 × 1.5 cm Auricular and Parotid Defect with Patient on Dialysis (Figs. 2.253, 2.254, 2.255, 2.256, 2.257, 2.258, 2.259, 2.260, 2.261, 2.262, 2.263, 2.264, 2.265, 2.266, 2.266 and 2.267)

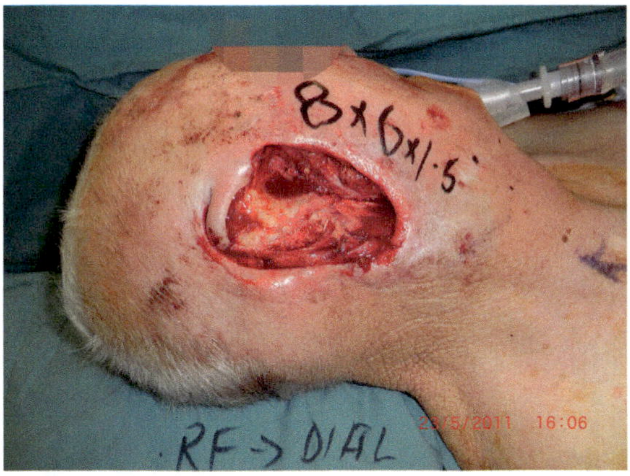

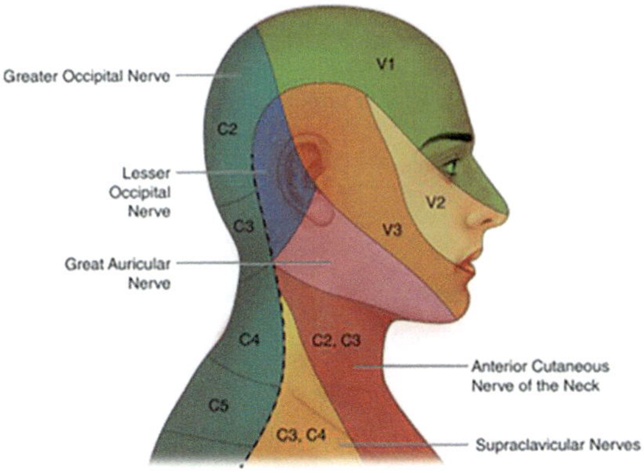

Fig. 2.253 The 8 × 6 × 1.5 cm surgical defect down to the external canal, showing the exposure of the ascending ramus. The dermatomal mark outs become the line of incision of the dermis and epidermis, ensuring that one-third deeply is attached with only partial undermining to facilitate the closure and vascular integrity of the defect. (Reprinted with permission from Atlas, *Reconstructive Technique in Melanoma Management* (p. 19), by Felix Behan, Springer Nature 2023)

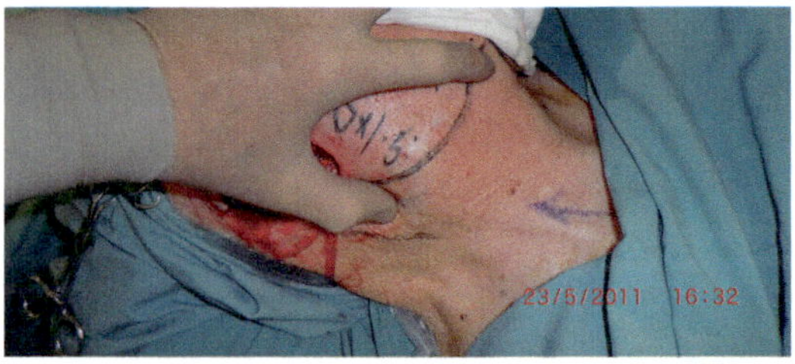

Fig. 2.254 The dotted mark out of the cervico-submental Keystone flap

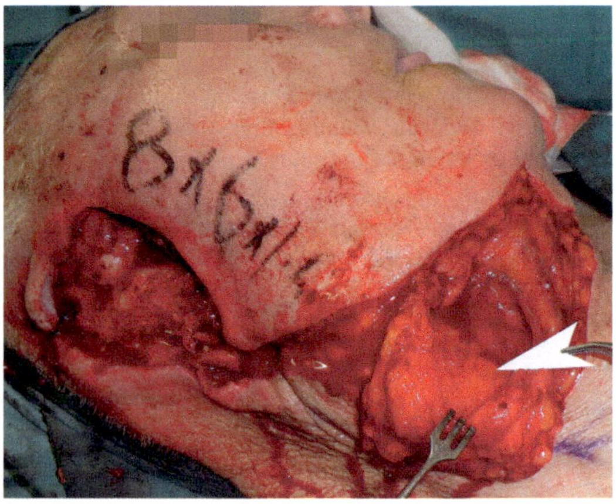

Fig. 2.255 The flap being retracted at the level of the fascia, showing the perfusion in the suprafascial plane—the lifeline for the hyperaemia effect

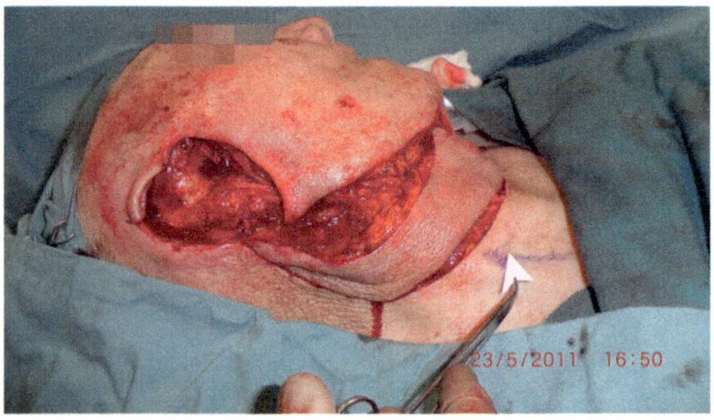

Fig. 2.256 The hyperaemia has taken 12 min to become evident (timestamped)

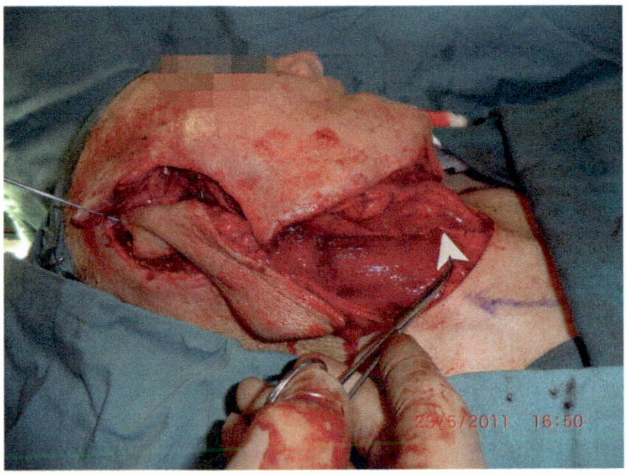

Fig. 2.257 Any vascular points are clipped with haemostatic microclips

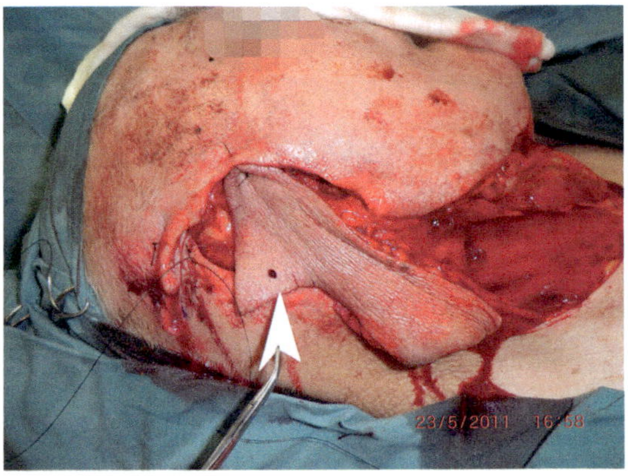

Fig. 2.258 The red dot sign (arrowed) in the hyperaemic Keystone flap rotated on the sternomastoid perforators

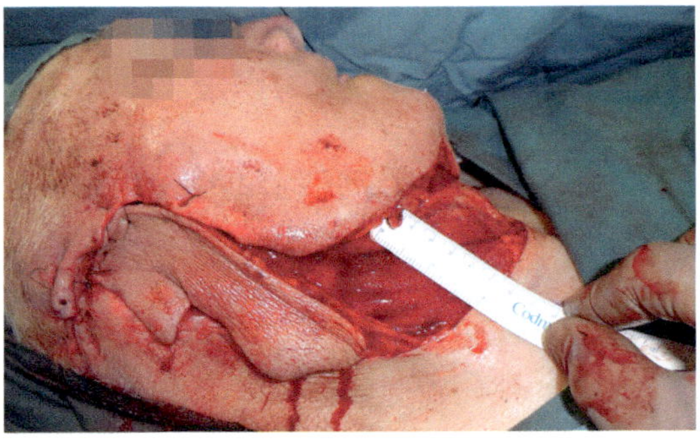

Fig. 2.259 A 5.5 cm gap in the neck, representing the secondary defect in the cervico-submental flap, which is closed directly. An absolute imperitive here is the use locking mattress sutures at the apex, and these are left in for 3 weeks; otherwise, wound breakdown will be a natural consequence, causing extra morbidity

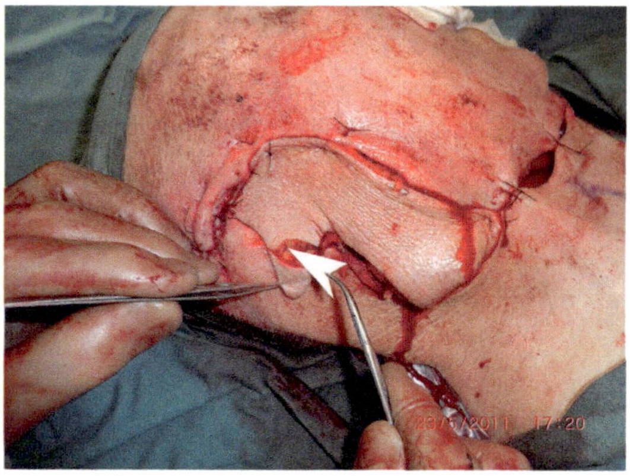

Fig. 2.260 The dog ear is trimmed in the acute phase because of the reliable vascularity (arrowed) and closed directly with locking mattress sutures because of the element of tension thus created

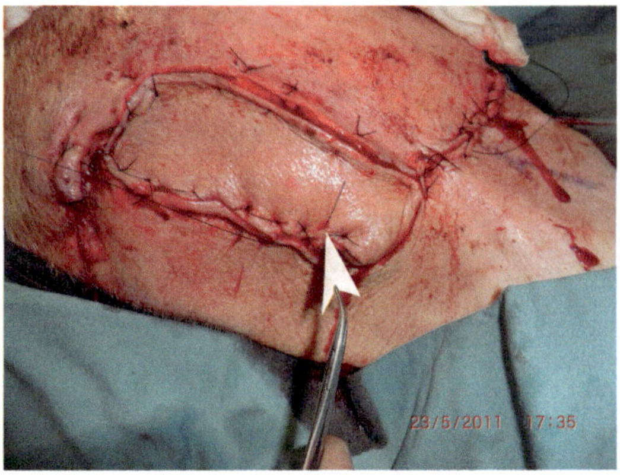

Fig. 2.262 The red dot sign is evident, confirming hypervascularity to ensure sound healing and direct neck closure with locking mattress sutures

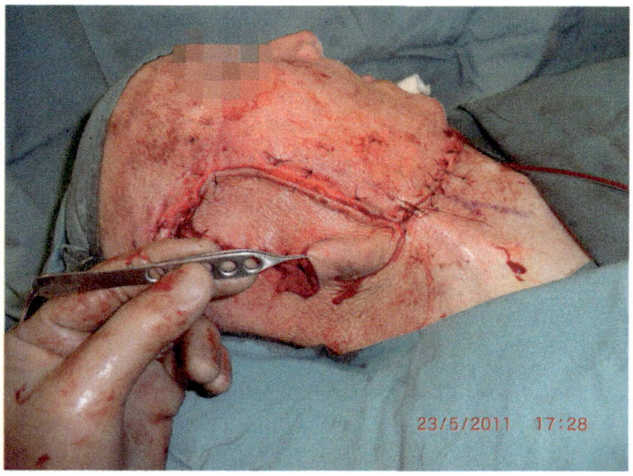

Fig. 2.261 Removal of an additional dog ear

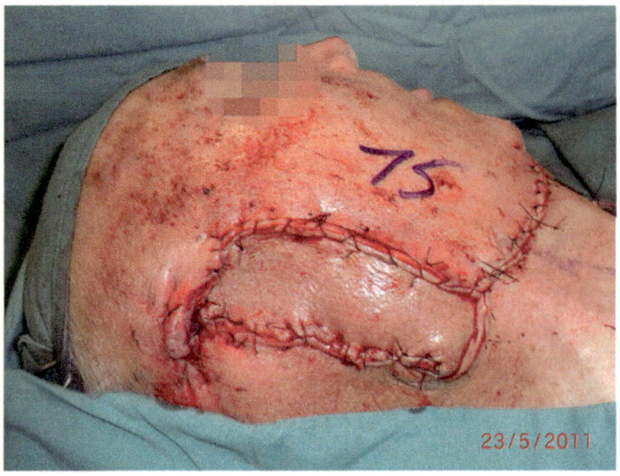

Fig. 2.263 Closure in 75 min

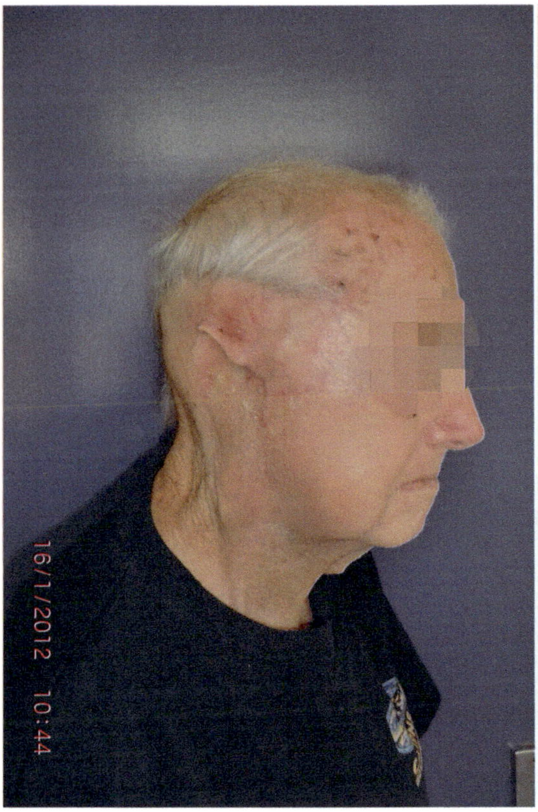

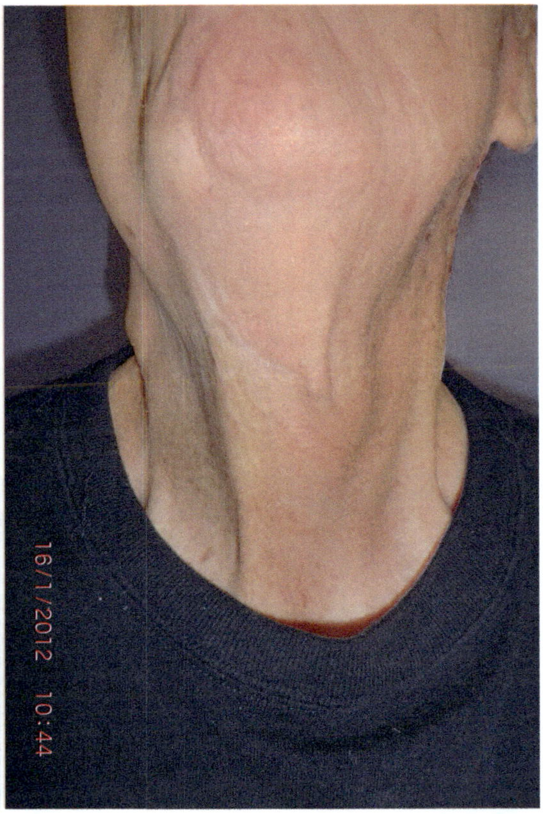

Fig. 2.264 The apperance at 7 months is shown, and the patient is totally satisfied with his appearance and tumour excision without any sign of recurrence. Scars are barely discernable when using the standard three-phase locking mattress suture technique

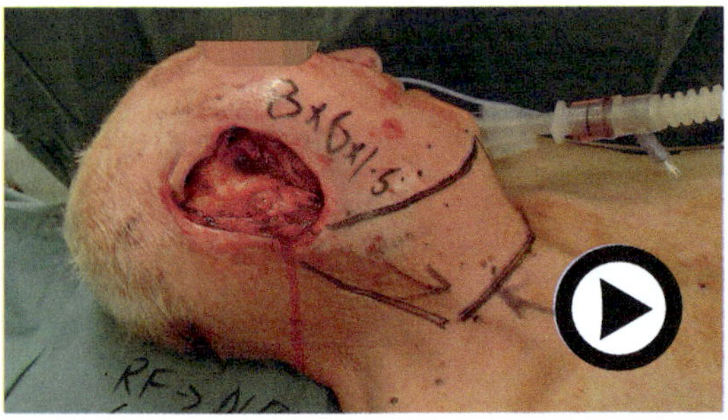

Fig. 2.265 Video 2.34 A closure of a large parotid defect using a cervico-submental Keystone based on random sternomastoid perforators (▶ https://doi.org/10.1007/000-k6z)

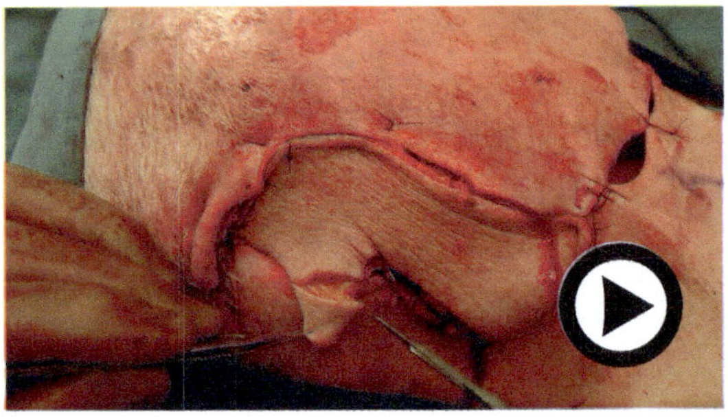

Fig. 2.266 Video 2.35 The trimming of a dog ear, reliably done because of the hypervascularity of the Keystone (▶ https://doi.org/10.1007/000-k70)

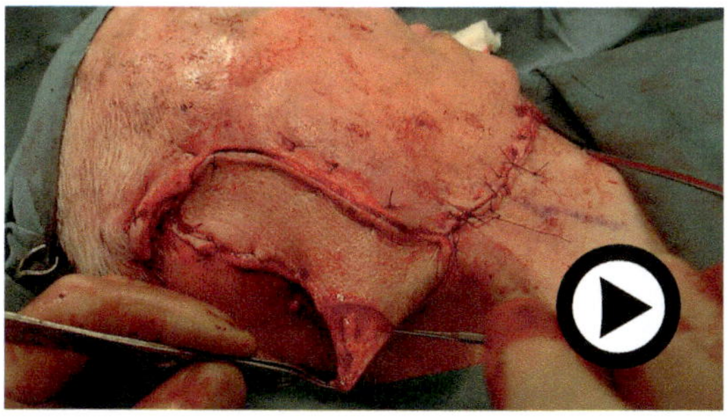

Fig. 2.267 Video 2.36 The trimming of the dog ear in the acute phase, reliably performed because of the hypervascularity in the Keystone design with cervical fascia support (▶ https://doi.org/10.1007/000-k71)

The PACES characteristics were all exemplified: pain-free, aesthetic, no vascular complications, economical in terms of time and sensory recovery with the resolution of oedema.

2.1.1.27 Case 27—Total Auriculectomy for an SCC down the External Canal (Figs. 2.268, 2.269, 2.270, 2.271, 2.272 and 2.273)

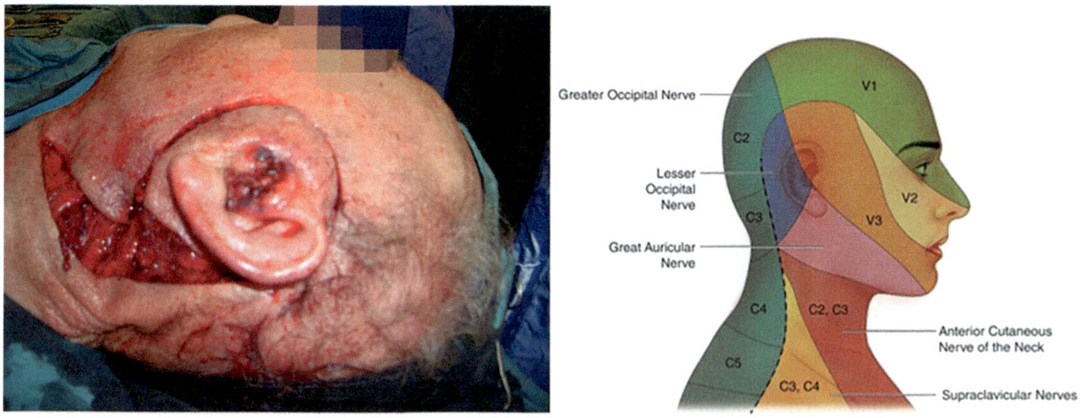

Fig. 2.268 The surgical defect outlined with neck dissection was done by Professor Sizeland. The dermatomal mark outs become the line of incision of the dermis and epidermis, ensuring that one-third deeply is attached with only partial undermining to facilitate the closure and vascular integrity of the defect. (Reprinted with permission from Atlas, *Reconstructive Technique in Melanoma Management* (p. 19), by Felix Behan, Springer Nature 2023)

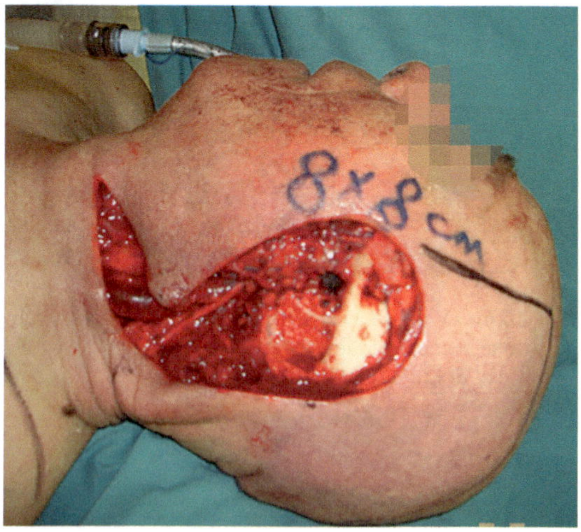

Fig. 2.269 A scalp Keystone outlined based on occipital perforators

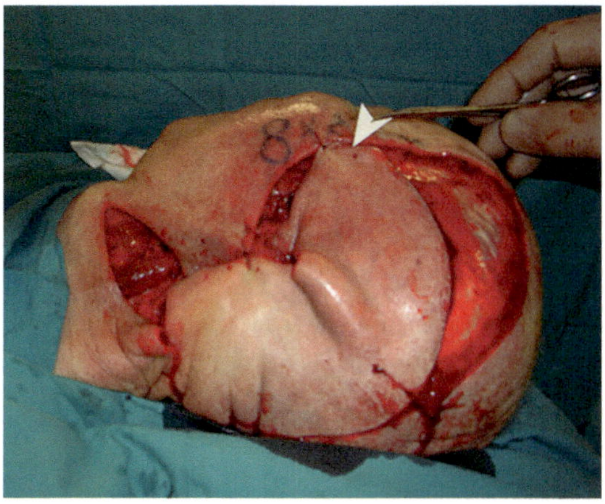

Fig. 2.270 Keystone has been inserted. The red dot signs of vascularity are arrowed prior to complete closure with a fenestrated full-thickness graft to the scalp

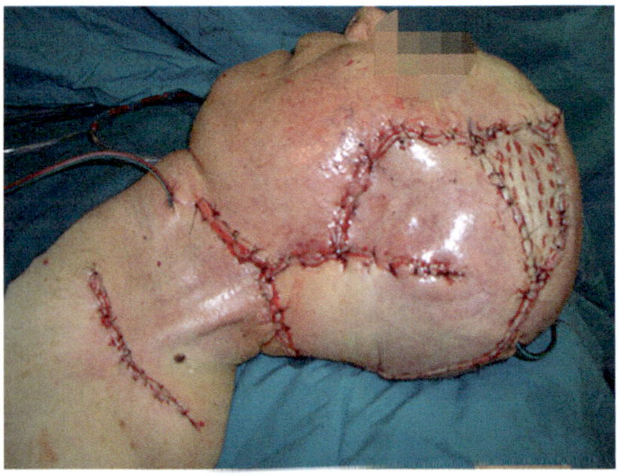

Fig. 2.271 On completion, the supraclavicular incision facilitates another Keystone design to allow the upward advancement of the neck tissue to close the first Keystone based on temporal circulation. Note that the vascular flare under Redivac drainage and the direct closure of the cervical wound covering the external jugular vein thanks to supraclavicular perforators is related to an additional Keystone in the neck. The fenetrated full-thickness graft on the skull is noted

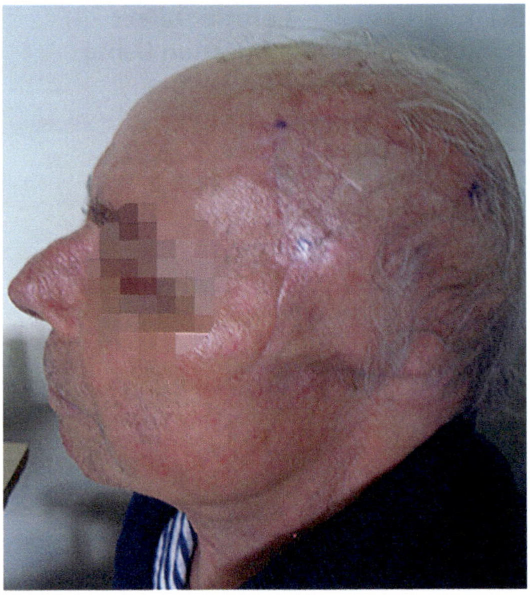

Fig. 2.273 The completion after radiation and a delayed tarrsorrophy completes the operation

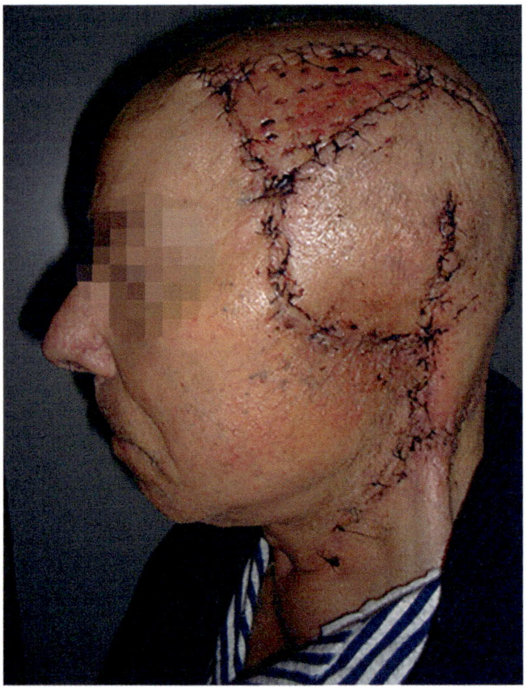

Fig. 2.272 The healed wound before the removal of the three-phase locking mattress sutures

The PACES characteristics were all exemplified: pain-free, aesthetic, no vascular complications, economical in terms of time and sensory recovery with the resolution of oedema.

2.1.1.28 Case 28—Parotid Defect and Ear Amputation Using the DRAPE Procedure with the Keystone (Figs. 2.274, 2.275, 2.276, 2.277, 2.278, 2.279, 2.280, 2.281, 2.282, 2.283, 2.284, 2.285, 2.286, 2.287, 2.288, 2.289, 2.290, 2.291 and 2.292)

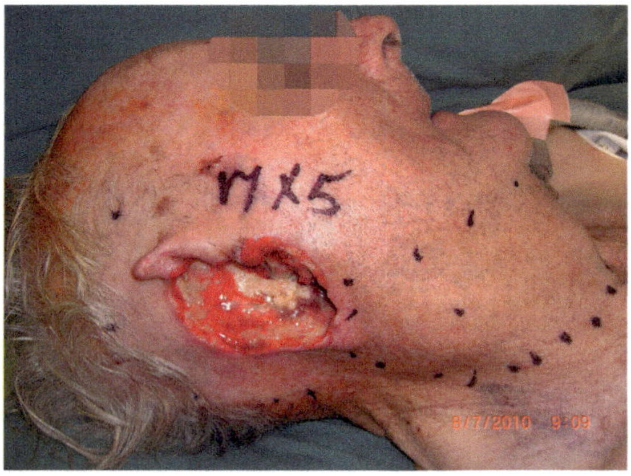

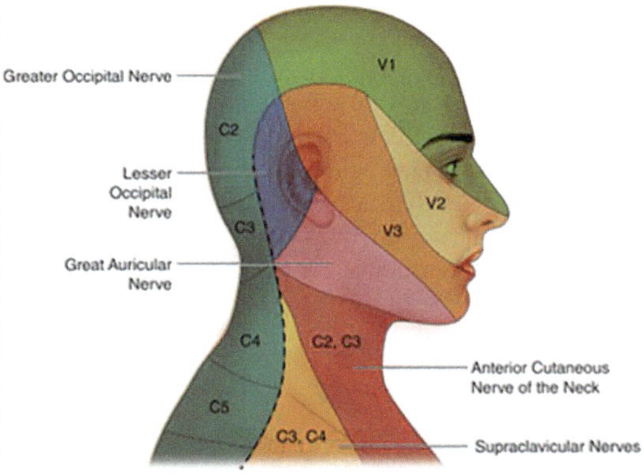

Fig. 2.274 The DRAPE procedure is shown. The cervico-submental Keystone that is marked out to close the auricular defect is illustrated, and the neck defect is closed directly with locking mattress sutures. The dermatomal mark outs become the line of incision of the dermis and epidermis, ensuring that one-third deeply is attached with only partial undermining to facilitate the closure and vascular integrity of the defect. (Reprinted with permission from Atlas, *Reconstructive Technique in Melanoma Management* (p. 19), by Felix Behan, Springer Nature 2023)

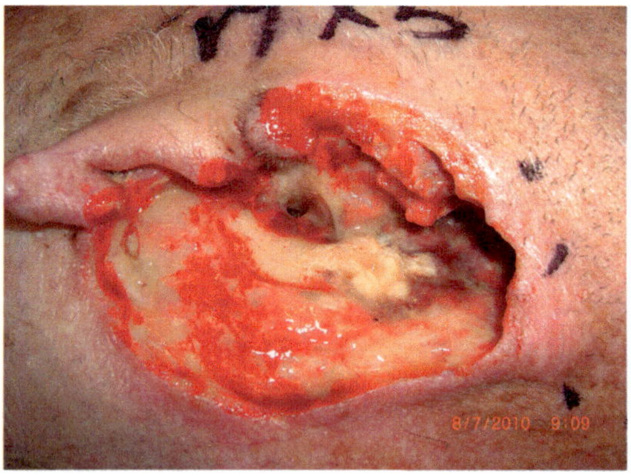

Fig. 2.275 The external canal excision from the lobule to the supra-auricular region

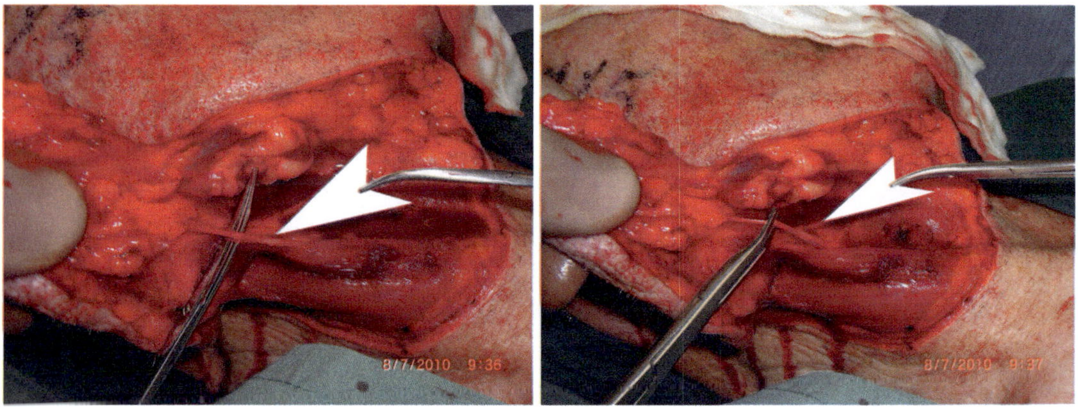

Fig. 2.276 Visible structures in the block dissection constitute a teaching mechanism. Part of the nodal II, III and IV clearance (Professor Sizeland) shows the accessory nerve

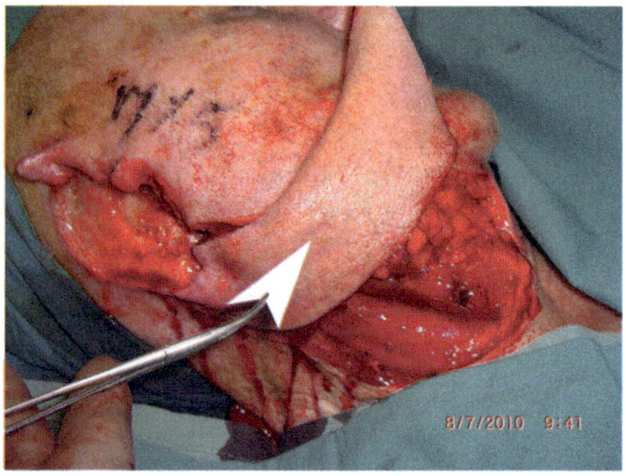

Fig. 2.277 The hyperaemia of the Keystone developing in 30-plus min

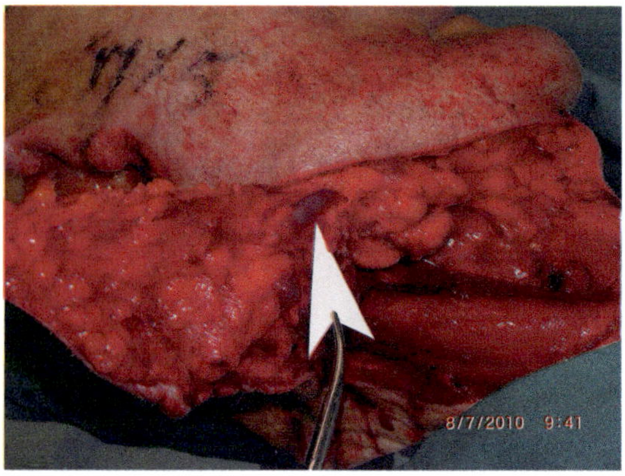

Fig. 2.278 The plane of the cervical fascia (arrowed)

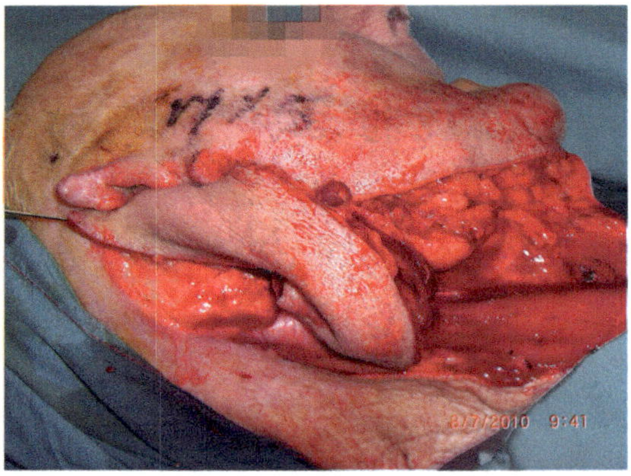

Fig. 2.279 The preinsertion of the cervico-submental flap rotated in the vicinity of the sternomastoid insertion using microperforators to produce the hyperaemic appearance

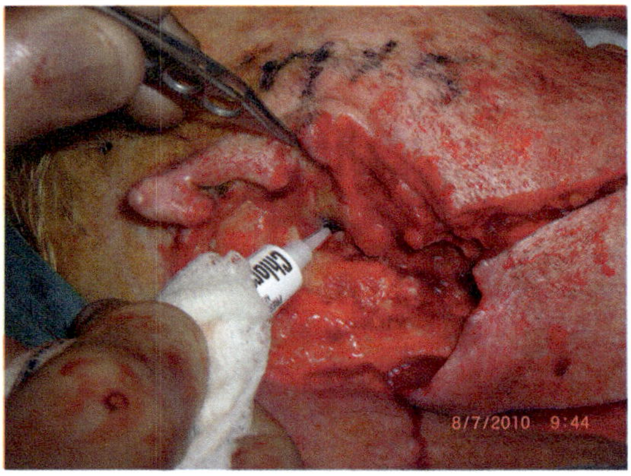

Fig. 2.280 Eye ointment is in the external canal, but no reconstruction is done here in the acute phase because it jeopardises the circulation

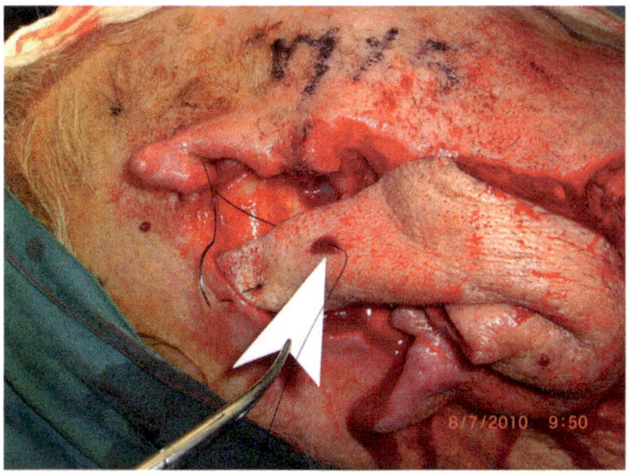

Fig. 2.281 The red dot sign confirms perfusional dynamics, and the pink flare is noted

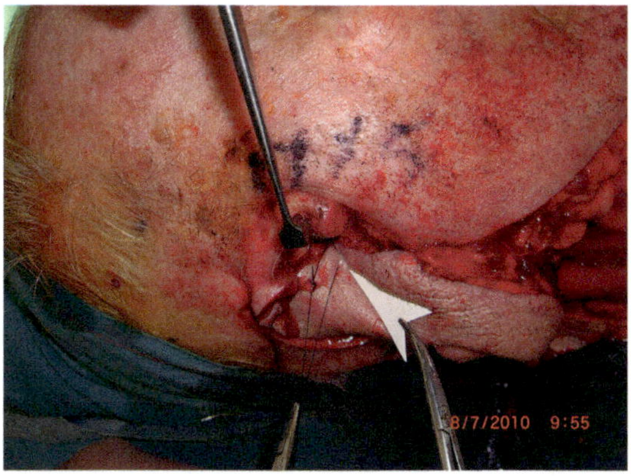

Fig. 2.282 Another red dot sign at the suture point

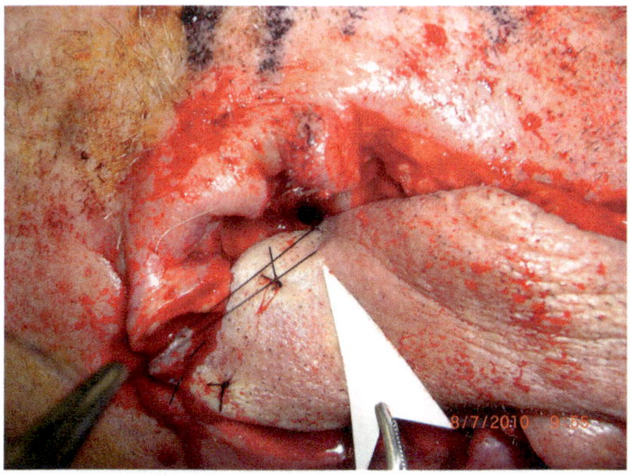

Fig. 2.283 The insertion is being finalised. No evidence of any vascular impedance appears here, confirmed by the pink flare

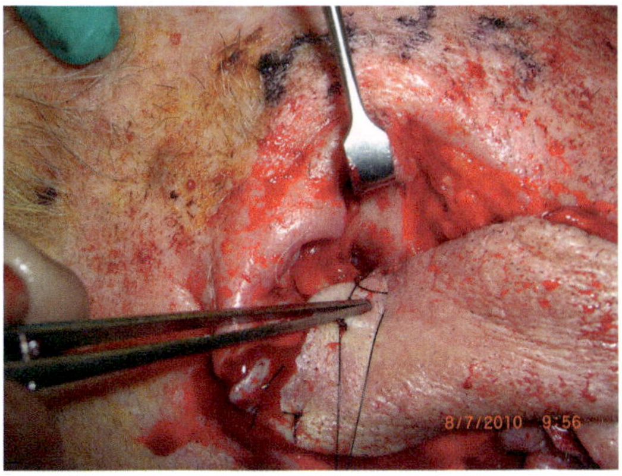

Fig. 2.284 Final stages of closure

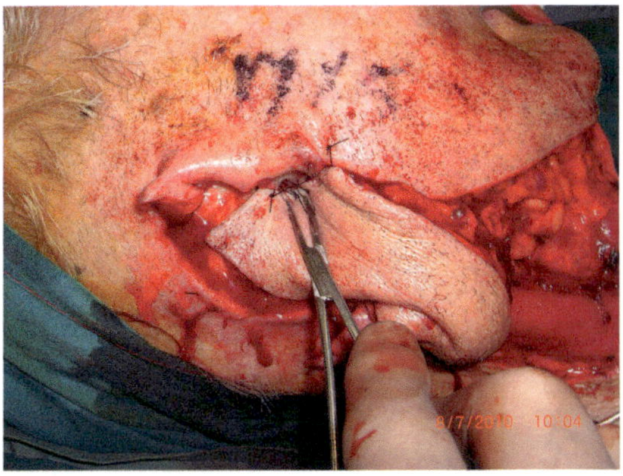

Fig. 2.285 Sealing the knot

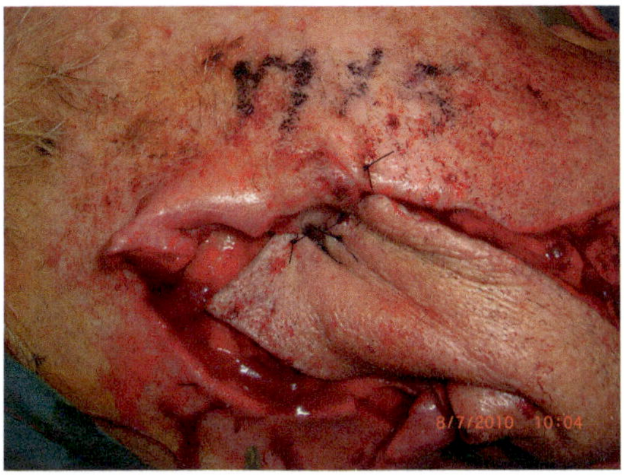

Fig. 2.286 Almost complete

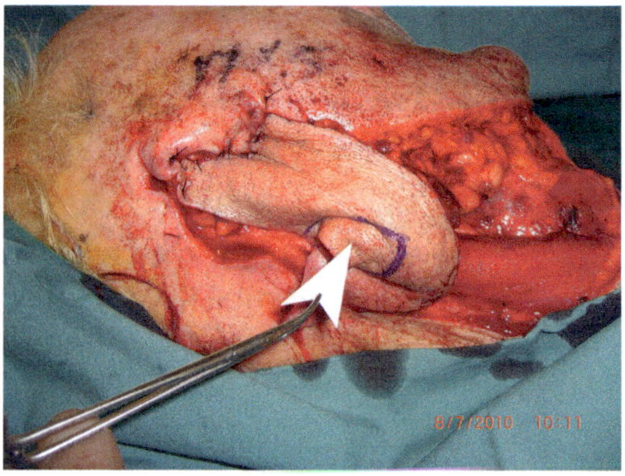

Fig. 2.287 The arrow indicating the site of rotation prior to trimming the dog ear because of the reliable perfusion

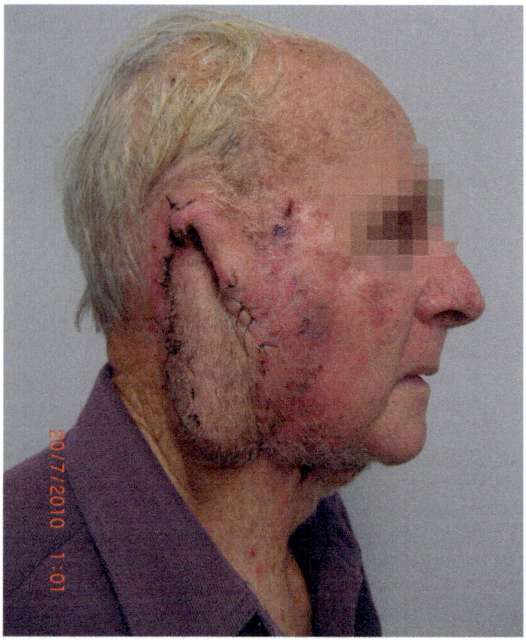

Fig. 2.288 On completion and appearance at 12 days with no element of anxiety in the patient's face, because he was quite satisfied with the pain-free outcome

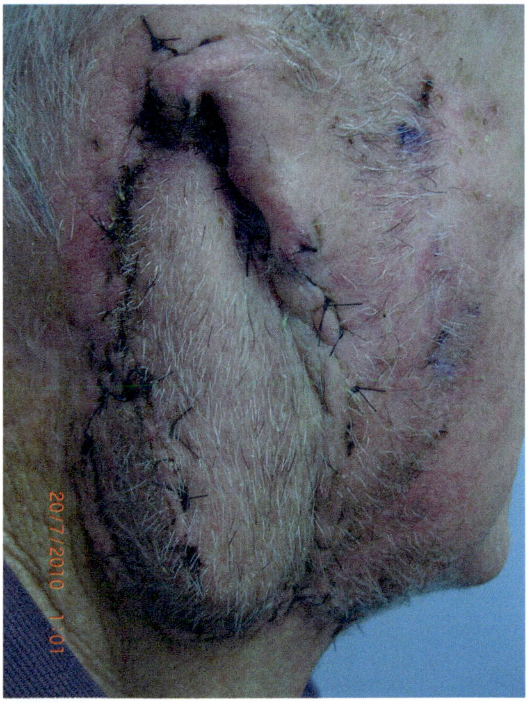

Fig. 2.289 A closeup at 12 days, with the locking mattress suture closing the neck defect

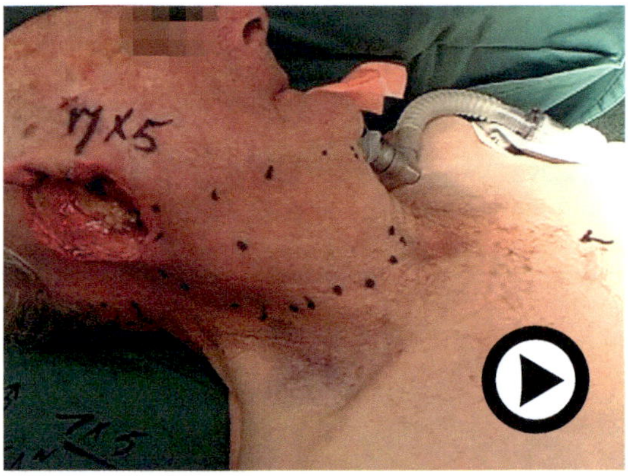

Fig. 2.290 Video 2.37 Planned operative reconstruction with a cervico-submental Keystone (▶ https://doi.org/10.1007/000-k72)

The PACES characteristics were all exemplified: pain-free, aesthetic, no vascular complications, economical in terms of time and sensory recovery with the resolution of oedema.

2.1.1.29 Case 29—Parotid and Ear Defect Closed with a, 8 × 5 cm Cervico-submental Keystone Defect After XRT (Figs. 2.293, 2.294, 2.295, 2.296, 2.297, 2.298, 2.299, 2.300, 2.301, 2.302, 2.303 and 2.304)

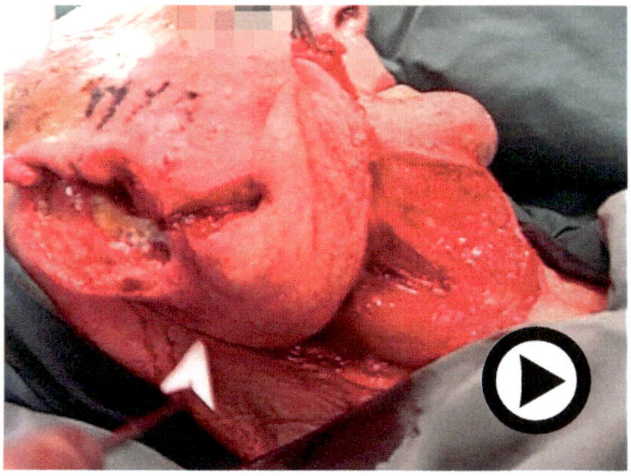

Fig. 2.291 Video 2.38 Raising the Keystone of the neck and retaining the cervical fascia using the blunt dissection technique (▶ https://doi.org/10.1007/000-k73)

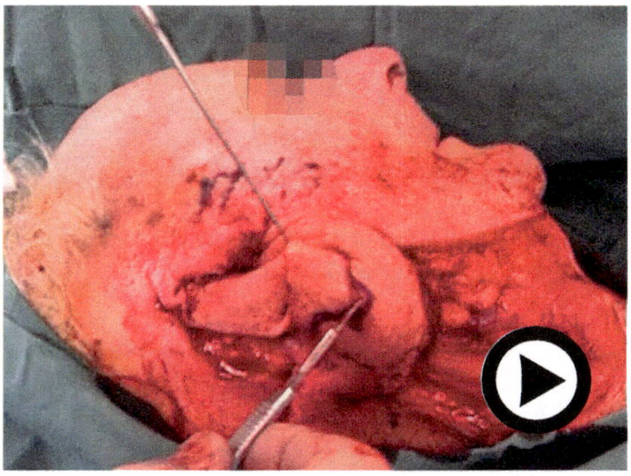

Fig. 2.292 Video 2.39 The trimming of the dog ear at the level of the subdermis (▶ https://doi.org/10.1007/000-k74)

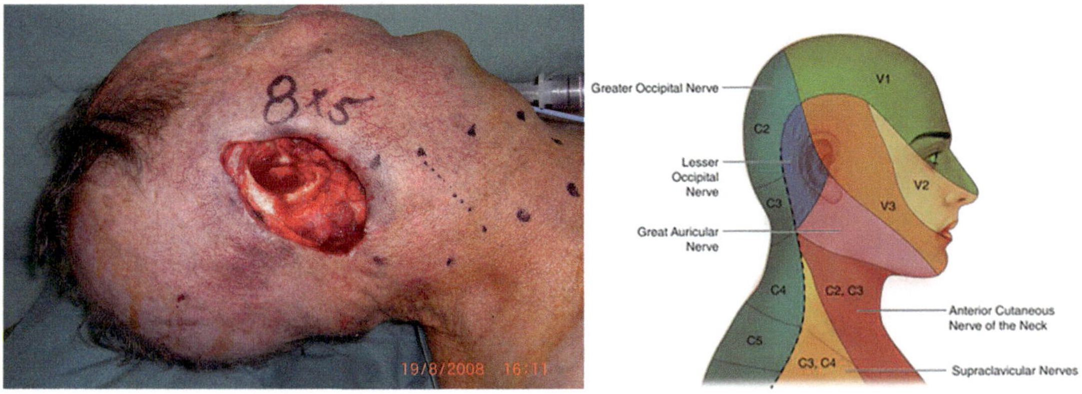

Fig. 2.293 The cervico-submental Keystone mark out for this 8 × 5 cm auricular defect is shown. The dermatomal mark outs become the line of incision of the dermis and epidermis, ensuring that one-third deeply is attached with only partial undermining to facilitate the closure and vascular integrity of the defect. (Reprinted with permission from Atlas, *Reconstructive Technique in Melanoma Management* (p. 19), by Felix Behan, Springer Nature 2023)

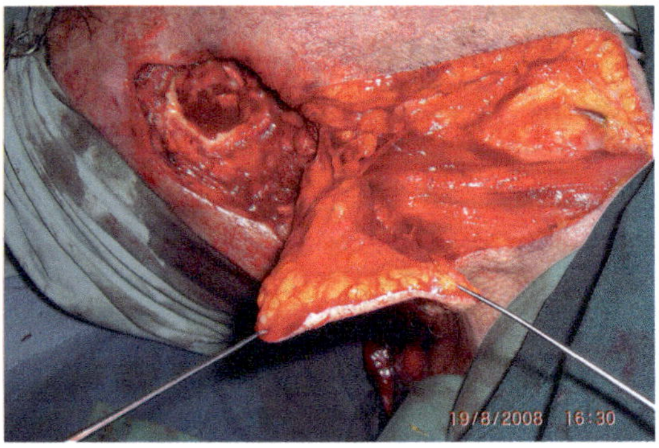

Fig. 2.294 Raising the cervico-submental flap with a fascial base

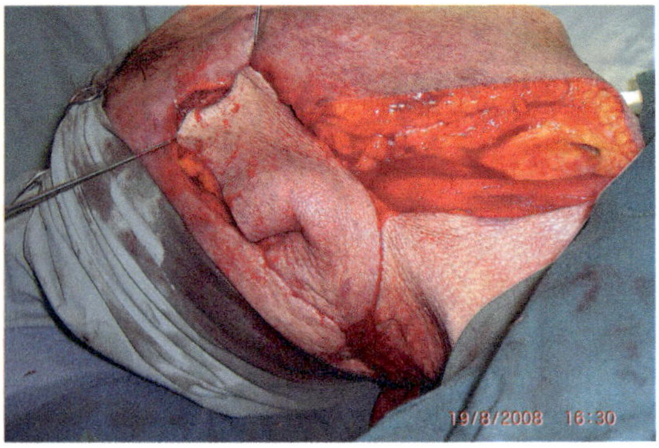

Fig. 2.295 Rotation on the sternomastoid axes to close the auricular defect before the direct closure of the cervical defect

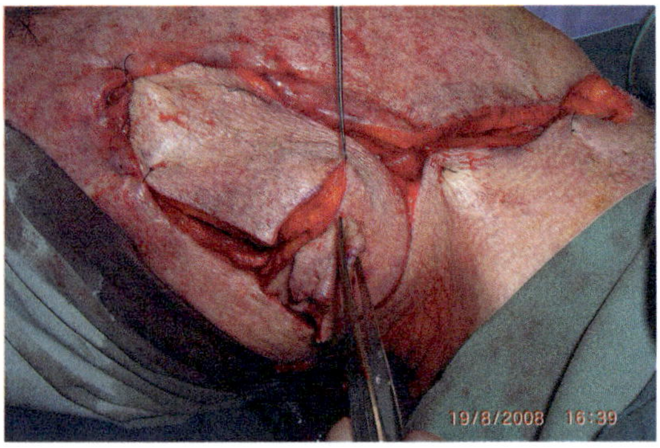

Fig. 2.296 Again, the excision of the dog ear at the dermal-epidermal level is carried out to avoid a secondary procedure

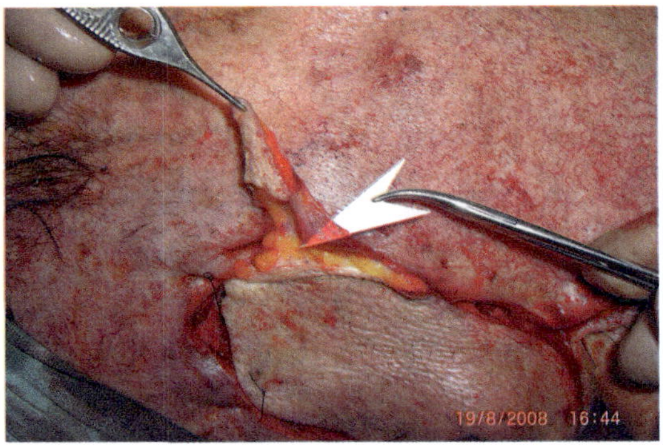

Fig. 2.297 The fascial base supporting this dog ear excision from a vascular perspective

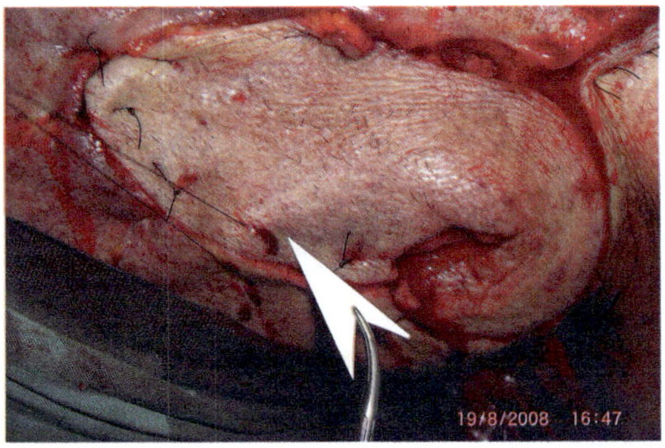

Fig. 2.298 The red dot sign marks the confirmation of its vascularity

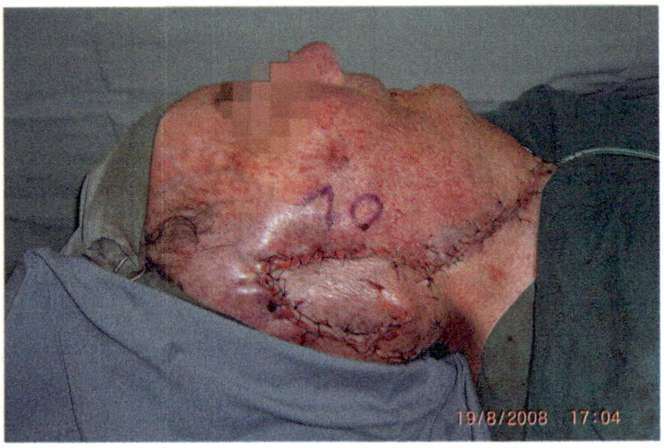

Fig. 2.299 Closure in 40 min in this 85-year-old patient

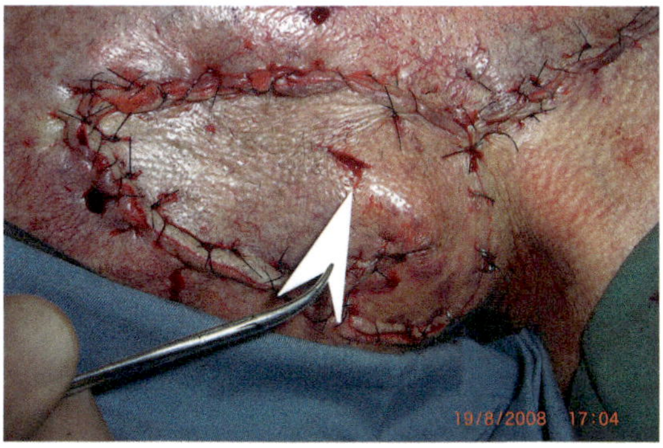

Fig. 2.300 Arrow indicating hypervascularised perfusion

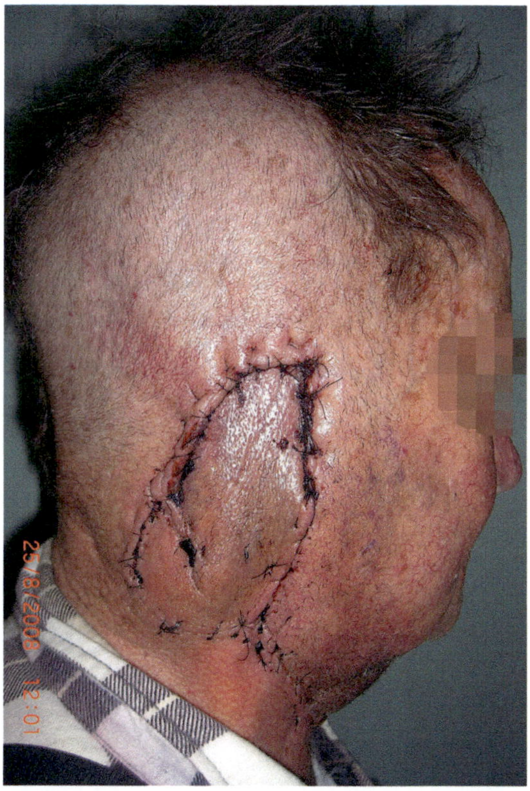

Fig. 2.301 The apearance at 6 days is shown, as time-stamped. The standard three-phase locking mattress suture technique is used throughout

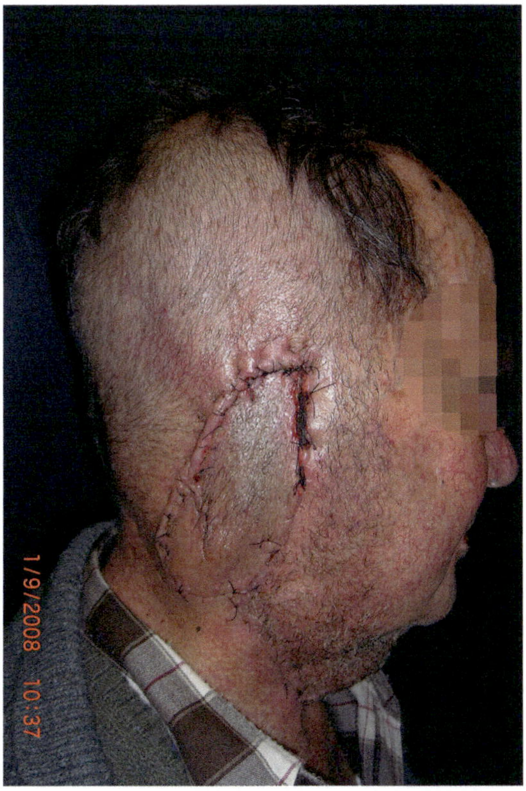

Fig. 2.302 Appearance at 13 days—no vascular impedence and fully healed

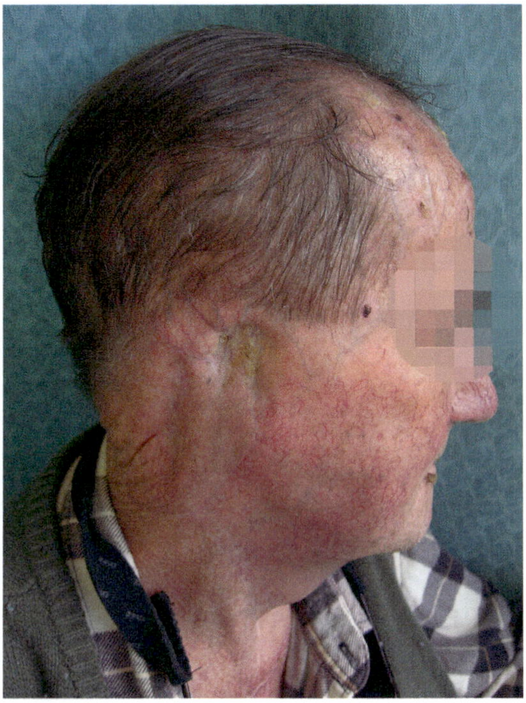

Fig. 2.303 Appearance at 12 months

The PACES characteristics were all exemplified: pain-free, aesthetic, no vascular complications, economical in terms of time and sensory recovery with the resolution of oedema.

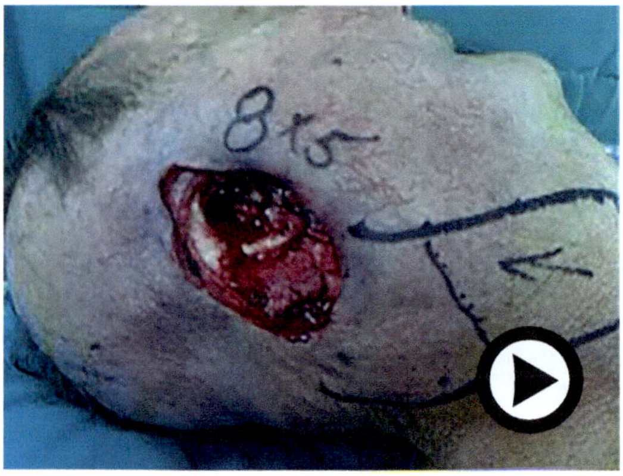

Fig. 2.304 Video 2.40 The planned operative reconstruction (▶ https://doi.org/10.1007/000-k75)

2.1.1.30 Case 30—A Simple Postauricular Trap Door Closure Using the Keystone Principle on Random Perforators from the Scalp (Figs. 2.305, 2.306, 2.307, 2.308, 2.309, 2.310, 2.311, 2.312, and 2.313)

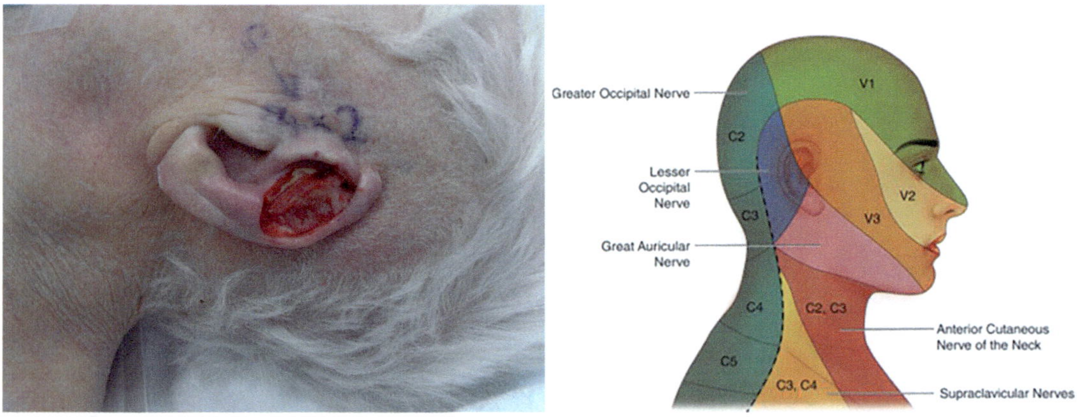

Fig. 2.305 A 4 × 2 cm surgical defect over the scaphoid fossa for a mitotic lesion is shown. The dermatomal mark outs become the line of incision of the dermis and epidermis, ensuring that one-third deeply is attached with only partial undermining to facilitate the closure and vascular integrity of the defect. (Reprinted with permission from Atlas, *Reconstructive Technique in Melanoma Management* (p. 19), by Felix Behan, Springer Nature 2023)

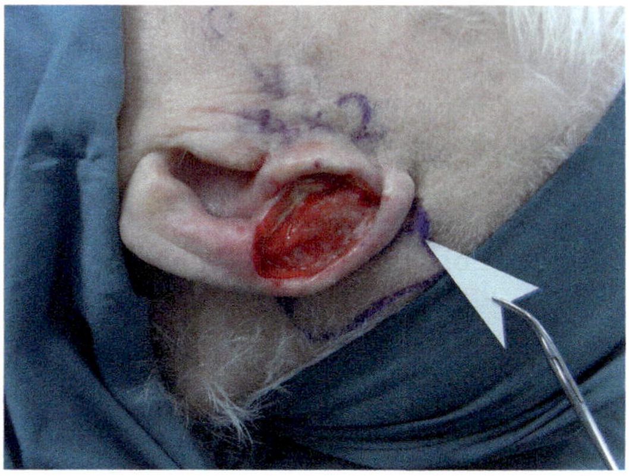

Fig. 2.306 The postauricular Keystone is delineated. The ear is flexed forward to facilitate the insertion of the Keystone from the postauricular alignment in the C2 and C3 dermatomes

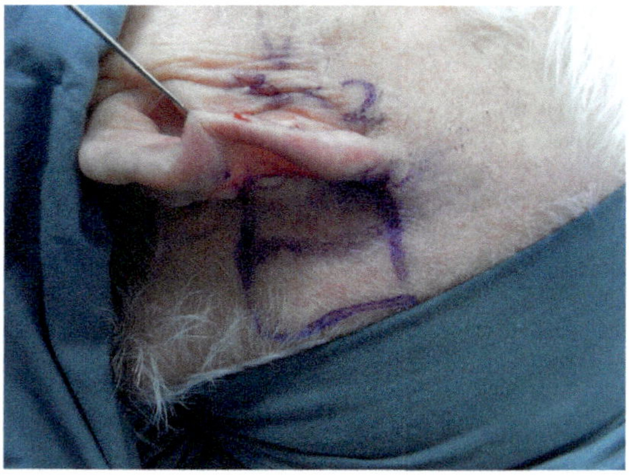

Fig. 2.307 With the mark out of the Keystone, the transverse line creates the island that enables going into the scaphoid fossa, and the helix falls back into the divided segment to give wound closure over the mastoid into the postauricular groove

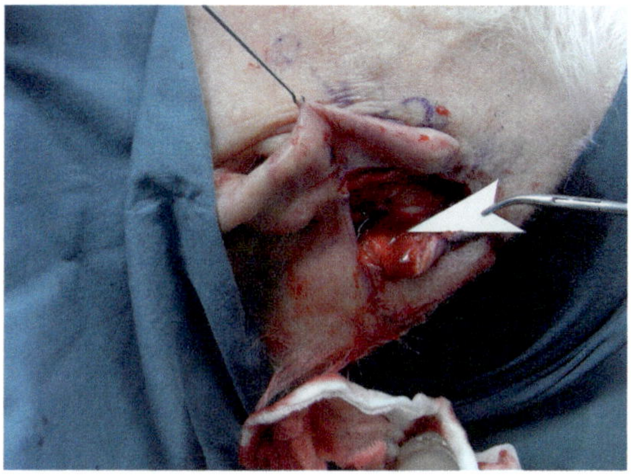

Fig. 2.308 Creating the island of tissue for the scaphoid insertion

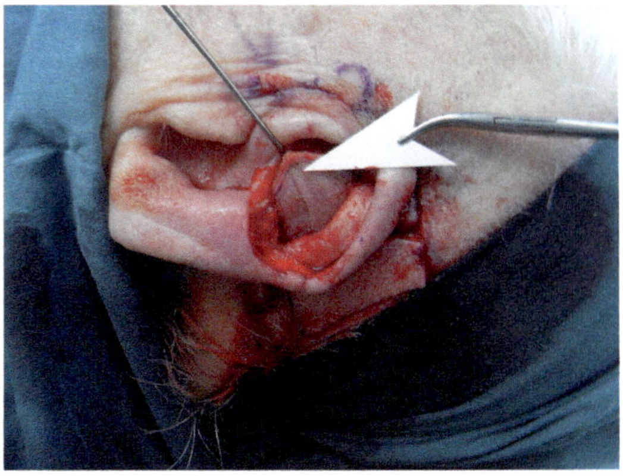

Fig. 2.309 The island flap in situ and sewn into position before the helix is sewn back into the divided Keystone

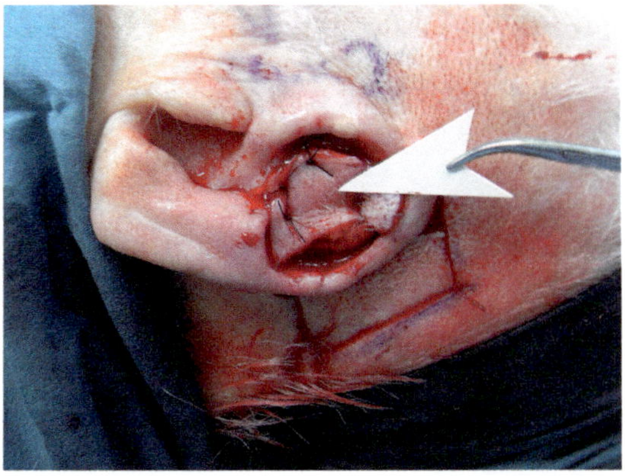

Fig. 2.310 The island flap is fully vascularised and hypervascularised in the Keystone manner, and the helix covers the division that created the island to ensure sound healing

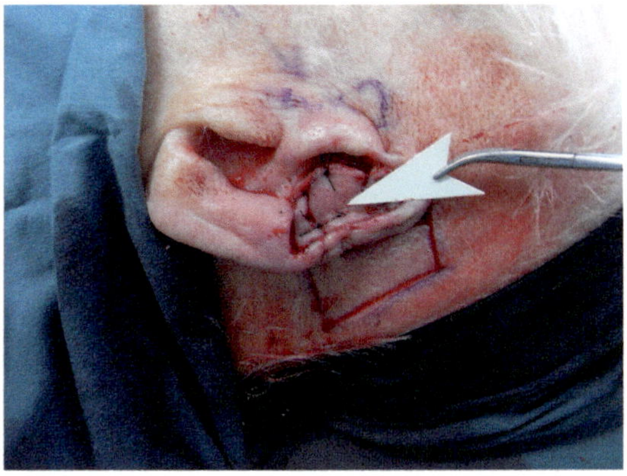

Fig. 2.311 The postauricular incision of the skin creates the Keystone design and ensures hypervascularity—a Keystone characteristic. The postauricular incision is just closed directly

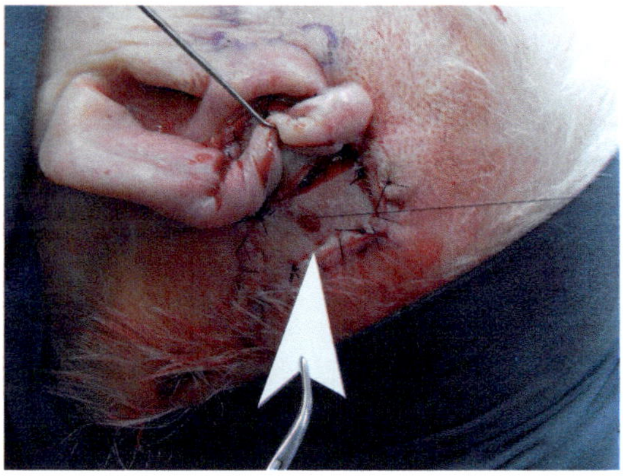

Fig. 2.312 The red dot sign confirms the hypervascularity when closing the postauricular incision

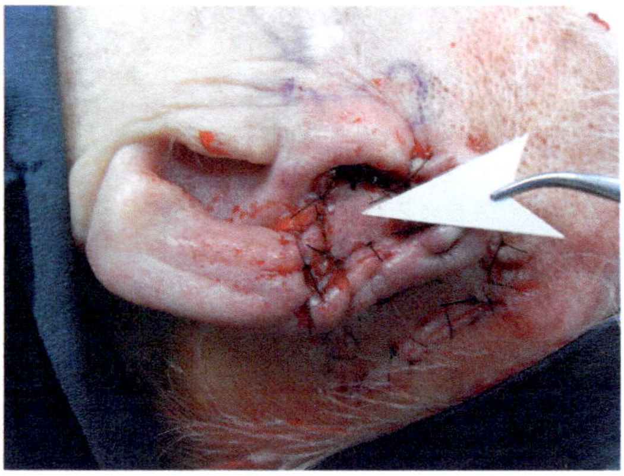

Fig. 2.313 The finished procedure, fully vascularised with all the PACES characteristic exemplified

The PACES characteristics were all exemplified: pain-free, aesthetic, no vascular complications, economical in terms of time and sensory recovery with the resolution of oedema.

2.1.2 Forehead

The Keystones in the forehead are based on the main vessels, including the supratrochlear, supraorbital and superficial temporal artery neurovascular structures. The associated sensory supply, when included in the Keystone, provides contact and protective sensation in the vicinity of the repair. One must be aware of the facial nerve innervation of the frontalis muscle and exercise caution in the reconstruction of such defects in such significant areas. However, the relative inelasticity of any tissue [12] is a well-recognised restriction in reconstruction in this region. Simple techniques such as A-to-T flaps are part of the reconstructive options. The Bezier neurovascular island flap [13] is an ellipsoidal V-Y design that uses V-Y principles as originally documented [14] (Figs. 2.314 and 2.315). Using local tissue for local tissue has the advantage of an aesthetic outcome with the surrounding tissues. Various locational sites will be part of the presentation.

Free tissue transfer is reserved for larger defects, but the Keystone has a remarkable proclivity for spreading tension throughout the distribution of the delineated fascial island flap, which seems, on the basis of the dermatomes, to make closure a reasonable alternative and allows for bypassing microsurgical reconstructions from a time and aesthetic point of view. I offer you the appearance of a free flap reconstruction compared with the Keystone, and the likes of latissimus dorsi and radial forearm compare quite unfavourably from a tissue match point of view, never mind the bulky protuberance.

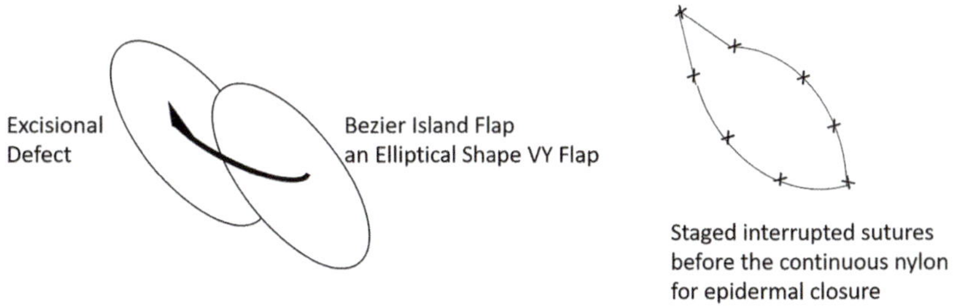

Fig. 2.314 An excisional defect with the Bezier markout is shown. The curvilinear lines ease the reconstruction and avoid tension points. Surgical closure is carried out with V-Y apposition

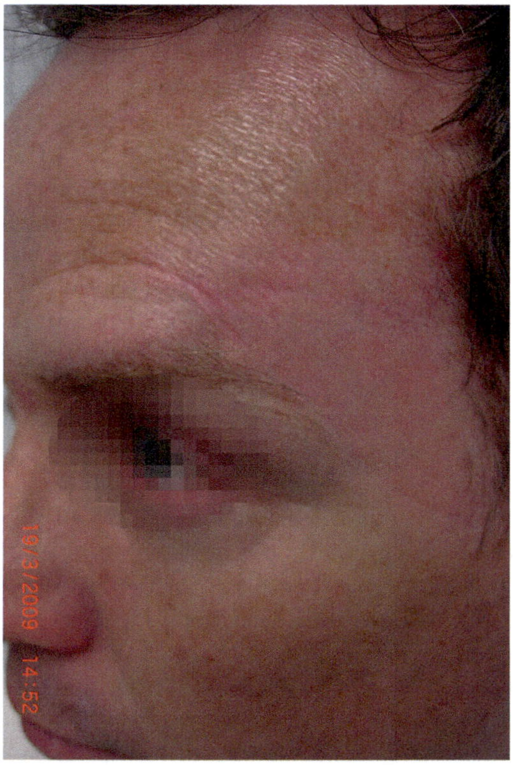

Fig. 2.315 A clinical exmaple of the Bezier curvilinear V-Y island flap—appearance at 6 months, with a good aesthetic appearance

2.1.2.1 Case 31—Bezier Flap for a Mitotic Lesion of the R Temple (Figs. 2.316, 2.317, 2.318, 2.319, 2.320, 2.321 and 2.322)

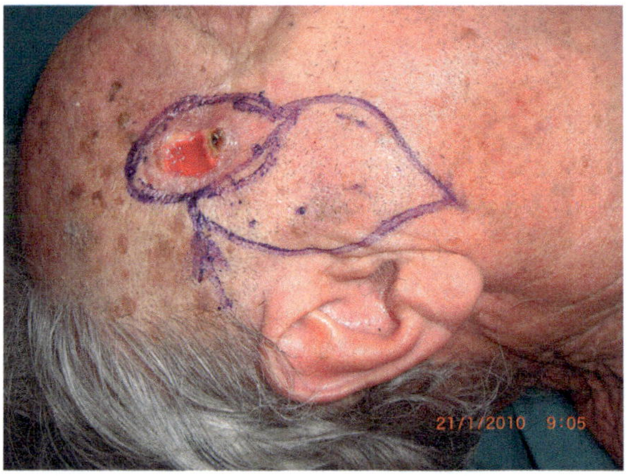

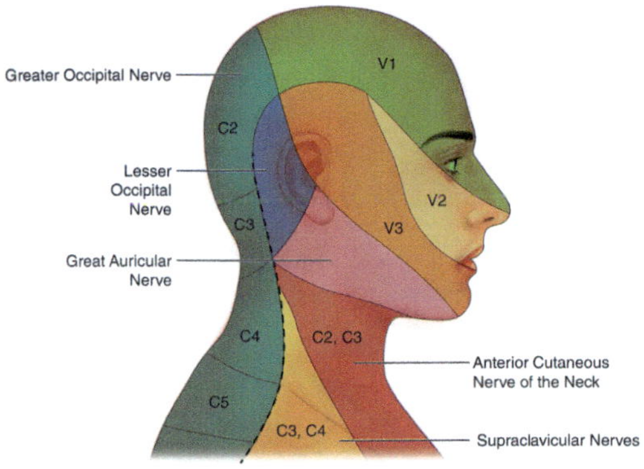

Fig. 2.316 The 6 × 4 cm excisional defect is closed via the curvilinear Bezier flap, by employing the same V-Y principles. The Bezier design is also suitable over the zygomatic arch. The dermatomal mark outs become the line of incision of the dermis and epidermis, ensuring that one-third deeply is attached with only partial undermining to facilitate the closure and vascular integrity of the defect. (Reprinted with permission from Atlas, *Reconstructive Technique in Melanoma Management* (p. 19), by Felix Behan, Springer Nature 2023)

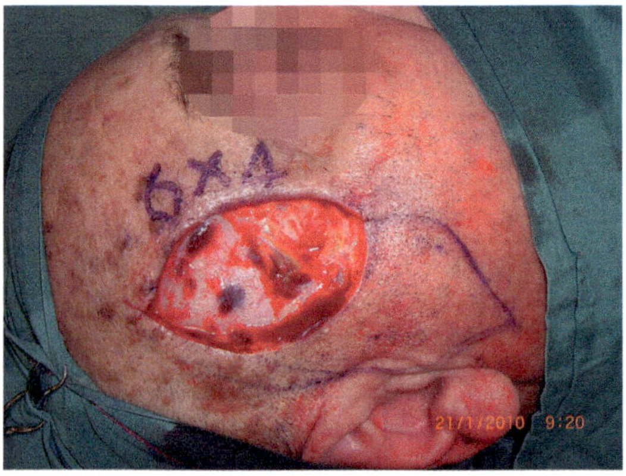

Fig. 2.317 The size of the excisional defect: 6 × 4 cm

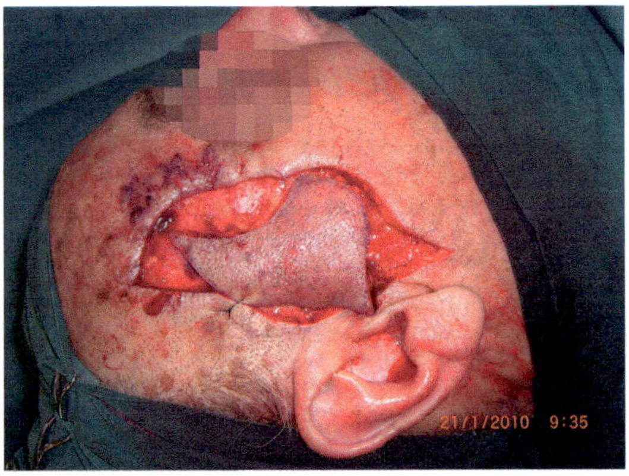

Fig. 2.318 Blunt dissection around the periphery of the flap preserves the integrity of the facial nerve branches without individually defining them, leaving one-third deep attachment

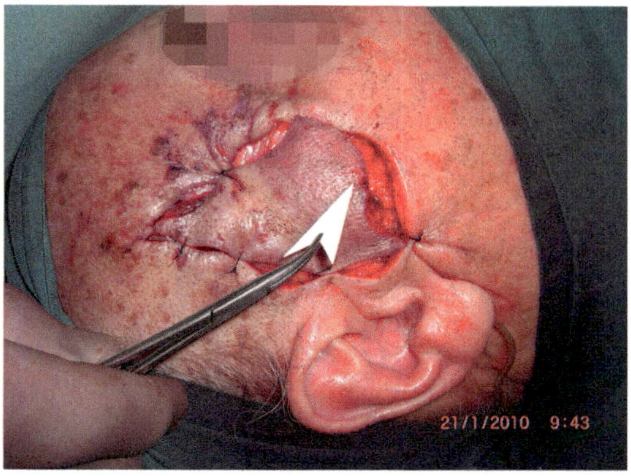

Fig. 2.319 The arrow sits on a red dot sign, indicating it is in the hyperaemic phase, confirming Keystone principles

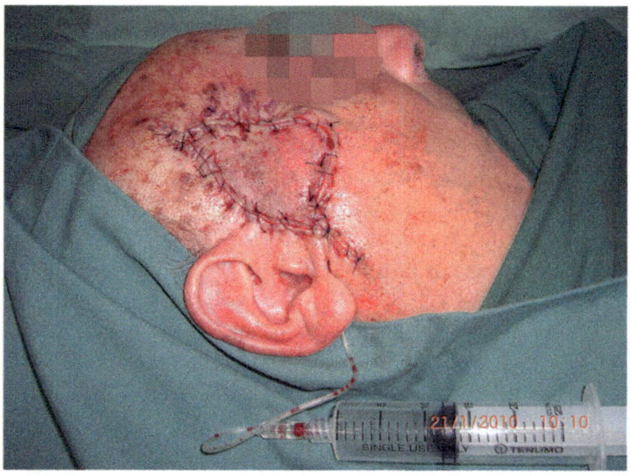

Fig. 2.320 Completed closure is shown. Note the hyperaemia consistent with the Keystone principles, without undue tension at the outer canthus. The drainage technique uses a 20 ml syringe: Fenestrated plastic tubing attached to a 20 ml syringe that is held out to length by the needle protector sheath. The volume of the drainage is measured, then suction is reapplied

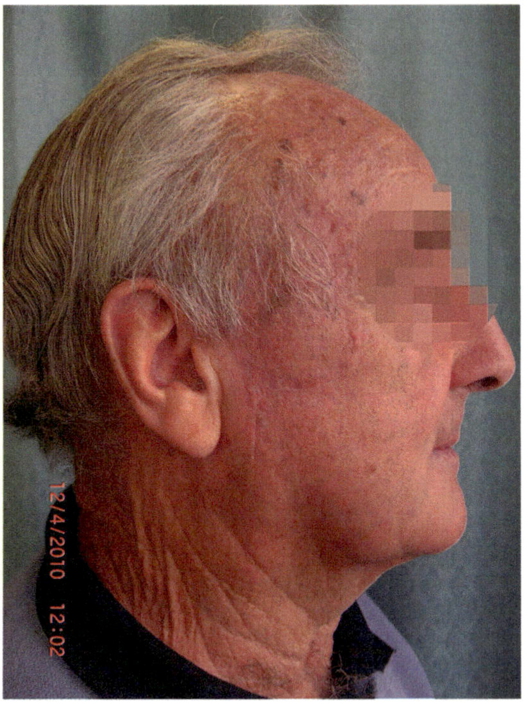

Fig. 2.321 Appearance at 3 months

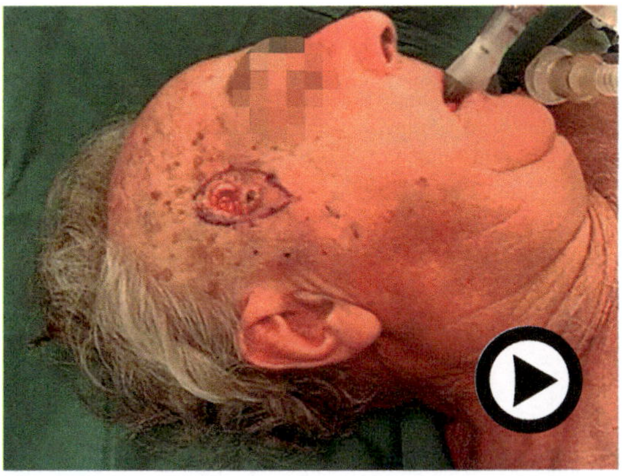

Fig. 2.322 Video 2.41 Operative sequence (▶ https://doi.org/10.1007/000-k76)

The PACES characteristics were all exemplified: pain-free, aesthetic, no vascular complications, economical in terms of time and sensory recovery with the resolution of oedema.

2.1.2.2 Case 32—Level II Melanoma in a Hutchinson Melanotic Freckle of the R Supraorbital Region

In Case 32, the 75-year-old male farmer had an HMF of the R forehead, which was surgically excised, and reconstruction was delayed awaiting pathology (the DRAPE [15] procedure). Further surgical excision confirmed the clearance histologically (Figs. 2.323, 2.324, 2.325, 2.326, 2.327, 2.328, 2.329, 2.330, and 2.331).

In summary, all the PACES characteristics of the Keystone were evident throughout the procedure. It was done as a duet procedure with Professor Andrew Sizeland at the Peter McCallum Cancer Centre.

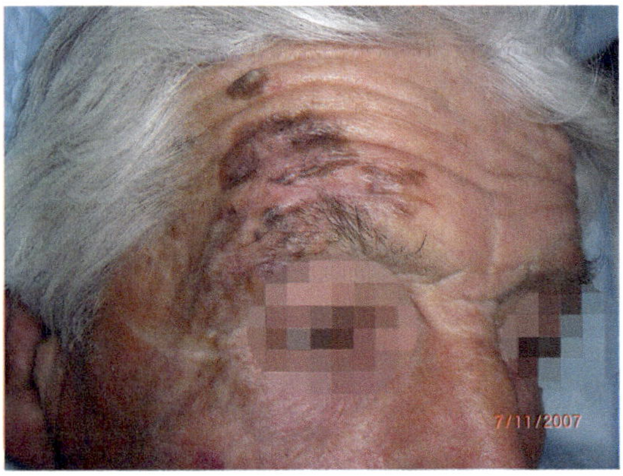

Fig. 2.323 Level II melanoma in an Hutchinson melanotic freckle is shown. The Hutchinson melanotic freckle extended over a 6 × 6 cm distance of the R supraorbital region

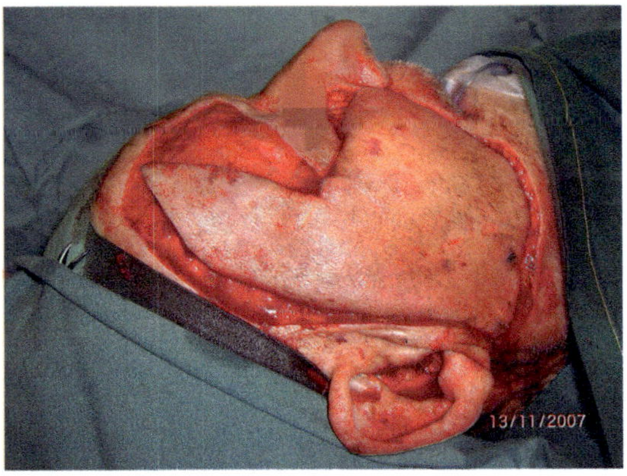

Fig. 2.325 This quadrangular Keystone is advanced towards the midline of the forehead with blunt dissection around the posterior and superior limits of the flap. The inferior limits (neck) and anterior limits (nasolabial) are just closed directly. Islanding a flap creates hyperaemia – an observational finding. It takes 10–15 min to show this vascular change

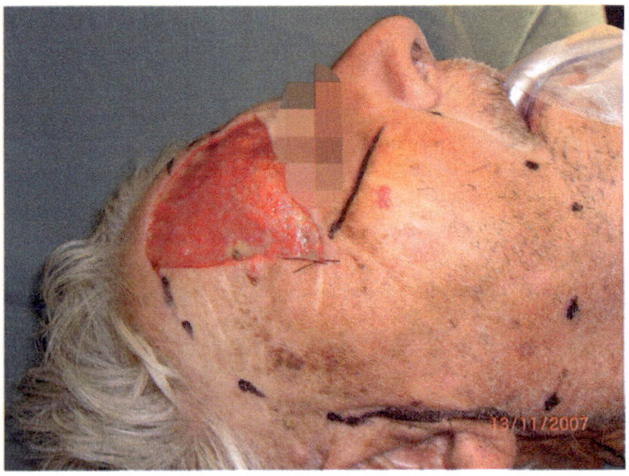

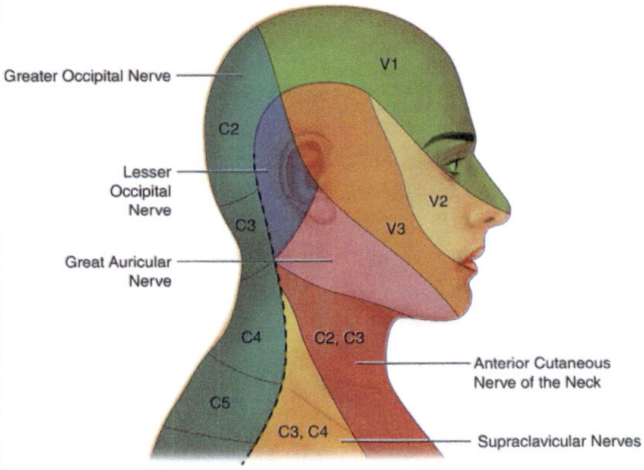

Fig. 2.324 The 6 × 6 cm surgical defect is revealed, including supraorbital nerves, to avoid any perineural dissemination. The Keystone flap mark out is dotted around the R cheek and infraorbital region. The oblique incision along the lower eyelid region is done to avoid ectropion. The skin island incision from the nasolabial region around to the angle of the jaw is not part of the flap advancement or rotation. This nasolabial incision creating the island is closed directly. Creating the hyperaemic phase in the island flap is absolutely necessary to avoid necrosis and lying within the V2 and V3 dermatomes. The dermatomal mark outs become the line of incision of the dermis and epidermis, ensuring that one-third deeply is attached with only partial undermining to facilitate the closure and vascular integrity of the defect. (Reprinted with permission from Atlas, *Reconstructive Technique in Melanoma Management* (p. 19), by Felix Behan, Springer Nature 2023)

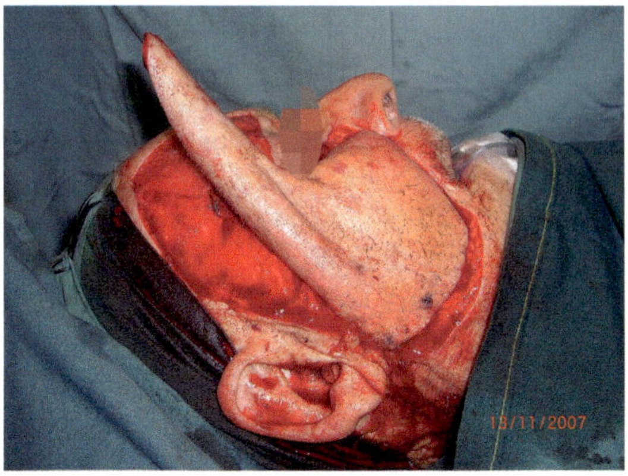

Fig. 2.326 The posterosuperior margins of the flap are undermined, leaving approximately one-third attached in the region of the infraorbital nerve and the neurovascular bundle on the V2 dermatome. As long as at least one-third deep attachment is in the infraorbital and nasolabial regions, the viability of the flap is ensured

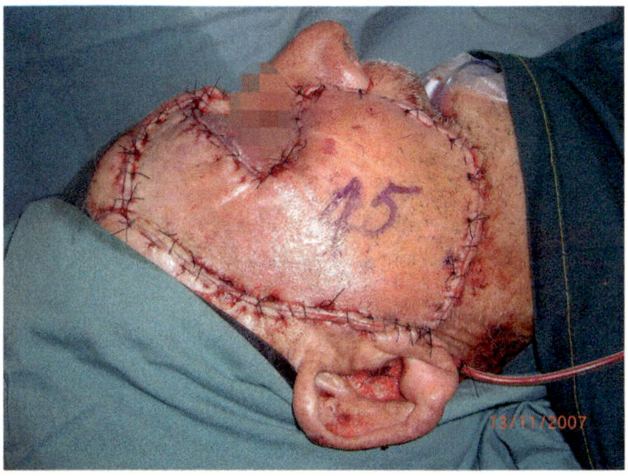

Fig. 2.327 The three-phase closure technique is shown: locking mattress sutures at the points of maximum tension, ordinary mattress sutures for tissue alignment and a continuous nylon suture to get epidermal seal. Suture removal comes out at 1-, 2- and 3-week intervals

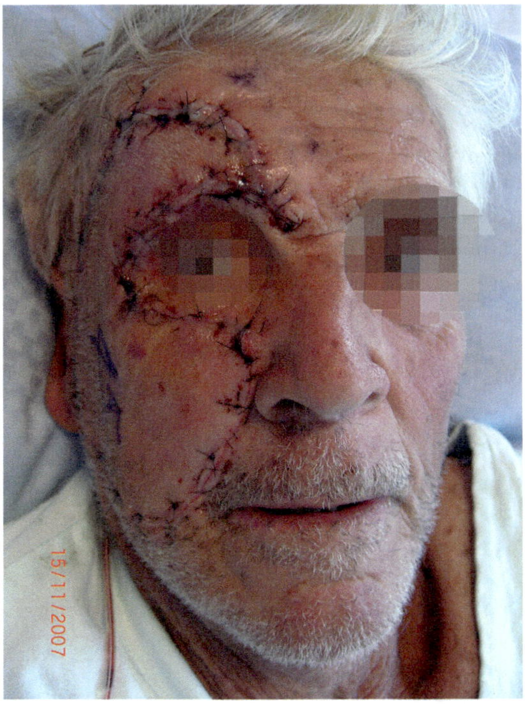

Fig. 2.328 Appearance at 2 days showing no evidence of impending flap necrosis with the Redivac still in situ

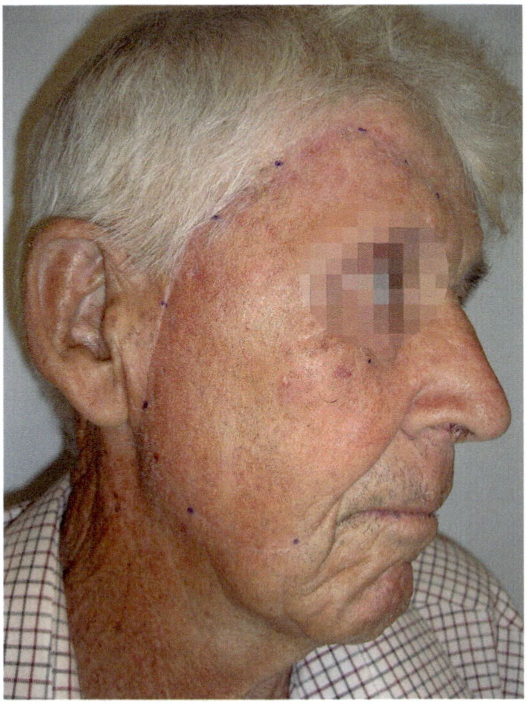

Fig. 2.329 The appearance at 6 months shows the quality of the wound healing. The suture outline has been dotted to show the outcome without necrosis

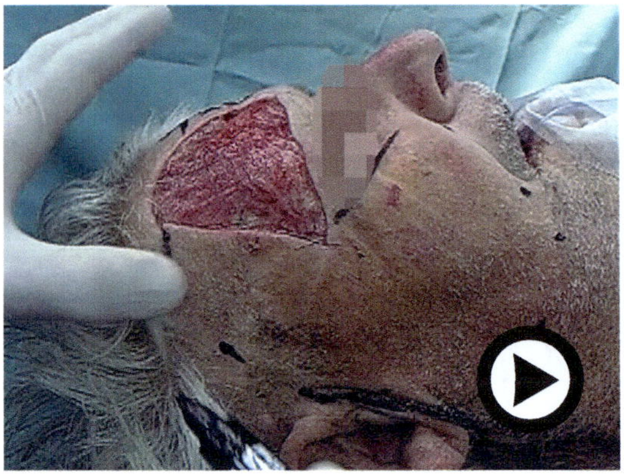

Fig. 2.330 Video 2.42 Planned operative reconstruction (▶ https://doi.org/10.1007/000-k77)

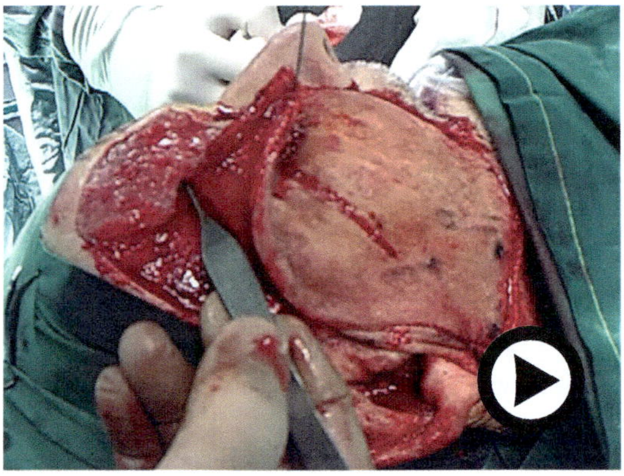

Fig. 2.331 Video 2.43 Operative sequence (▶ https://doi.org/10.1007/000-k78)

2.1.2.3 Case 33—Forehead Reconstruction Using the Keystone

Multifocal mitotic skin lesions are shown on the L forehead. The supraorbital Keystone design, preserving the integrity of the supraorbital vascular complex, is achieved via blunt dissection using the scissor technique, stretching the tissue, visualising the nerve and closing in the routine Keystone manner (Figs. 2.332, 2.333, 2.334, 2.335 and 2.336).

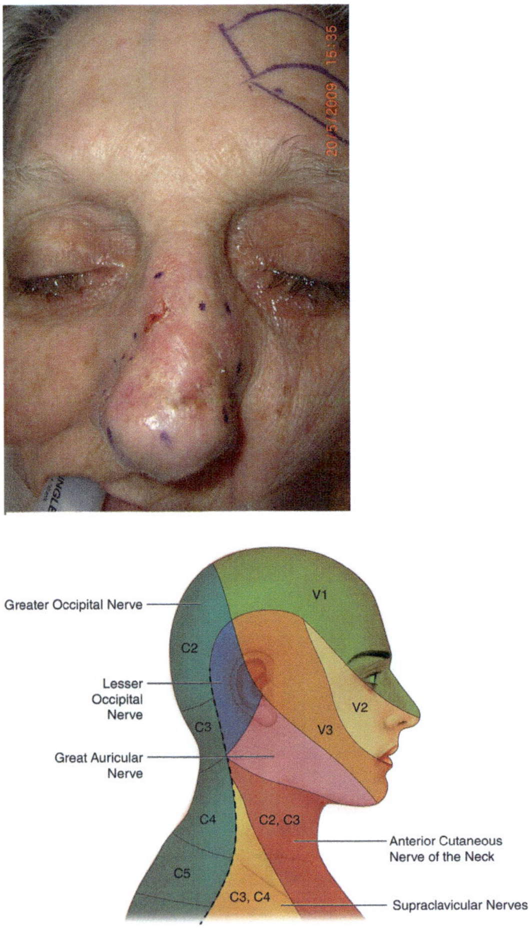

Fig. 2.332 Keystone repair of the forehead defect is shown. The excision of the L supraorbital region is followed by a superior supraorbital Keystone, and the blunt dissection is part of the technique, as illustrated in Fig. 2.333. The dermatomal mark outs become the line of incision of the dermis and epidermis, ensuring that one-third deeply is attached with only partial undermining to facilitate the closure and vascular integrity of the defect. (Reprinted with permission from Atlas, *Reconstructive Technique in Melanoma Management* (p. 19), by Felix Behan, Springer Nature 2023)

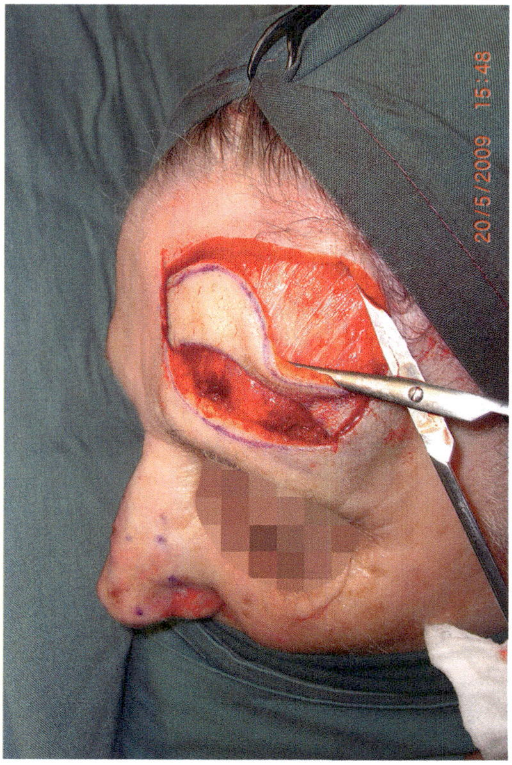

Fig. 2.333 The tissue displacement with surgical scissors preserves the integrity of the supraorbital nerve with blunt dissection. It is another application of intrinsic expansion [16], where the flap is made to fit the defect through stretching

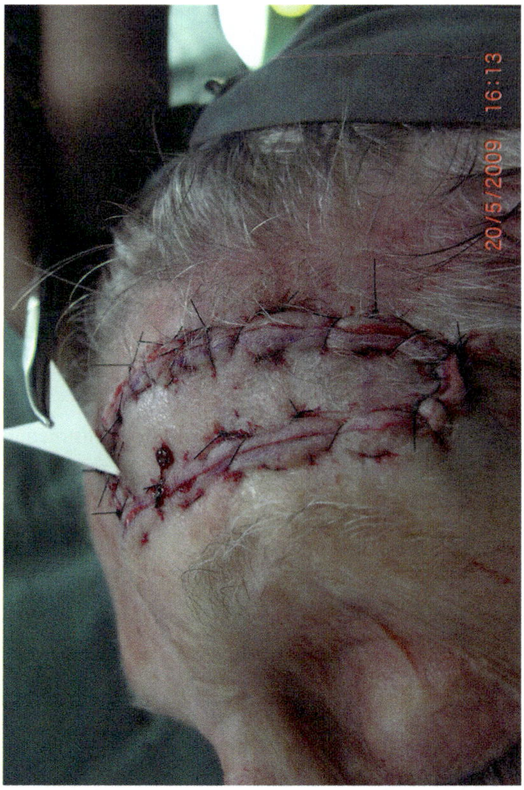

Fig. 2.334 The completion of the Keystone reconstruction is shown. Note the red dot sign on the arrow confirming its vascular integrity

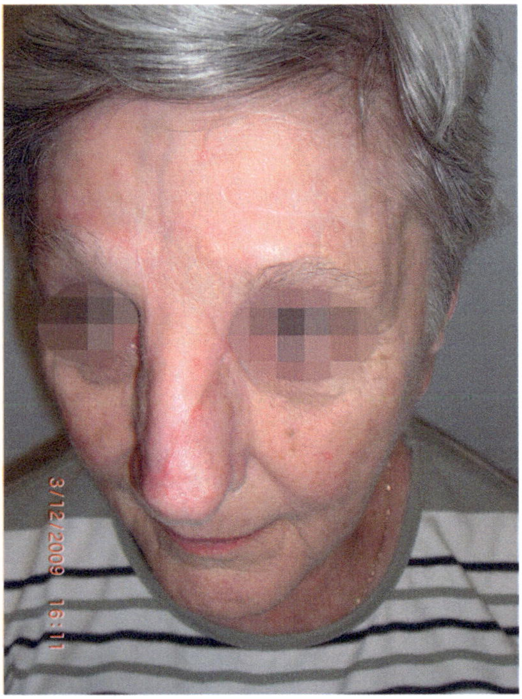

Fig. 2.335 Postoperative appearance at 6 months, where the aesthetic appearance fully acceptable to the patient while maintaining full neural sensation from the supraorbital complex

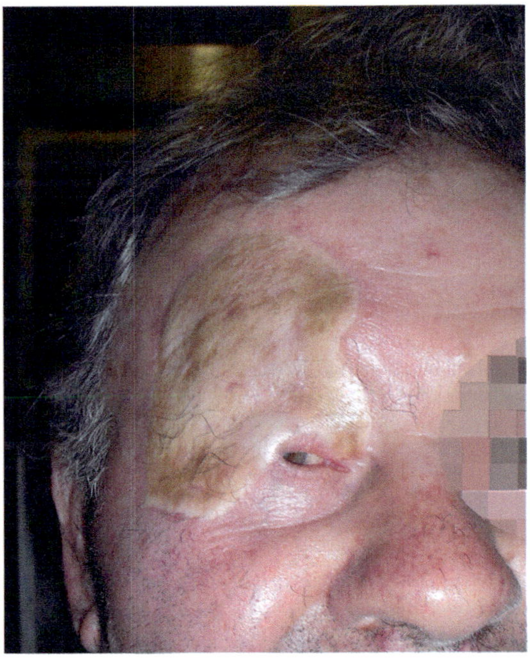

Fig. 2.336 Microsurgical reconstruction done by another unit is illustrated here for a comparison of the repair of a similar defect. Dare I say that this is a bad aesthetic outcome when the Keystone solution with the techniques above has produced an acceptable alternative reflecting its characteristics

2.1.2.4 Case 34—Keystone of the Glabella Based on Supraorbital Neurovascular Supply (Figs. 2.337, 2.338, 2.339, 2.340, 2.341, 2.342, 2.343, 2.344 and 2.345)

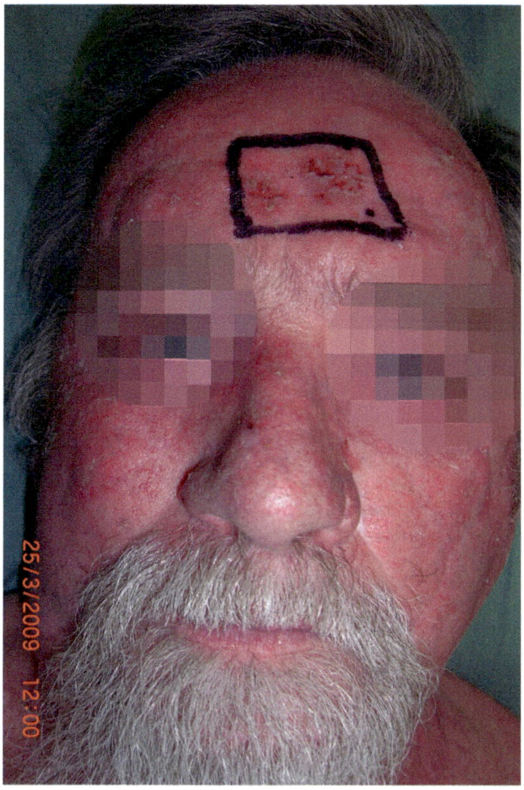

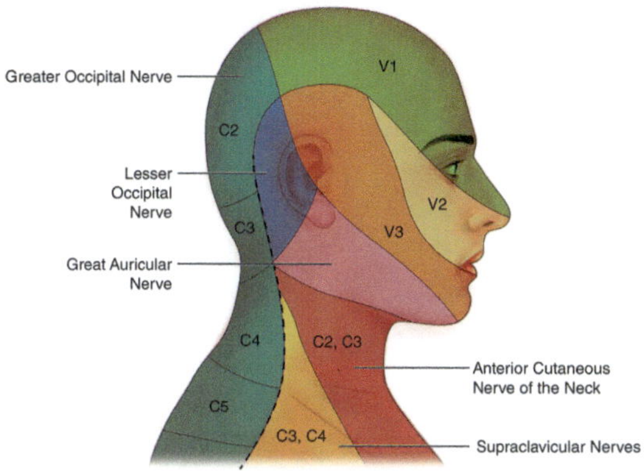

Fig. 2.337 Patient on presentation is showing the multifocal lesion. The dermatomal mark outs become the line of incision of the dermis and epidermis, ensuring that one-third deeply is attached with only partial undermining to facilitate the closure and vascular integrity of the defect. (Reprinted with permission from Atlas, *Reconstructive Technique in Melanoma Management* (p. 19), by Felix Behan, Springer Nature 2023)

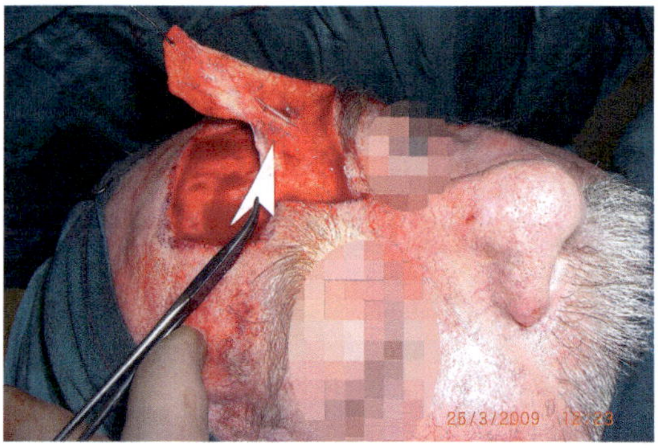

Fig. 2.338 The arrow indicates the neurovascular support, which is just teased from the surrounding tissues to be inserted into the surgical defect

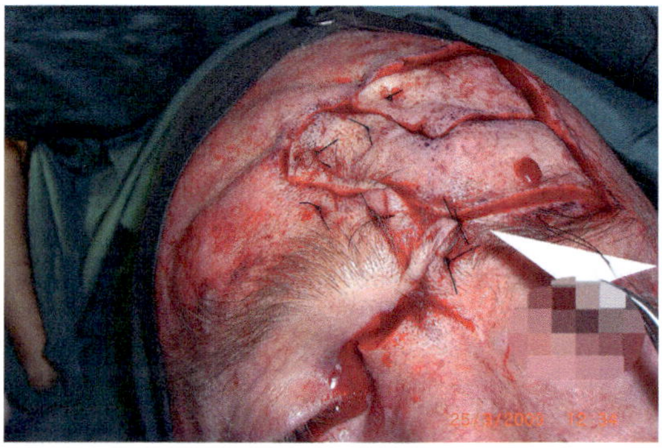

Fig. 2.339 Staged insertion is shown, and the red dot signs confirm its vascular integrity

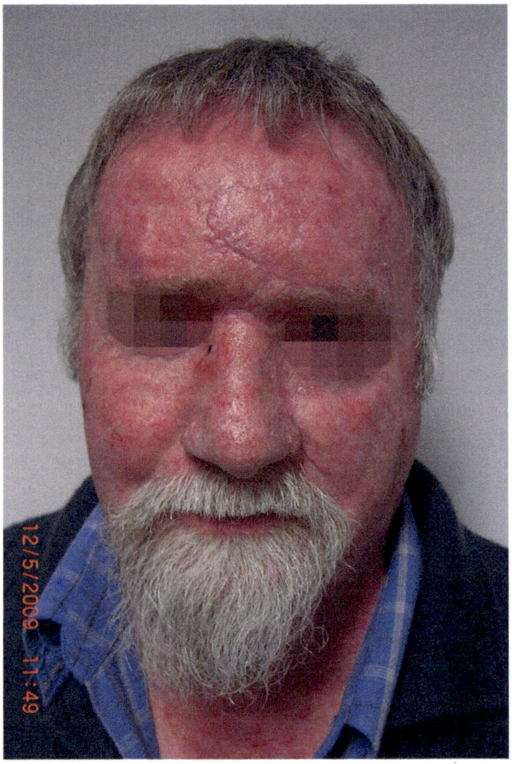

Fig. 2.340 Appearance at 2 months after the staged removal of sutures

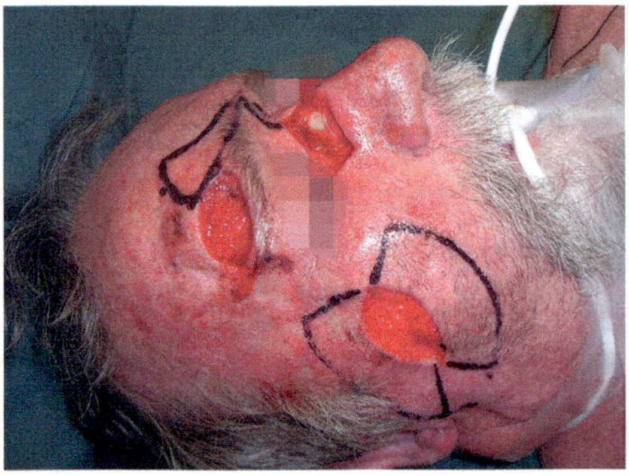

Fig. 2.341 Further Keystones to the supraorbital region and the R malar eminence

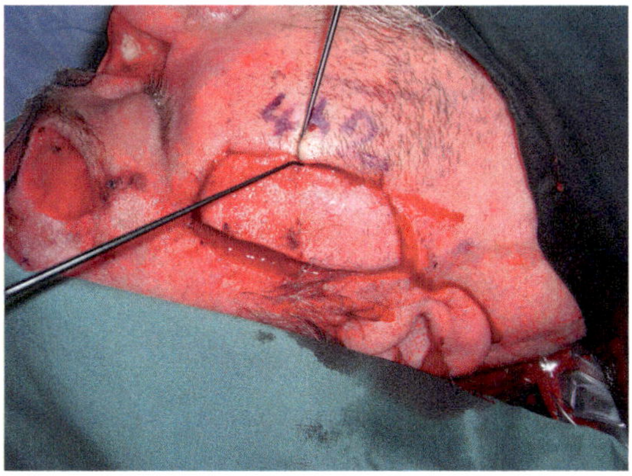

Fig. 2.342 Closure of the wounds under tension is shown. Note the hyperaemic flare

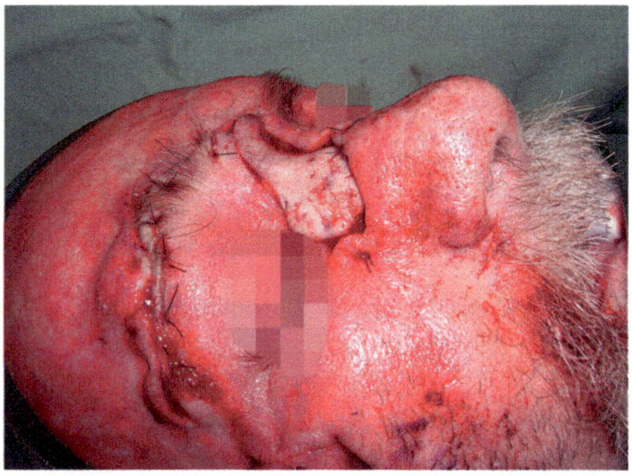

Fig. 2.343 On completion

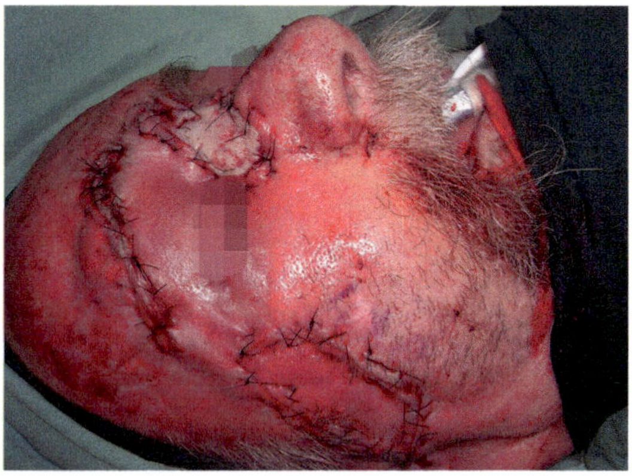

Fig. 2.344 On completion with a complementary graft to the R inner canthus to avoid tension

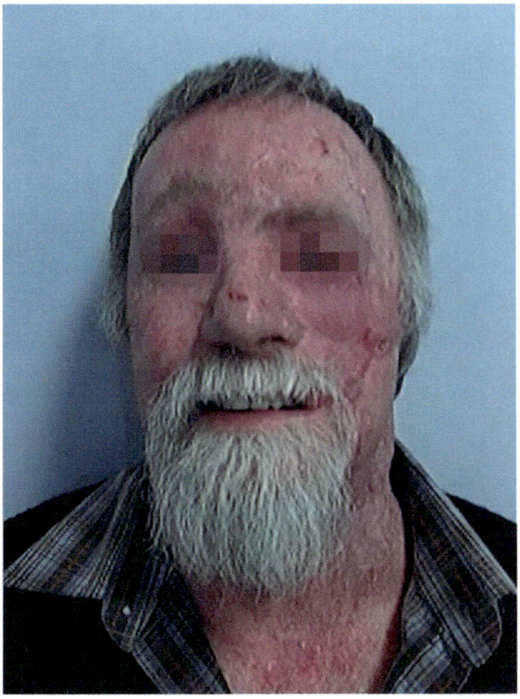

Fig. 2.345 Video 2.44 The patient's satisfaction with the outcome, exemplifying all the Keystone characteristics (PACES). People are commenting on how well the patient looked (▶ https://doi.org/10.1007/000-k79)

The PACES characteristics were all exemplified: pain-free, aesthetic, no vascular complications, economical in terms of time and sensory recovery with the resolution of oedema.

2.1.3 Lip

The topical landmarks of a normal lip involve the external or dry vermilion, the wet mucosal approaching the oral lining and the total commissure with the philtral columns and are governed by the orbicularis oris muscle. The inputs of the superior and inferior labial arteries are noted, and the trigeminal nerve and neural nerve input V2 for the upper (infraorbital innervation) and V3 for the lower (mental innervation).

Traditionally, direct closure is possible with a loss of 30% of the lip, but most prefer 25% with a layered approximation of the various components: muscle, mucosa internally, vermilion superiorly and cutaneous externally.

The triangulate defect—A-shaped—creates a T image on direct closure. Bilateral advancements of the upper or lower create triangular remnants, and the trimming of Burow's triangle is essential in the lateral extremes, simplistically (removing dog ears).

In the case of a total vermilionectomy, closing the mucosal defect is wrong in principle in that this brings hair-bearing tissue into the vermilion alignment in an internal direction. In this case, creating a Keystone design of the mucosa of the internal lining of the lower lip, which allows external wet vermilion alignment to sit as it formerly did along the dry margin, is wiser, and the secondary defect in the buccal sulcus is allowed to mucosalise as a secondary procedure, taking up to 10 days. Grafting is avoided because of the dissimilarity between mucosal structures and the external integument, and the clinical inconvenience of intraoral skin grafts needs no elaboration.

Multiple flaps are used to fix full-thickness lip loss, up to 50% (the Webster flap, the Gillies fan flap and the Karapandzic flap, which retains the neurovascular axis), and local tissues are generally inadequate for repairing lower lip defects exceeding 75% of lip length [17]. The Abbe flap is a manoeuvre for sharing part of one lip above to the defect below, based on neurovascular structures. This link is later divided at 2–3 weeks between the upper and lower lips, reconstituting lip continuity (S Lander a similar concept to the Abbe in that it takes tissue from the lateral aspect of the upper lip into a mirror image site of the lower lip). When tissues beyond these limits are needed, microvascular free flaps may be required.

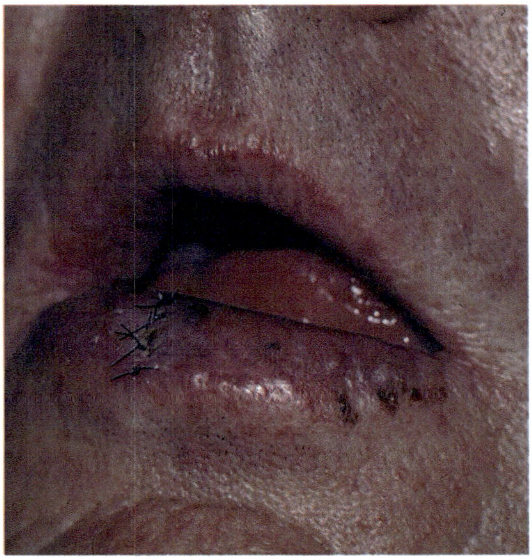

Fig. 2.346 The pathological confirmation of the HMF is noted with the suture line

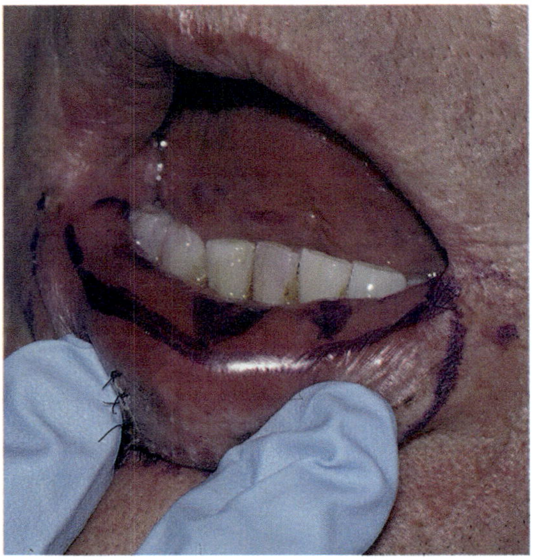

Fig. 2.347 The surgical excision of the total vermilionectomy from angle to angle of the lower lip is shown. Direct closure brings the hair-bearing tissue of the lower lip almost into an intraoral location, which has an adverse effect on shaving comfort

2.1.3.1 Case 35—Hutchinson Melanoma of the Lower Lip

An HMF of the lower lip in a farmer features a path diagnosis, confirming the clinical appearance (Figs. 2.346, 2.347, 2.348, 2.349, 2.350 and 2.351).

In summary, the PACES charactristics of the Keystone were all exemplified in this island flap repair. The mucosalisation of the secondary defect precludes the problems of tight closure and of bringing in hair-bearing tissue of the integument to achieve lip seal. The new vermilion has a normal alignment with the hair-bearing tissue of the lower lip.

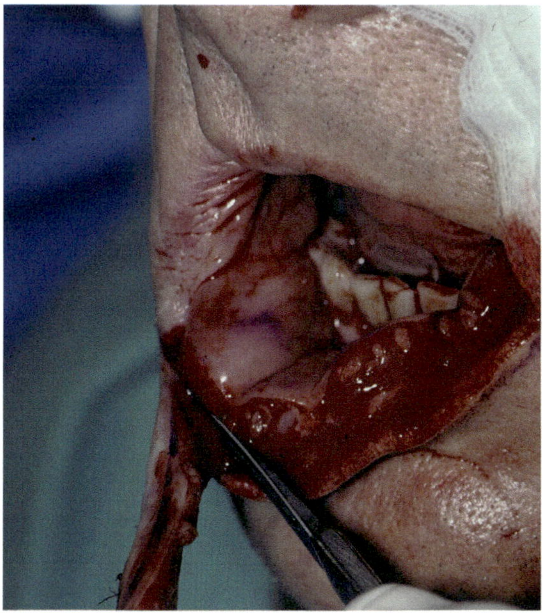

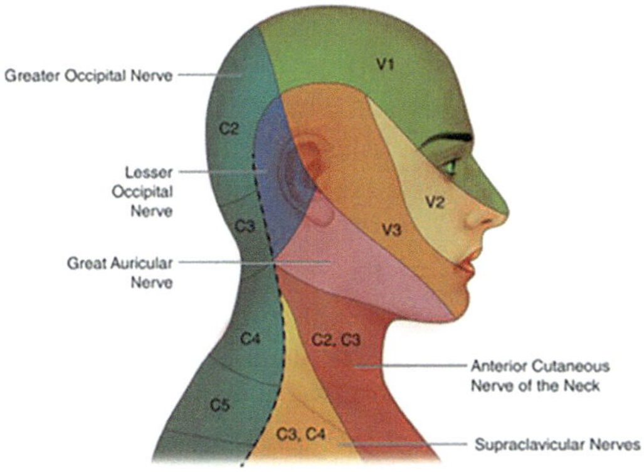

Fig. 2.348 The in-transit procedure for the removal of the lower lip vermilion margin is shown. The dermatomal mark outs become the line of incision of the dermis and epidermis, ensuring that one-third deeply is attached with only partial undermining to facilitate the closure and vascular integrity of the defect. (Reprinted with permission from Atlas, *Reconstructive Technique in Melanoma Management* (p. 19), by Felix Behan, Springer Nature 2023)

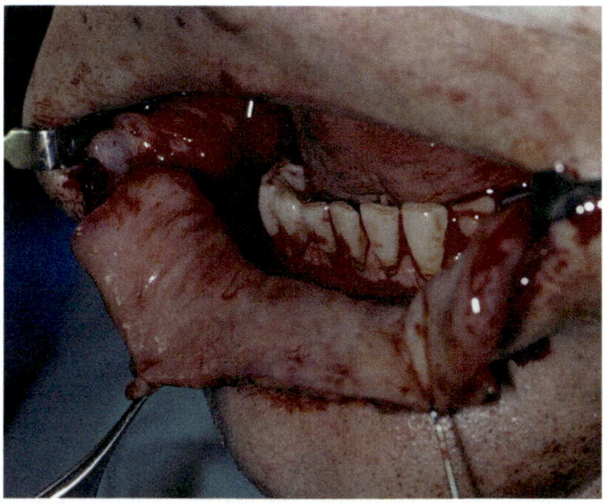

Fig. 2.349 The advancement as a Keystone of the internal lining of the lower lip creates the new vermilion. The secondary defect in the internal lining of the lower lip just above the buccal alveolar sulcus is left to mucosalise through secondary intention to avoid complications from having hair-bearing tissue being dragged into the intraoral arrangement

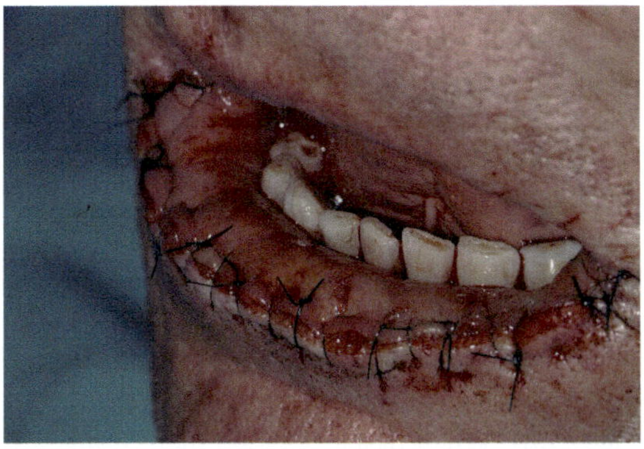

Fig. 2.350 The completed wound, with the secondary defect left unsutured in the buccal alveolar succus

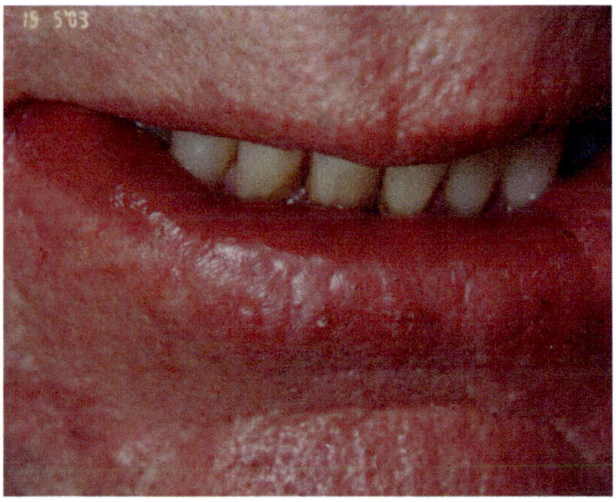

Fig. 2.351 The final appearance – lip seal achieved and the patient totally satisfied

2.1.3.2 Case 36—Mitotic Lesion Removing Two-Thirds of the Lower Lip with Neck Gland Clearances

Intrinsic expansion is exemplified in this technique, achieving tissue cover (Figs. 2.352, 2.353, 2.354, 2.355, 2.356, 2.357, 2.358, 2.359, 2.360, 2.361, 2.362, 2.363 and 2.364).

The video of the patient talking in the supplement, with full articulation and movement and functional mastication, shows a satisfactory outcome.

In summary, functional normality has been achieved in lip seal and articulation, reverting to the embryological mark outs of the V3 dermatome, and any microstoma is overcome by bringing a fresh island of mucosa from the lax tissue of the oral cavity. The PACES characteristics of the Keystone were all exemplified in this island flap repair.

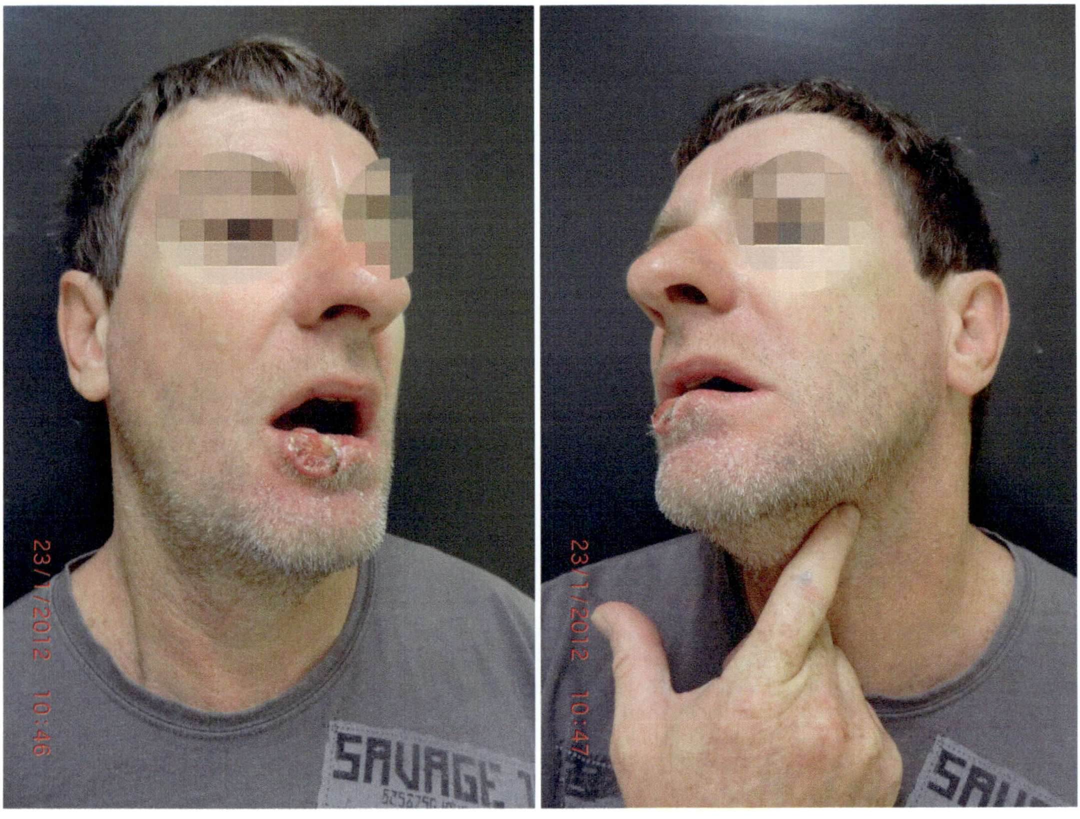

Fig. 2.352 A 2.5 cm lesion in the lateral side of the lower lip is shown. The patient gestures to the L submandibular nodal dissemination

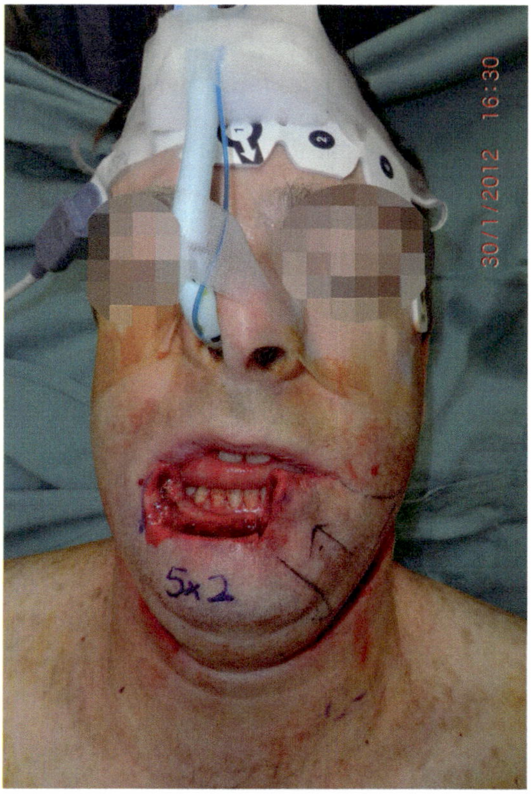

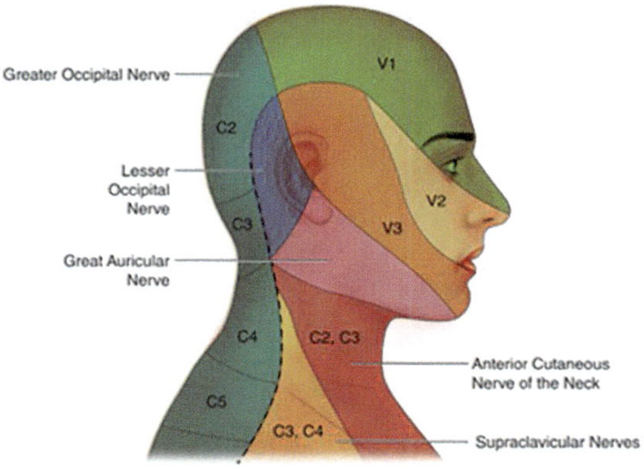

Fig. 2.353 The 5 × 2 cm full-thickness loss and on the L the vermilion on the L side, based on the Keystone design, along the L mental eminence has advanced to the right angle of the mouth. The dermatomal mark outs become the line of incision of the dermis and epidermis, ensuring that one-third deeply is attached with only partial undermining to facilitate the closure and vascular integrity of the defect. (Reprinted with permission from Atlas, *Reconstructive Technique in Melanoma Management* (p. 19), by Felix Behan, Springer Nature 2023)

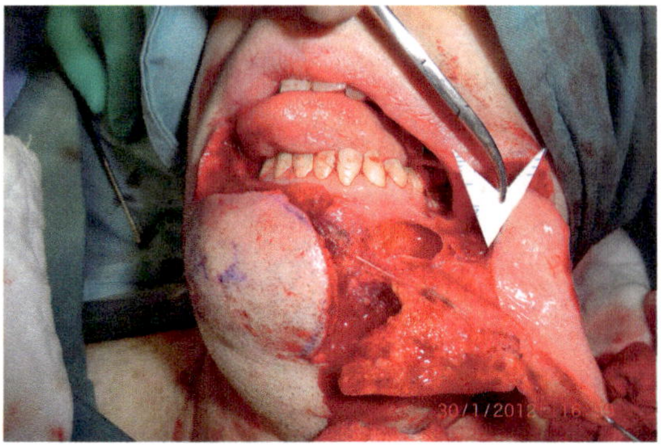

Fig. 2.354 The neurovascular structures emerging from the mental eminence in this mucosal lined lower lip reconstructive flap are based on a quadrangular Keystone design

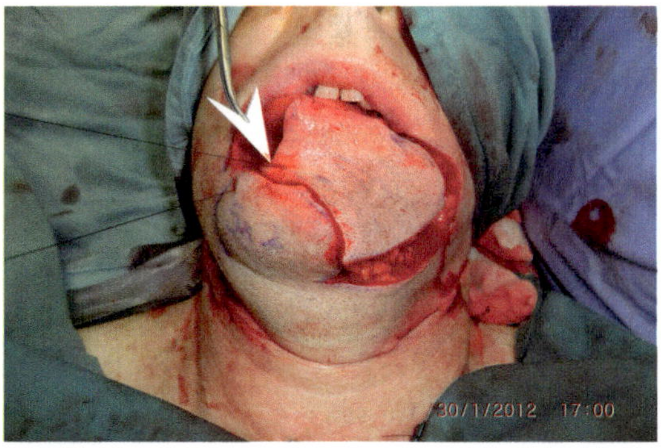

Fig. 2.355 Vermilion alignment at the right angle of the mouth as a layered closure, with mucosal, muscle and external epidermal alignment

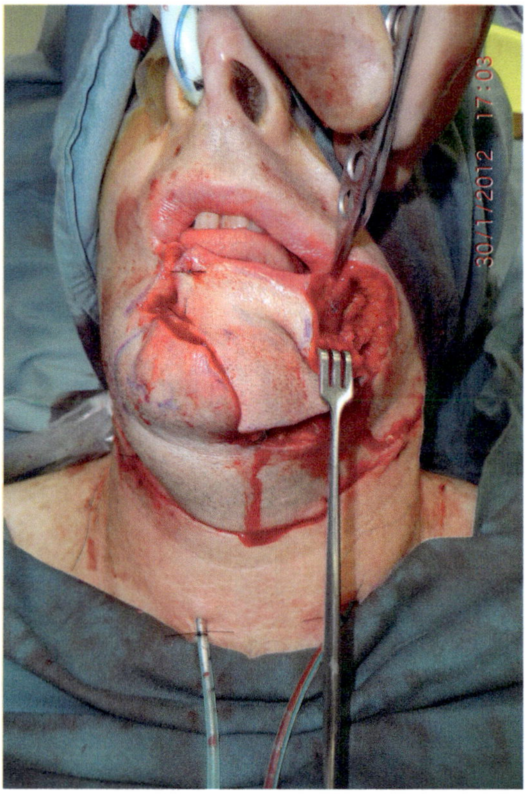

Fig. 2.356 Direct closure would have caused a microstoma, and the vermilion replacement of approximately 2 cm is achieved by bringing an intraoral mucosal island flap, adjacent to the parotid duct, to fill this space and avoid a microstoma, which would have occurred if direct closure had been employed

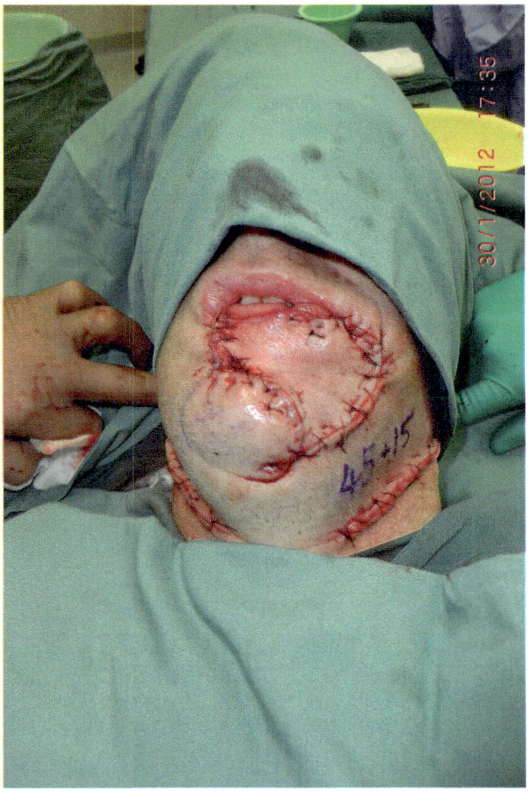

Fig. 2.357 Total timeframe for repair was 60 min, as indicated on the submandibular

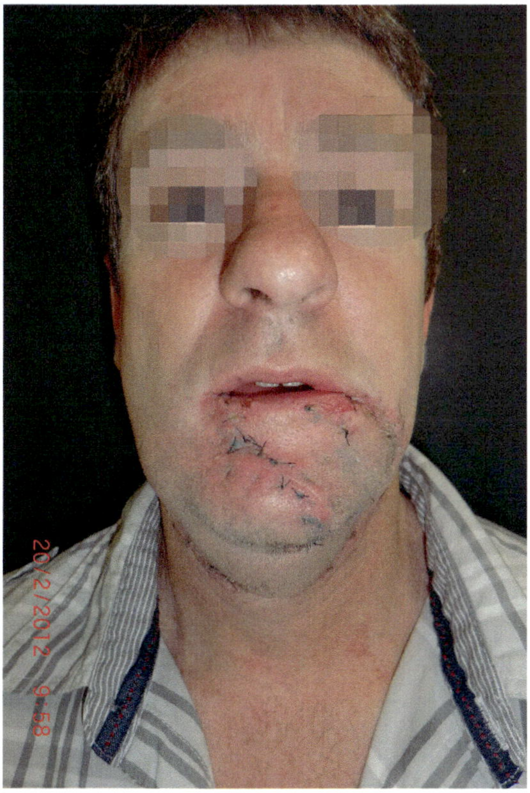

Fig. 2.358 The appearance at 2 weeks with two-thirds of the sutures removed is shown. Note the normal vermilion appearance and no microstoma

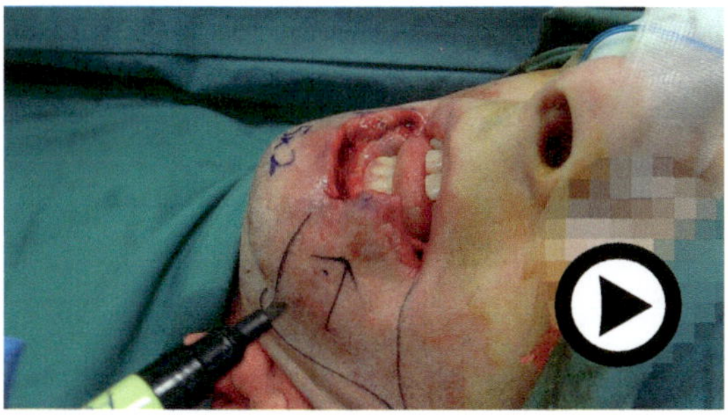

Fig. 2.359 Video 2.45 Operative sequence (▶https://doi.org/10.1007/000-k7a)

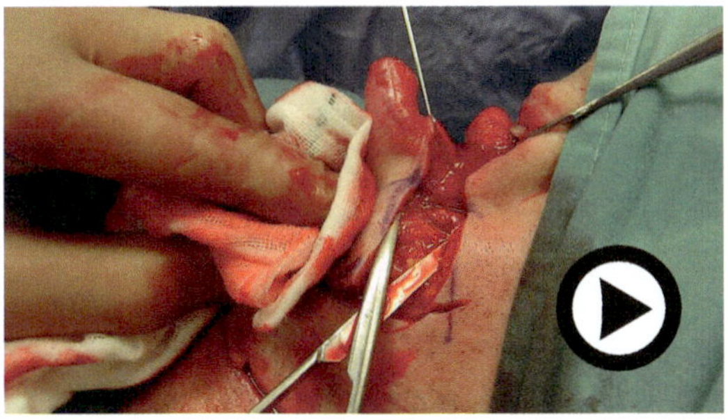

Fig. 2.360 Video 2.46 Operative sequence (▶ https://doi.org/10.1007/000-k7b)

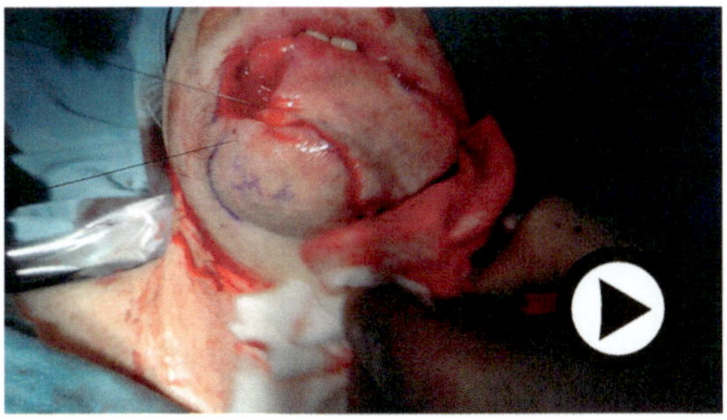

Fig. 2.361 Video 2.47 Operative sequence (▶ https://doi.org/10.1007/000-k7c)

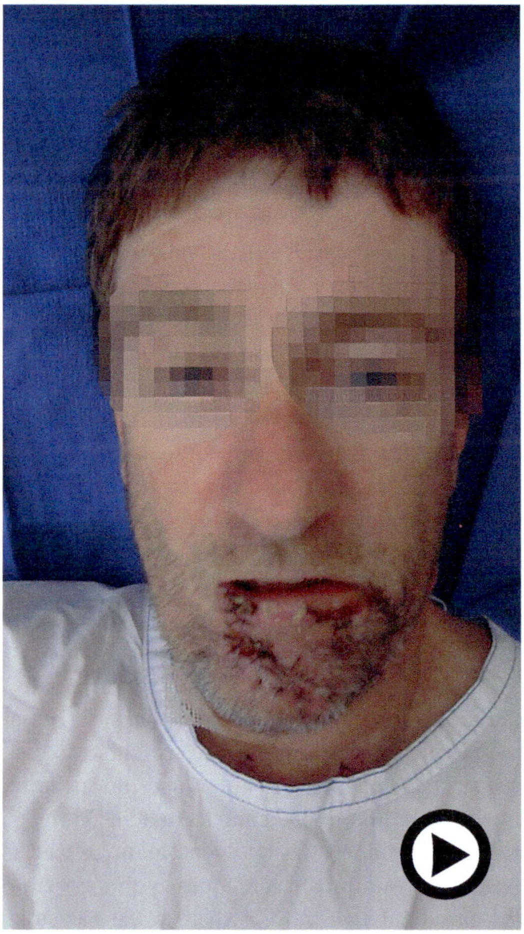

Fig. 2.362 Video 2.48 7-day postoperative patient perspective (▶ https://doi.org/10.1007/000-k7d)

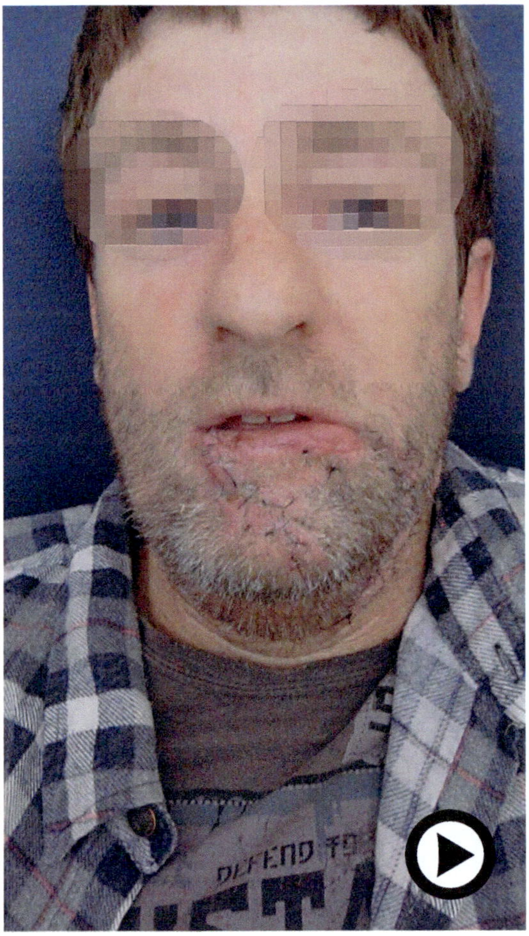

Fig. 2.363 Video 2.49 Postoperative patient perspective (▶ https://doi.org/10.1007/000-k7e)

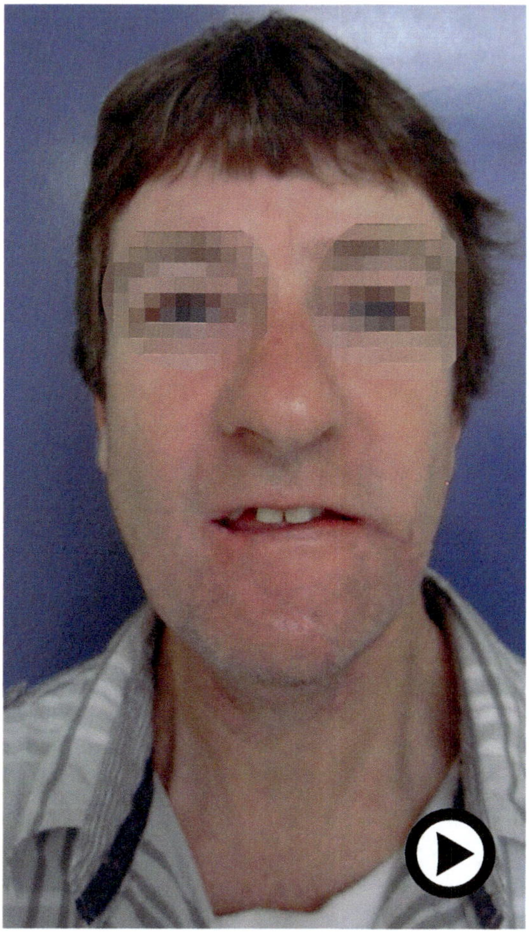

Fig. 2.364 Video 2.50 Postoperative patient perspective (▶ https://doi.org/10.1007/000-k7f)

2.1.4 Nose

This Keystone technique in nasal reconstruction for mitotic lesions has many applications. Incidentally, the multifocal skin lesions of the nasal bridge were excised, and once pathology clearance was achieved [18], a forehead island flap was used for closure. The standard vertical forehead flap is restricted by timeframes; when rotated to 180°, it often leaves a secondary defect at the hairline that needs grafting. This supraorbital forehead Keystone principle overcomes these deficiencies, in spite of closing under tension, a characteristic of the Keystone. Importantly, this patient wanted a secondary procedure done for another lesion during the healing phase of the L forehead lesion, again showing the reliability of the Keystone vascularity on the basis of anatomical norms using the dermatomal mark outs. In this case, the supratrochlear and supraorbital neurovascular structures produced an acceptable aesthetic outcome.

The principles of nasal reconstruction, referring to Burget and Menick's work [19], have a long tradition. In these cases, usually only skin cover is required, and the Keystone provides a vascular foundation in the nasal reconstruction of the cutaneous envelope. Free tissue transfer has no applications in this Keystone concept and has universal application in covering all elements of this nasal envelope. The Keystone provides excellent colour match, thickness and texture in the reconstruction.

The principal melanoma excision and closure by elements of secondary intention are not practiced by plastic surgeons, in spite of a 1 cm defect with restricted aesthetic drawbacks. Never forget that the grafting option is always a possibility.

The Keystone principle seems to universalise the collection of locoregional flaps in nasal reconstruction—too many are available to list, such as advancement, rotation and transposition types, including bilobed and the hatchet variants. Even Rohrich et al.'s 1999 nasal tip repair is based on traditional techniques with skin from the proximal two-thirds, whereas the Keystone design seems to incorporate this restriction.

The staged midline forehead flap variety [18, 19] has its drawbacks and may be necessary to achieve closure when one considers time, tightness and vascular impedance. Any defects in the hairline sometimes warrant surgical scar revision.

2.1.4.1 Case 37—Side of the Nose Recurrent Basal Cell Carcinoma (BCC)

The nasolabial line of reconstruction is based on random branches of the facial artery (Figs. 2.365, 2.366, 2.367, 2.368, 2.369, 2.370 and 2.371).

In summary, an aesthetically acceptable outcome comes from using the V-Y Dieffenbach flap based on random neurovascular perforators from the nasal branch of the facial artery. The tissues are teased with blunt dissection to facilitate the advancement of the flap into the defect.

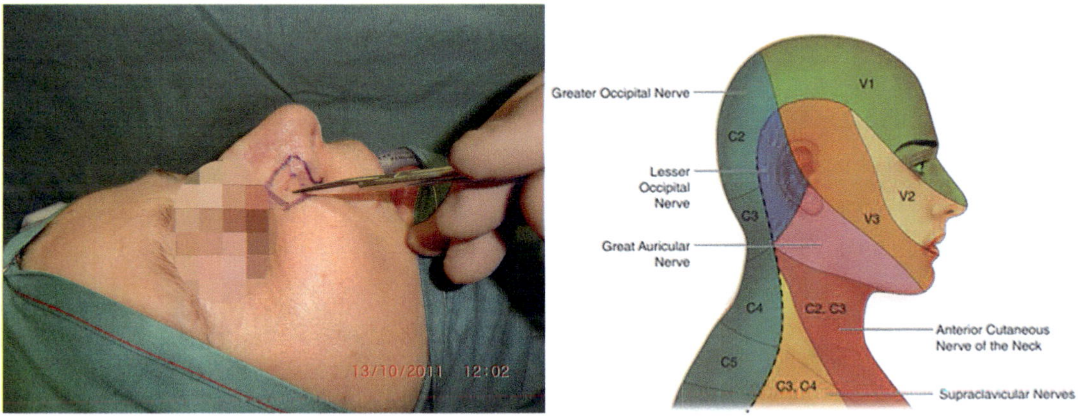

Fig. 2.365 Recurrent mitotic recurrence of the R side of the nose 6 months following initial surgery is shown. The dermatomal mark outs become the line of incision of the dermis and epidermis, ensuring that one-third deeply is attached with only partial undermining to facilitate the closure and vascular integrity of the defect. (Reprinted with permission from Atlas, *Reconstructive Technique in Melanoma Management* (p. 19), by Felix Behan, Springer Nature 2023)

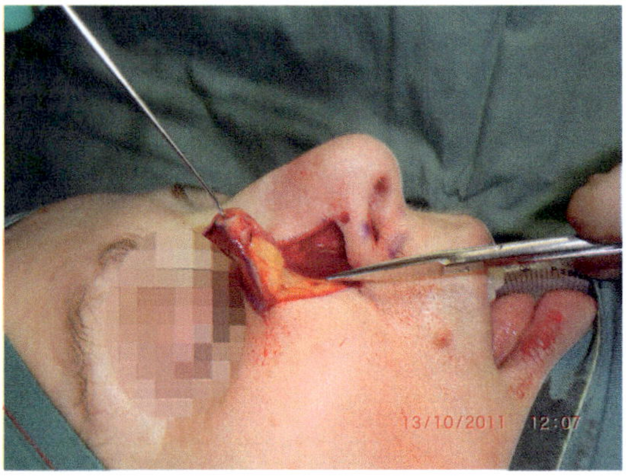

Fig. 2.366 The removal of the tumour is shown. The underlying neurovascular axis (with the nasal branch of the facial artery) is evident but not skeletonised or stripped. The DRAPE procedure was applied again following pathology clearance, and the repair was completed

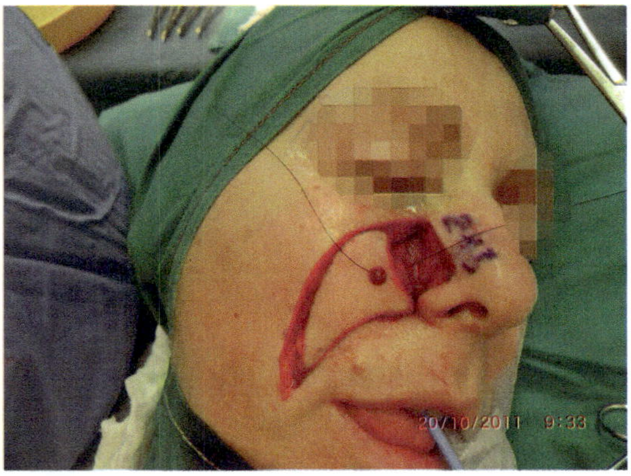

Fig. 2.367 The red dot sign at the suture point indicates the reflex hyperaemia evident in this V-Y island flap, as is also evident in the Keystone concept. The flap is supported by random perforators from the nasal branch of the facial artery, which explains the hyperaemia. None of vessels has been skeletonised because this unnecessary manoeuvre may strip autonomic fibres along the vessel. The blunt dissection using the scissor technique allows one to stretch the island flap on its axis to cover the defect, thus retaining any autonomic support

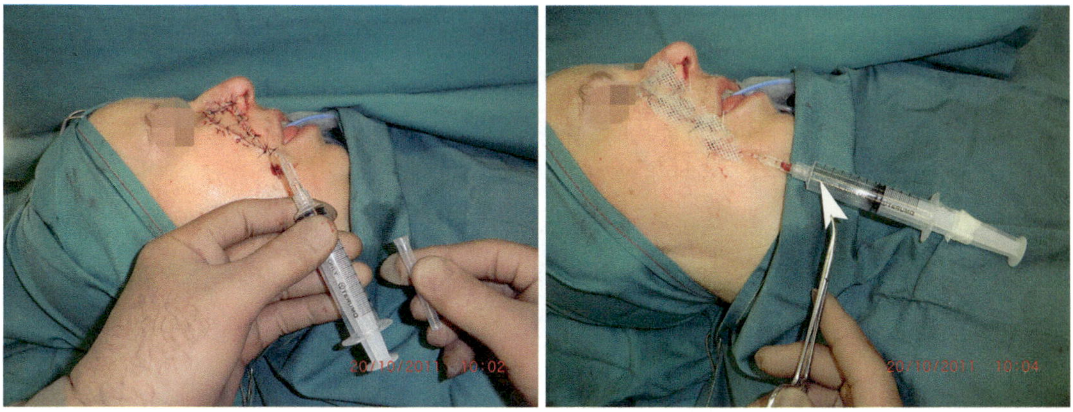

Fig. 2.368 Drainage technique using a 10 ml syringe with perforated plastic tubing attached is shown. It is held out to suction length and secured by using the plastic sleeve of the hypodermic needle. Suction is reinstated after release. The volume contained in the syringe is a measure of blood loss in millilitres. Reinstating the suction and reattaching the tubing allow ongoing drainage to be monitored until it is healed

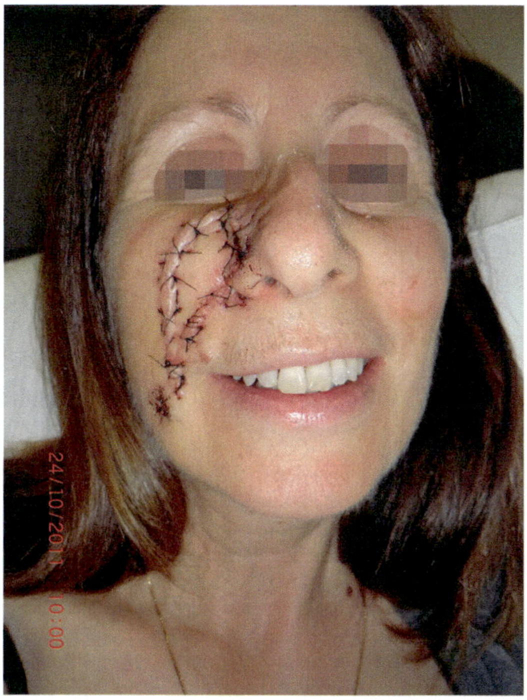

Fig. 2.369 The appearance at 24 h is shown. The wound is closed with the standard three-phase single-layer suture technique, and the nylon suture on the epidermis creates eversion to produce an excellent scar line, as in the Keystone. The PACES factors also apply (because this is comparable to a hemi-Keystone in design)

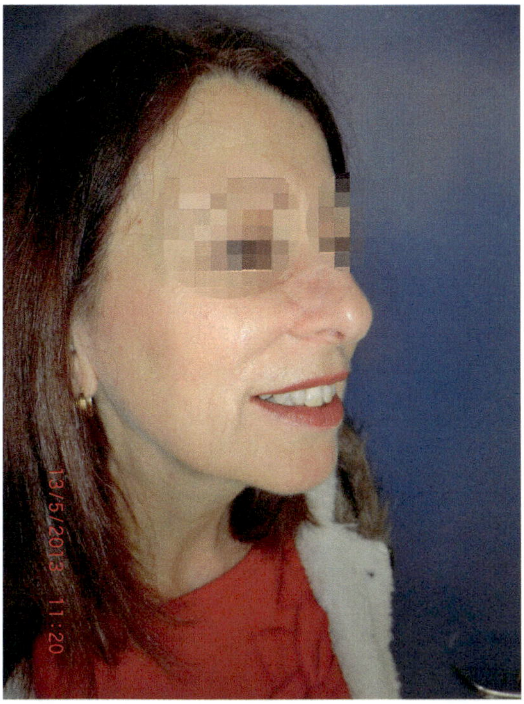

Fig. 2.370 The postoperative appearance at 2 years is shown, and the PACES characteristics have all been exemplified. This anxious patient appreciated the outcome of the modified Keystone, which is really a conjoined/double V-Y flap

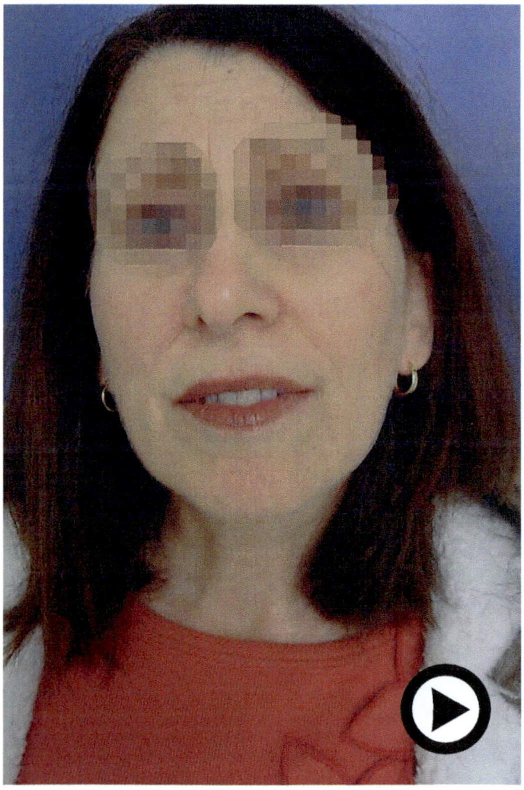

Fig. 2.371 Video 2.51 The patient's satisfaction with the V-Y flap. The Keystone design is really a design of two conjoined V-Ys, producing equal satisfaction in aesthetic outcome (▶ https://doi.org/10.1007/000-k7g)

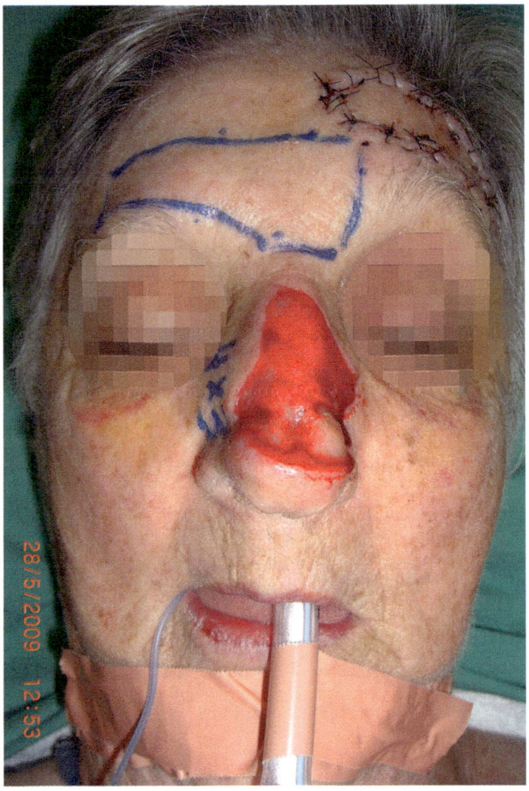

Fig. 2.372 The multifocal lesions of the nasal bridge are shown. The defect is 4 × 3 cm and awaiting pathology clearance (DRAPE). The forehead island flap mark out is based on the R supratrochlear and supraorbital neurovascular dermatome

The PACES characteristics were all exemplified: pain-free, aesthetic, no vascular complications, economical in terms of time and sensory recovery with the resolution of oedema.

2.1.4.2 Case 38—Total Nasal Cover Reconstruction Using a Transverse Keystone Design Variant from the Forehead, Avoiding a Two-Stage Operative Procedure of a Forehead Flap

Multifocal mitotic skin lesions of the nasal bridge make up the background pathology. The lesion over the L frontal eminence has successfully healed (Figs. 2.372, 2.373, 2.374, 2.375, 2.376, 2.377 and 2.378).

In summary, each reconstruction exemplified the PACES characteristics of the Keystone as applied to this variation of a forehead island flap. It is simpler to execute with upward closure over the R frontal eminence, no doubt sitting along the supraorbital and supratrochlear angiotome supply—V1.

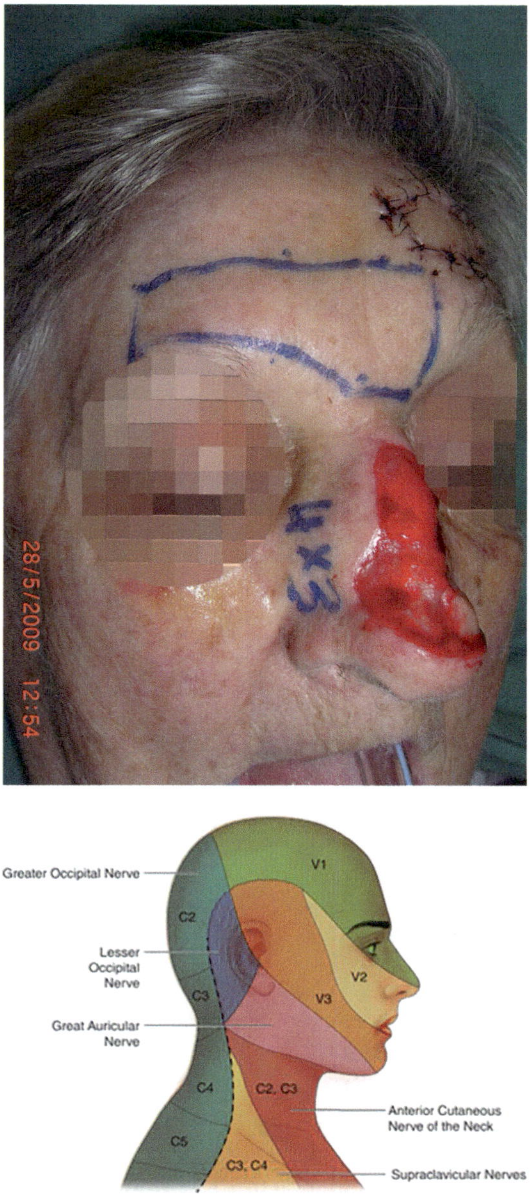

Fig. 2.373 The lateral view of the same defect in the V1 dermatome is shown. The dermatomal mark outs become the line of incision of the dermis and epidermis, ensuring that one-third deeply is attached with only partial undermining to facilitate the closure and vascular integrity of the defect. (Reprinted with permission from Atlas, *Reconstructive Technique in Melanoma Management* (p. 19), by Felix Behan, Springer Nature 2023)

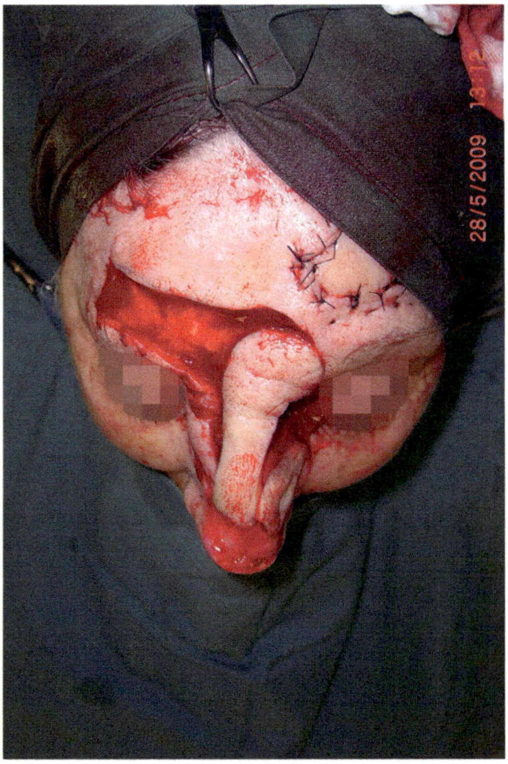

Fig. 2.374 The staged insertion of the transverse forehead Keystone island flap based on supratrochlear and supraorbital neurovascular systems to close the bridge

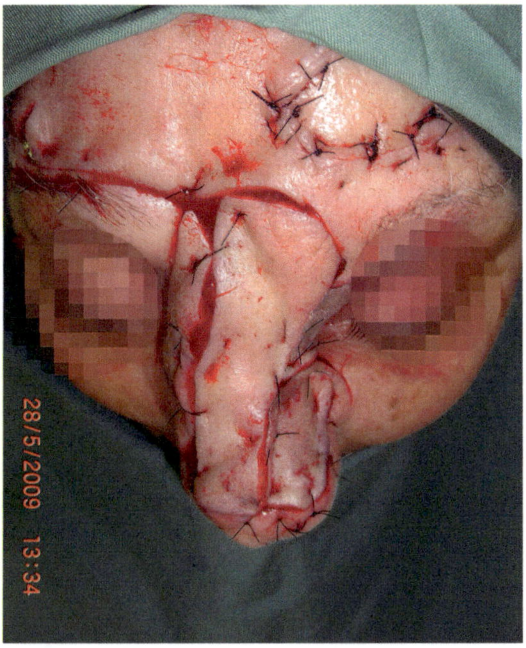

Fig. 2.375 The secondary defect is closed under tension. Note the viability of the nasal Keystone; the upper forehead Keystone has not been compromised; and the defect on the lateral side of the nose was full-thickness grafted

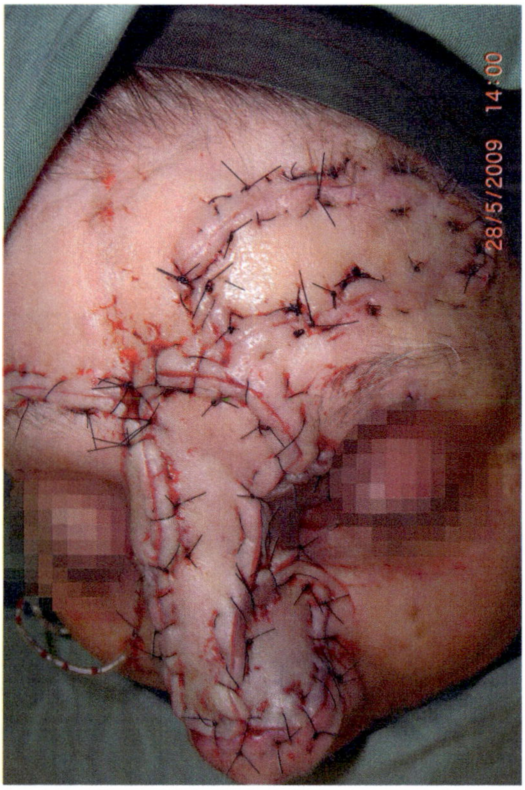

Fig. 2.376 The L forehead lesion with the staged removal of sutures is shown. The fenestrated full-thickness graft on the L side of the nose and the forehead island flap completes the closure

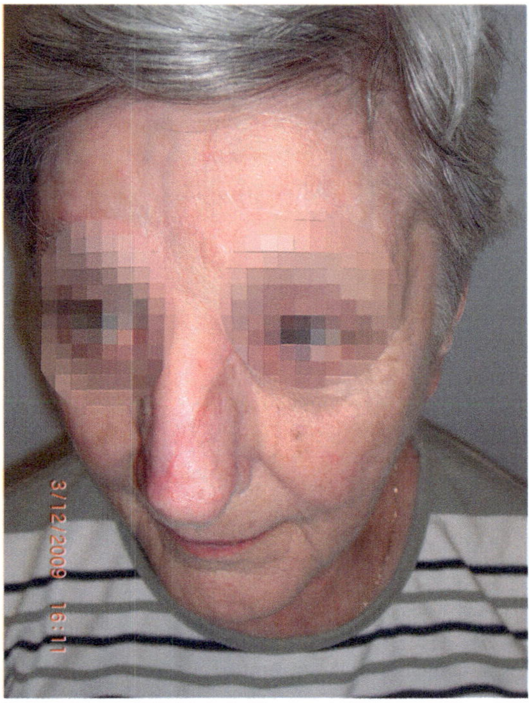

Fig. 2.377 Appearance at 6 months postoperative

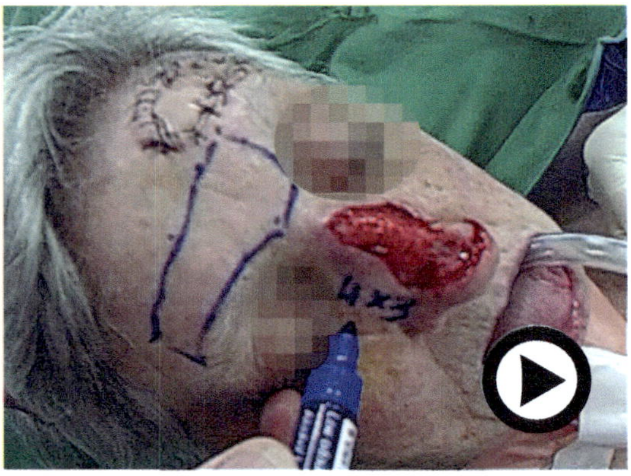

Fig. 2.378 Video 2.52 Planned operative procedure featuring a supraorbital Keystone, avoiding a forehead rhinoplasty, for the single-stage nasal reconstruction technique (▶ https://doi.org/10.1007/000-k7h)

2.1.4.3 Case 39—Nasal Tip Reconstruction

Case 39 features a 63-year-old woman with nasal tip melanoma in association with an adjacent BCC component, creating a defect 3 × 2 cm with 7 mm clearance achieved (Figs. 2.379, 2.380, 2.381, 2.382 and 2.383).

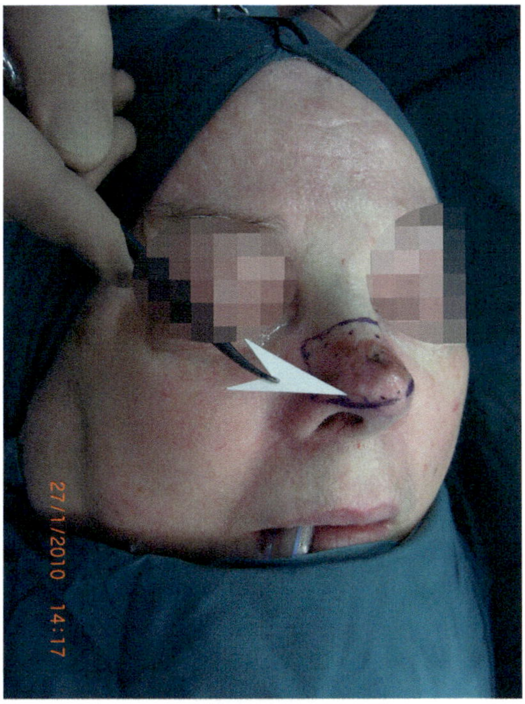

Fig. 2.379 The arrow indicates the planned tumour clearance incision. The dermatomal mark outs become the line of incision of the dermis and epidermis, ensuring that one-third deeply is attached with only partial undermining to facilitate the closure and vascular integrity of the defect. (Reprinted with permission from Atlas, *Reconstructive Technique in Melanoma Management* (p. 19), by Felix Behan, Springer Nature 2023)

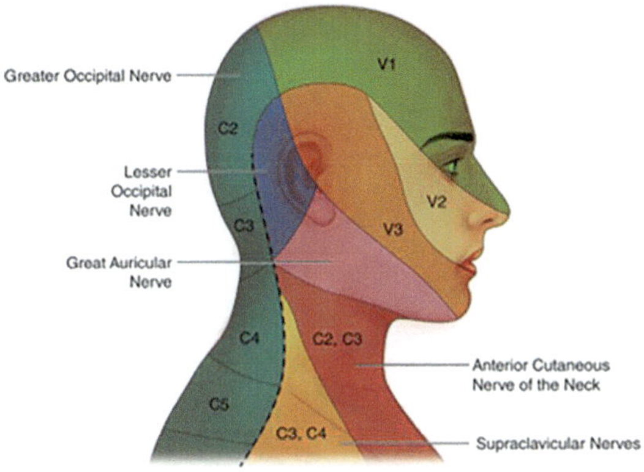

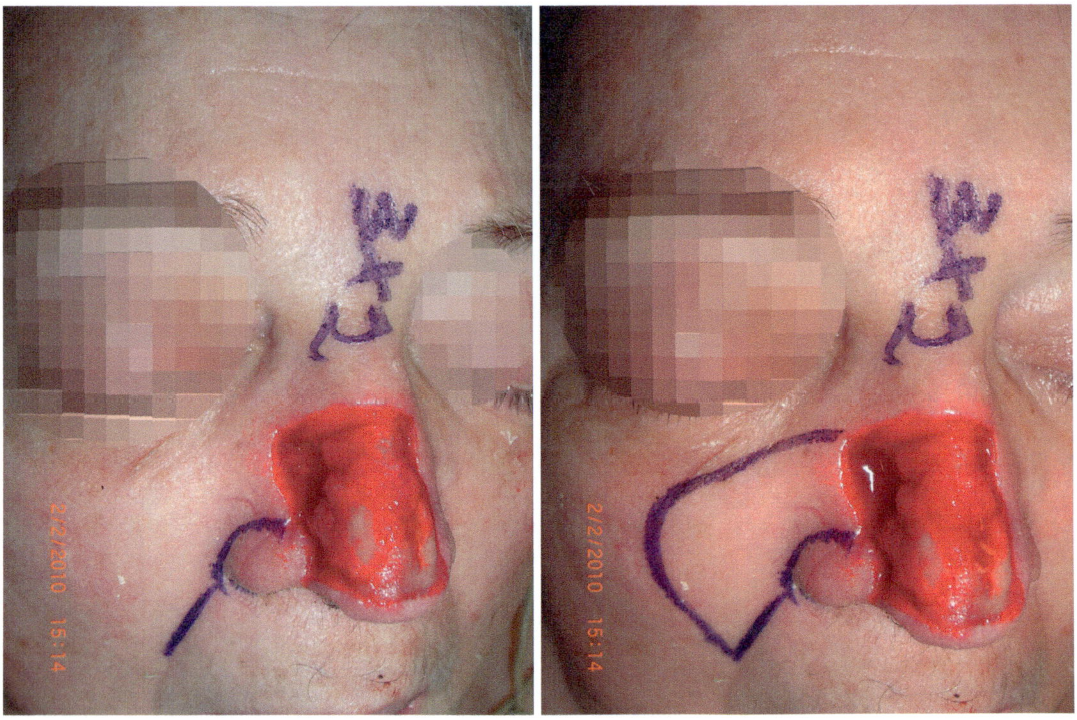

Fig. 2.380 A 3×2 cm oncological defect is shown. The Keystone flap repair was carried out on the infraorbital neurovascular axes and the nasal branch of the facial artery. The Keystone is outlined and raised with blunt dissection, ensuring one-third deep attachment at the flap origin to reach over the nasal defect, providing soft-tissue cover. Remnants from the infraorbital neurovascular axis and the nasal branch of the facial artery form a network of vascular circulation to allow the flaps to be placed at the nasal tip

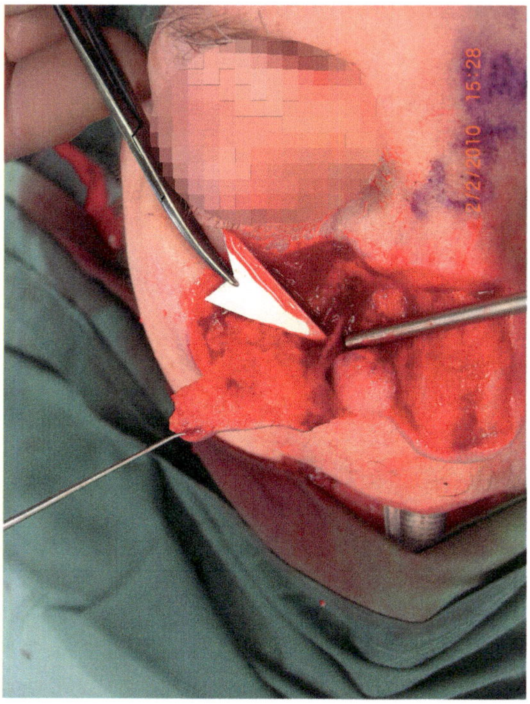

Fig. 2.381 The arrow indicates the nasal branch of the facial artery, which was been defined but not skeletonised, and the source of filamentous perforators ensures flap integrity

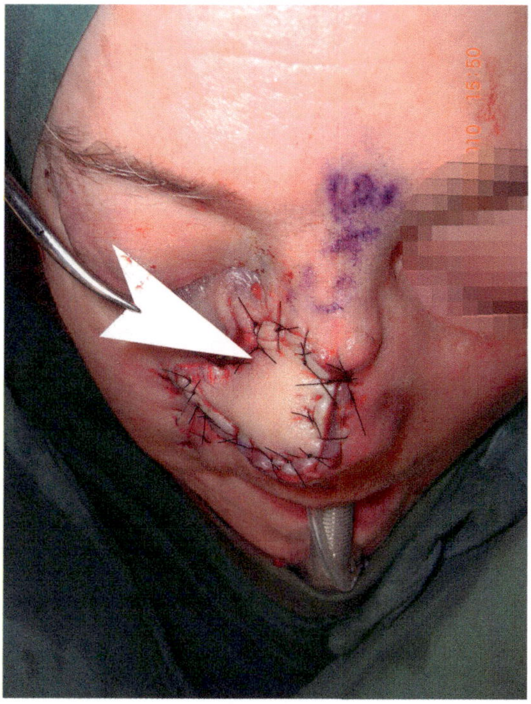

Fig. 2.382 The flap insertion using the standard three-phase single-layer suture technique

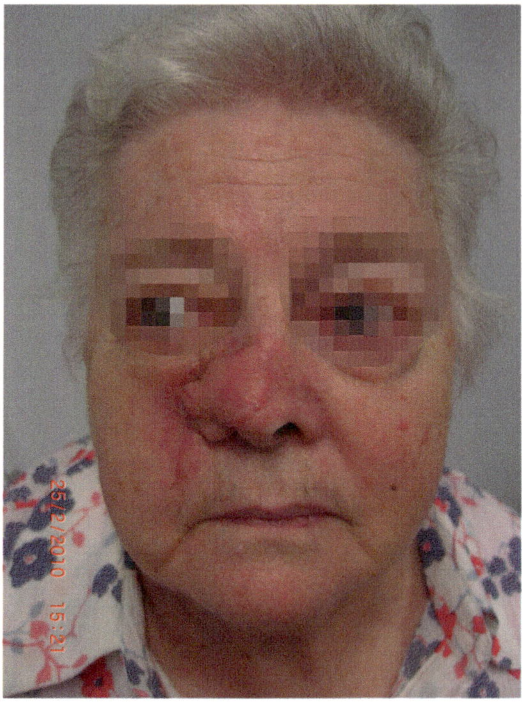

Fig. 2.383 Postoperative appearance at 2 weeks after the removal of sutures

The PACES characteristics were all exemplified: pain-free, aesthetic, no vascular complications, economical in terms of time and sensory recovery with the resolution of oedema.

2.1.4.4 Case 40—Infraorbital SCC Approaching the Orbital Margin and the Nasal Cavity (Figs. 2.384, 2.385, 2.386, 2.387, 2.388, 2.389, 2.390, 2.391, 2.392, 2.393, 2.394, 2.395, 2.396, 2.397 and 2.398)

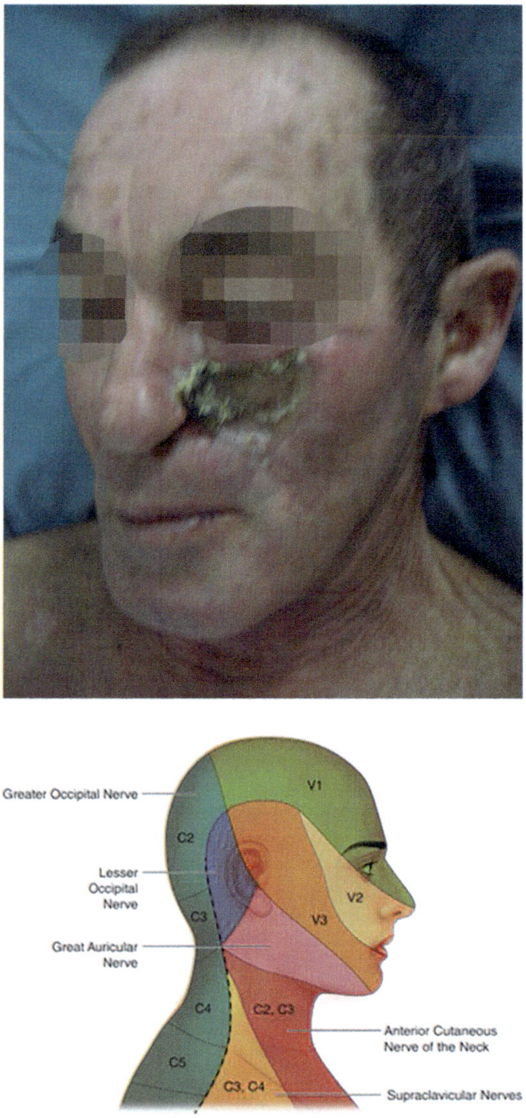

Fig. 2.384 This rural person was anxious about going to hospitals. The dermatomal mark outs become the line of incision of the dermis and epidermis, ensuring that one-third deeply is attached with only partial undermining to facilitate the closure and vascular integrity of the defect. (Reprinted with permission from Atlas, *Reconstructive Technique in Melanoma Management* (p. 19), by Felix Behan, Springer Nature 2023)

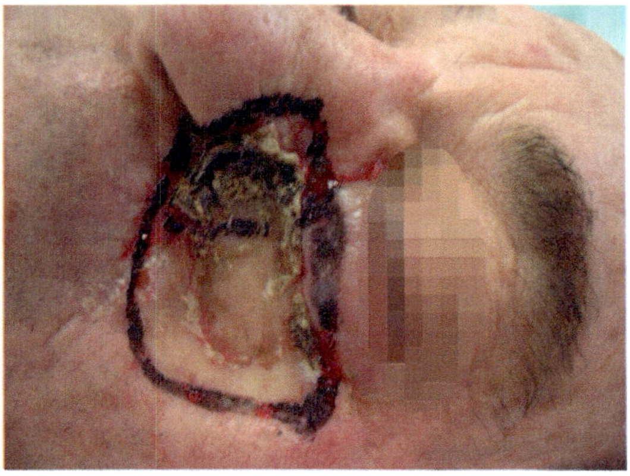

Fig. 2.385 This hemi-nasal defect with exposed mucosa was closed with a V2 cheek Keystone to hypervascularise it along the lines of tension, and the deep surface of the flap was left untouched so that it could mucosalise from the surrounding tissues

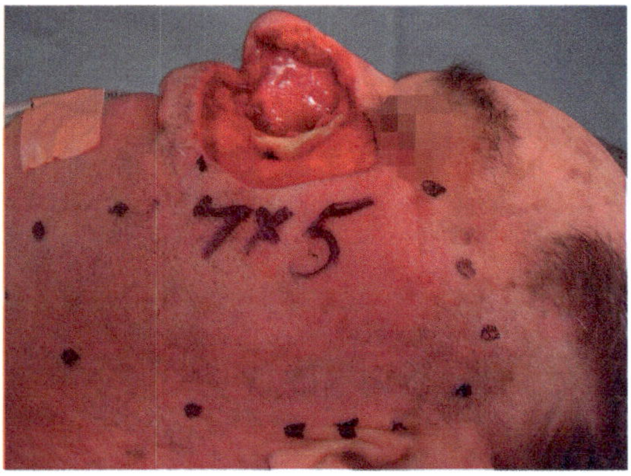

Fig. 2.386 The 7 × 5 cm surgical defect and the dotted outline of the proposed V2 Keystone reconstruction to be advanced upon being rotated to the bridge of the nose

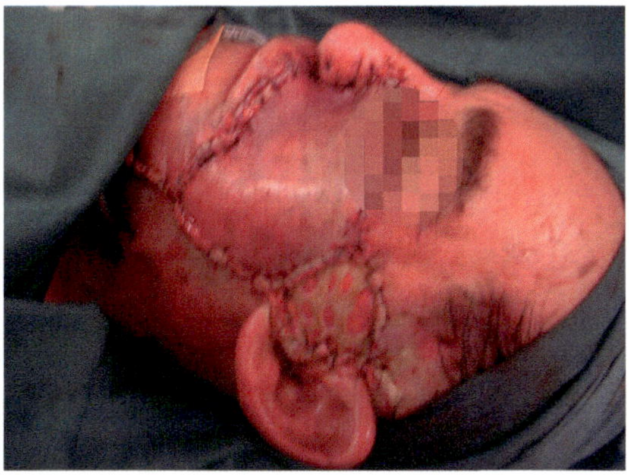

Fig. 2.387 The infraorbital margin was generously inserted with the Keystone to minimise any ectropion, and the secondary defect in the preauricular space could have been closed under tension, thus avoiding any ectropion of the lower eyelid. Therefore, a fenestrated full-thickness graft was installed into this secondary defect

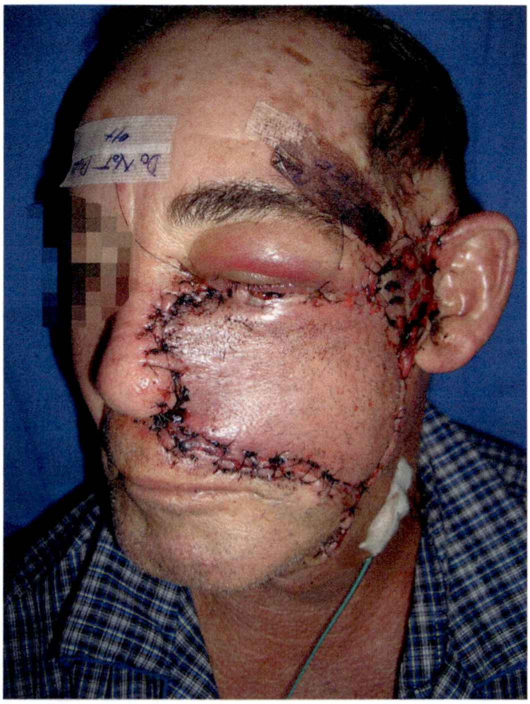

Fig. 2.388 Appearance at 24 h with suction drainage intact

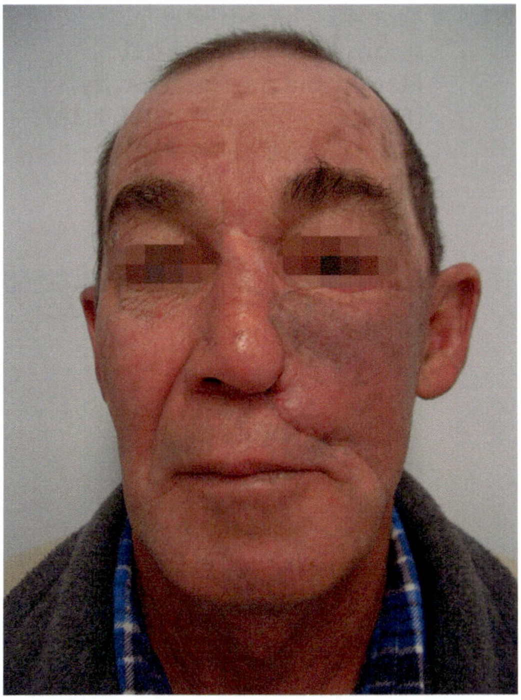

Fig. 2.389 Appearance at 2 months, where the redundant tissue in the L nasolabial line was earmarked for correction at the same time as the alar reconstruction of the nose

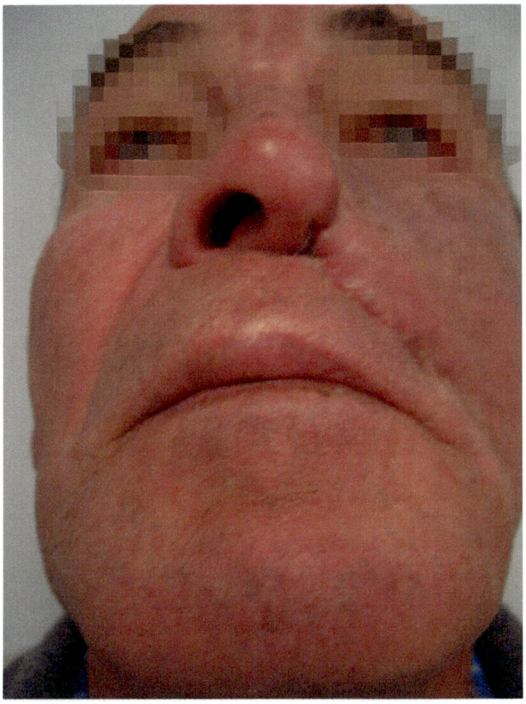

Fig. 2.390 The infranasal view shows the deformity of the nasal opening in the L. The solution was a composite graft from the opposite ear, including the alar rim

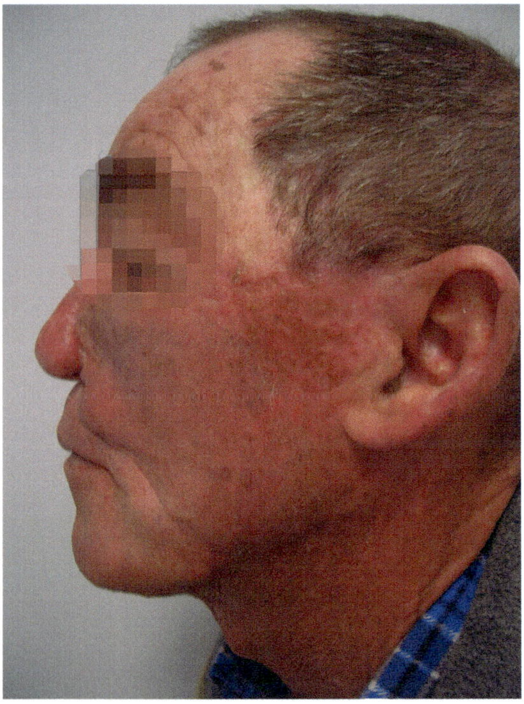

Fig. 2.391 Lateral view of the healed wounds

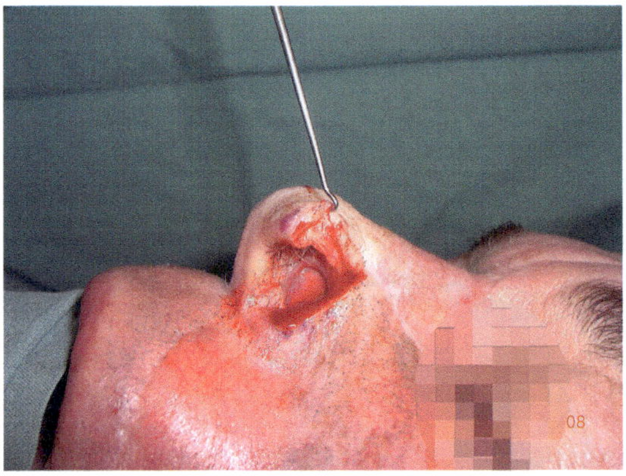

Fig. 2.392 Freshening the tissues for the composite graft

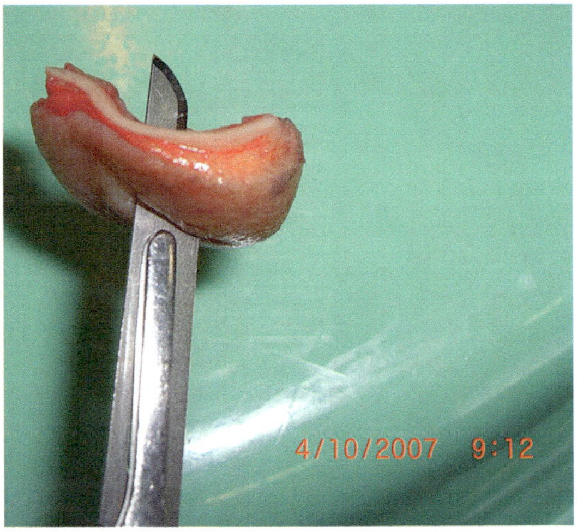

Fig. 2.393 The fenestration technique of the helix, with the tissue from the L ear being fenestrated to avoid venous stasis in alar rim reconstruction. This manoeuvre contributes to the success of the composite graft; it is otherwise a difficult area to reconstruct

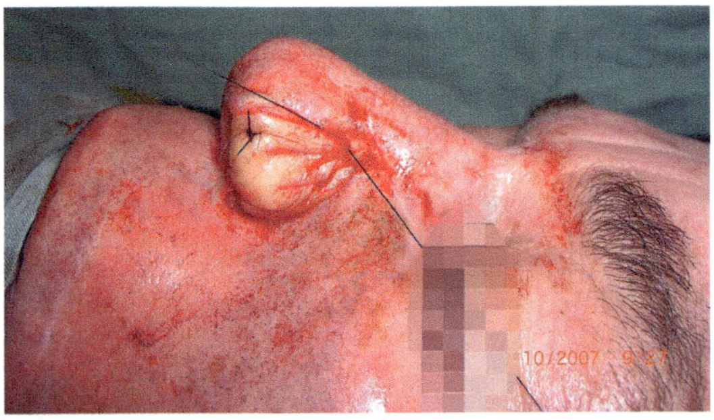

Fig. 2.394 Fenestrations filled with blood in the postoperative phase, indicating that flow is occurring from the sutured margin intranasally

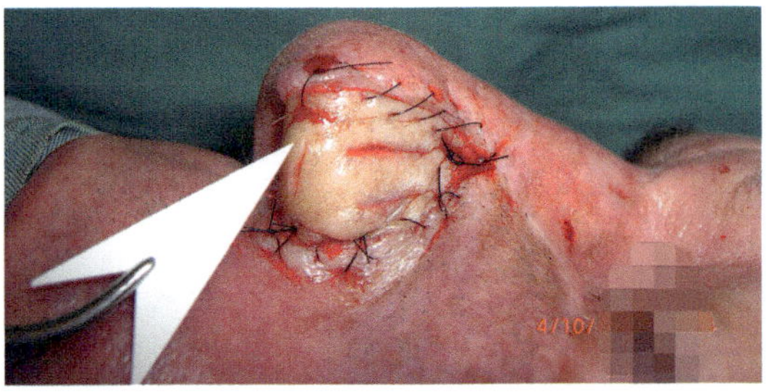

Fig. 2.395 More views of fenestrated oozing from the composite graft a keynote for success

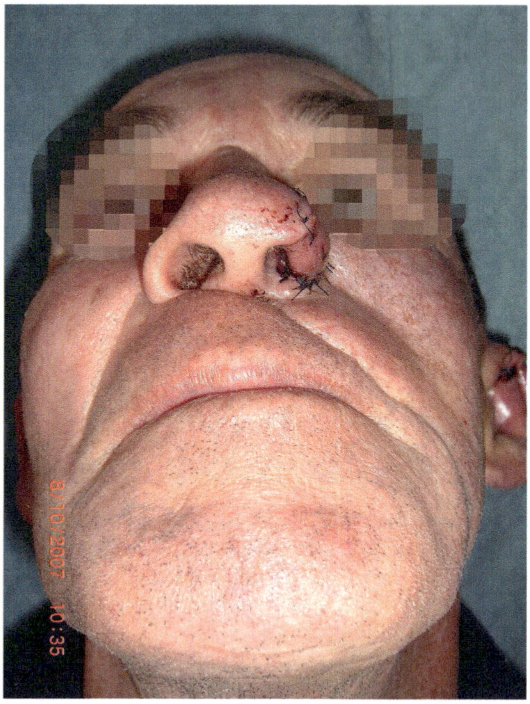

Fig. 2.396 Appearance at 4 days, showing that the vascularisation of the composite graft [20] is being completed by avoiding venous stasis

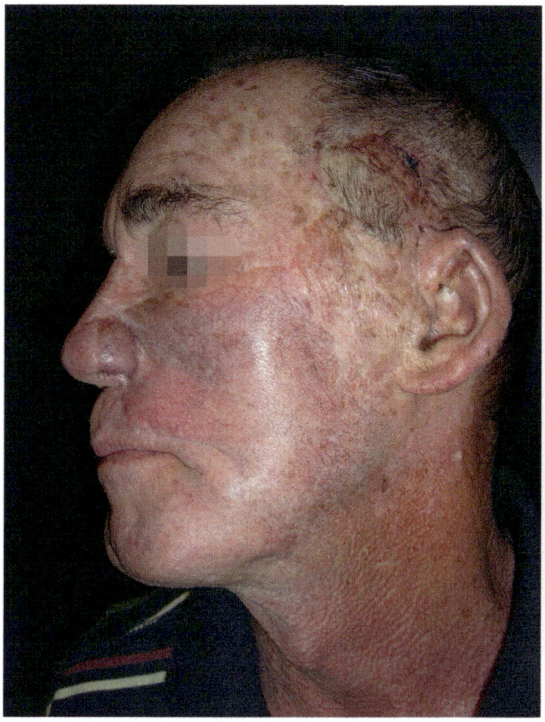

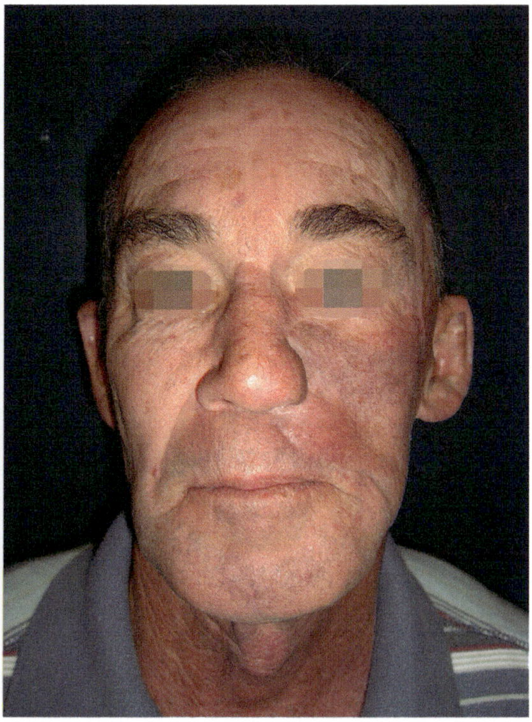

Fig. 2.397 The appearance of the nose with a healed composite graft is shown. The wedge excision of the ear is evident. The donor site from the L ear is barely discernible, for which the patient was grateful because he looked almost normal. The almost facial appearance on direct gaze is shown. The patient's hidden smile reflects his personal satisfaction

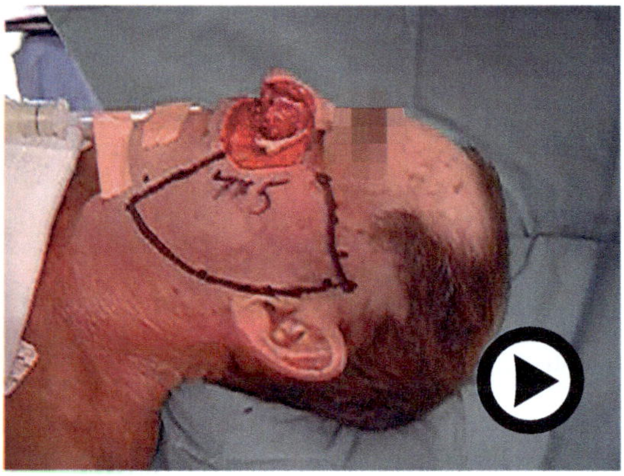

Fig. 2.398 Video 2.53 Outlining the planned Keystone reconstruction before the composite graft for the defect from the ear for the nasal margin (▶ https://doi.org/10.1007/000-k7j)

The PACES characteristics were all exemplified: pain-free, aesthetic, no vascular complications, economical in terms of time and sensory recovery with the resolution of oedema.

2.1.4.5 Case 41—SCC Recurrence L Wall of Nose (Figs. 2.399, 2.400, 2.401, 2.402, 2.403, 2.404, 2.405, 2.406, 2.407, 2.408 and 2.409)

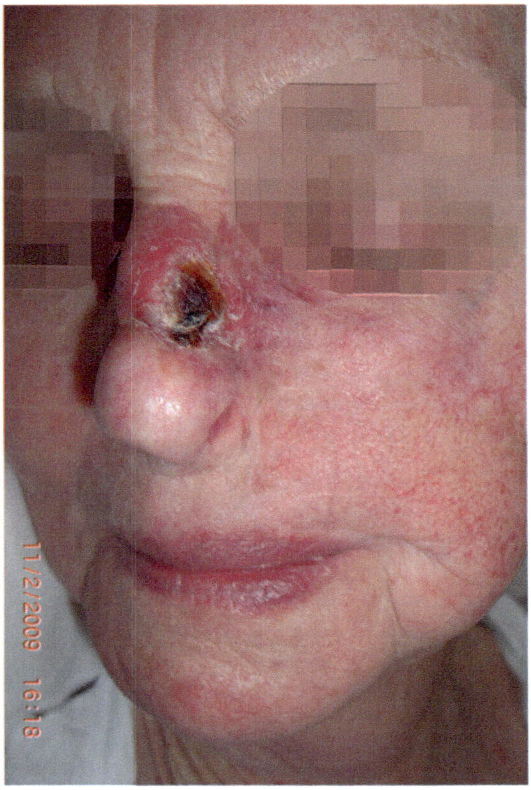

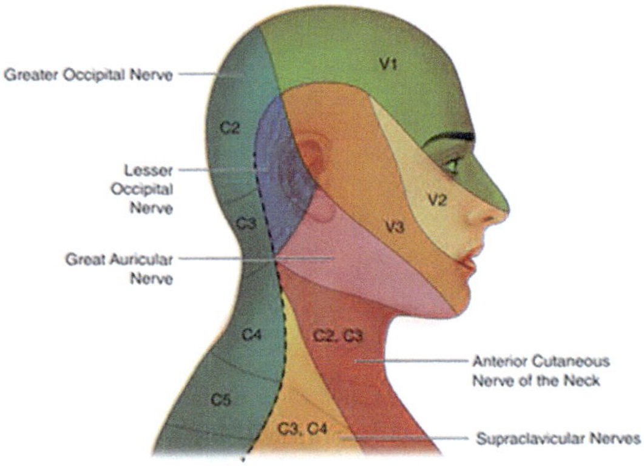

Fig. 2.399 A closeup with the peripheral oedema down the L side of the nose is shown, necessitating pathology clearance before reconstruction—a two-stage procedure (DRAPE). The dermatomal mark outs become the line of incision of the dermis and epidermis, ensuring that one-third deeply is attached with only partial undermining to facilitate the closure and vascular integrity of the defect. (Reprinted with permission from Atlas, *Reconstructive Technique in Melanoma Management* (p. 19), by Felix Behan, Springer Nature 2023)

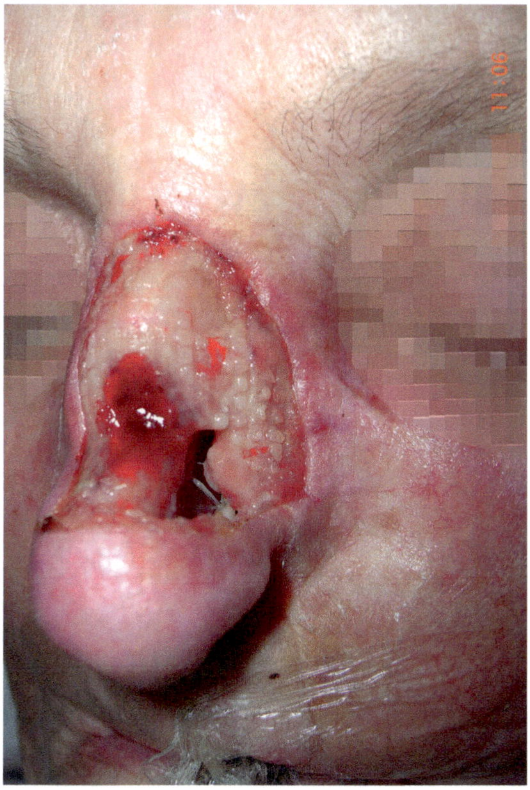

Fig. 2.400 The excisional defect

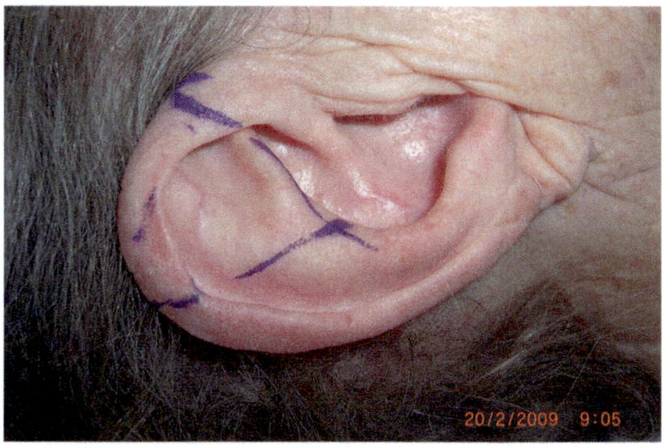

Fig. 2.401 The mark out from the donor site of the L ear is used to complete the reconstruction, using the ear as a fenestrated composite graft

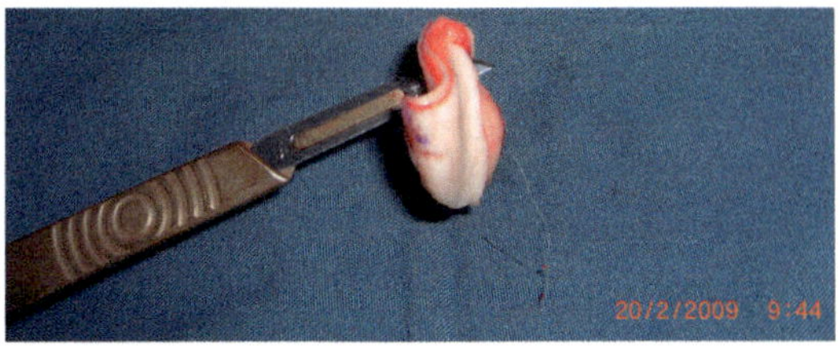

Fig. 2.402 The composite graft to be used in the lateral wall reconstruction in association with the supraorbital glabella island Keystone

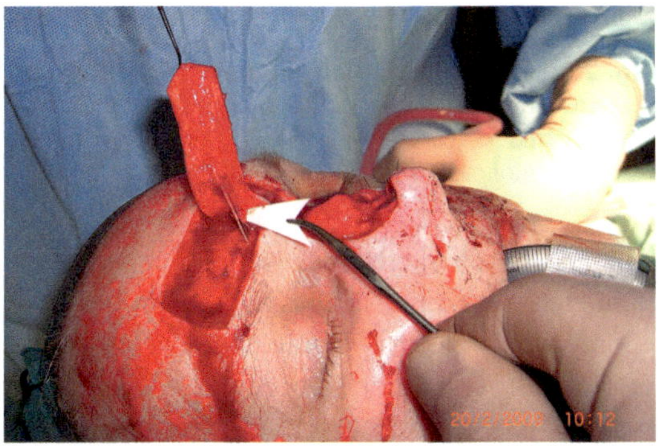

Fig. 2.403 Raising the supraorbital glabella island flap and the small neurovascular perforator support on which it is dependent (arrowed)

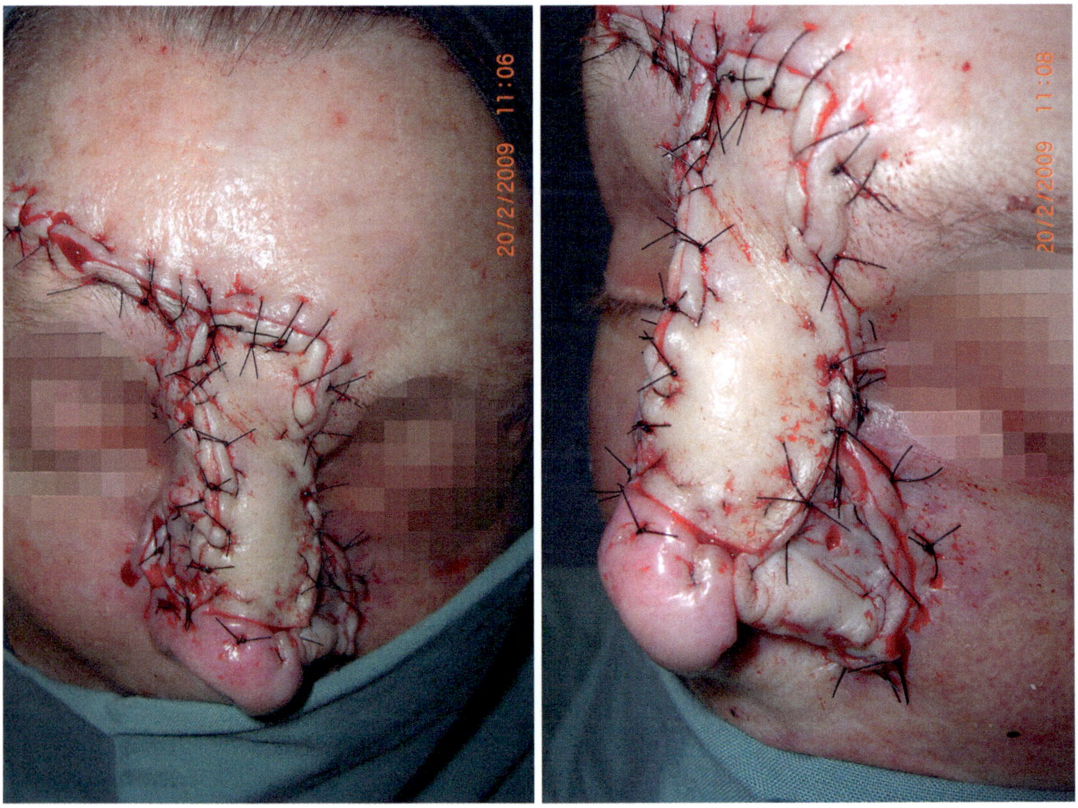

Fig. 2.404 The glabella island flap is inserted along the bridge of the nose, and the fenestrated composite graft from the L ear creates the helix margin to give it an alar rim

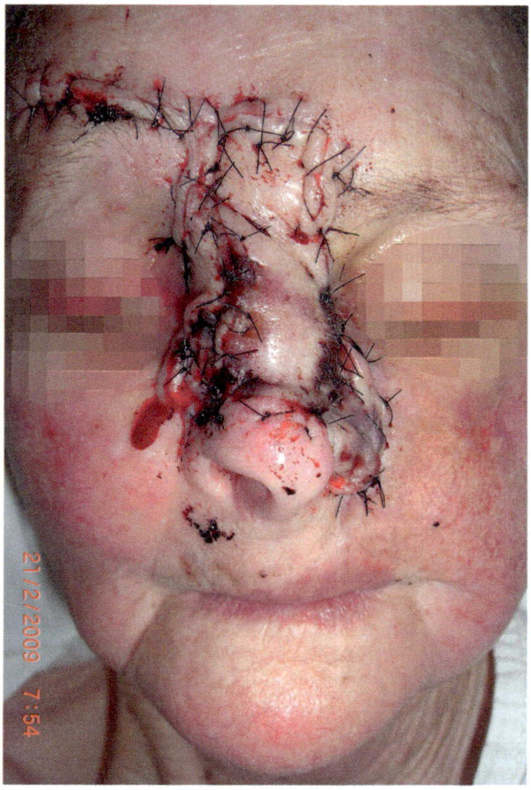

Fig. 2.405 The appearance at 24 h is shown, and the heparinised gauze is used to clean the fenestration sites to minimise any haematoma inside the composite grafts. The oozing is conducive to success and a characteristic of the fenestration technique for composite grafts

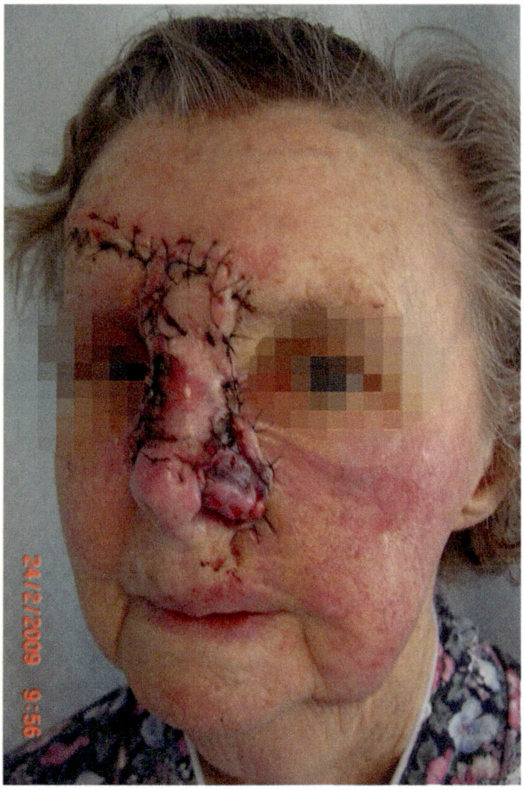

Fig. 2.406 The postoperative appearance at 4 days shows the success of the composite graft with revascularisation, and the fenestrations eliminate any haematoma formation

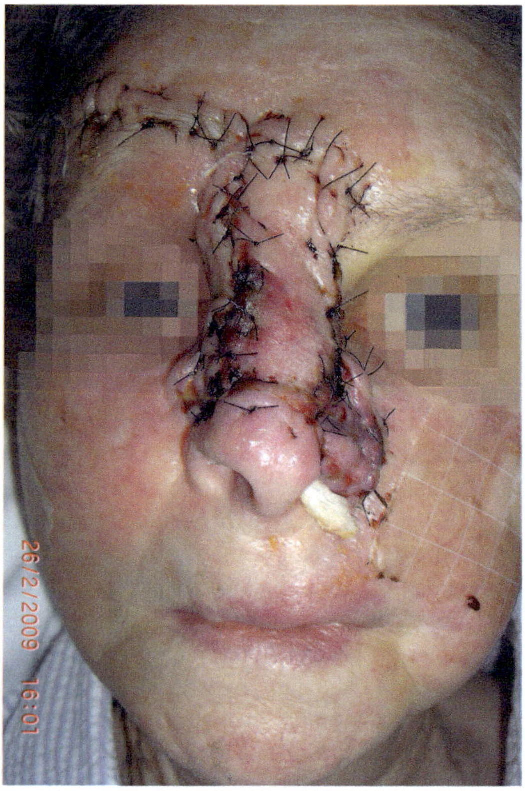

Fig. 2.407 Appearance at 6 days with ongoing heparinised gauze to facilitate ongoing drainage

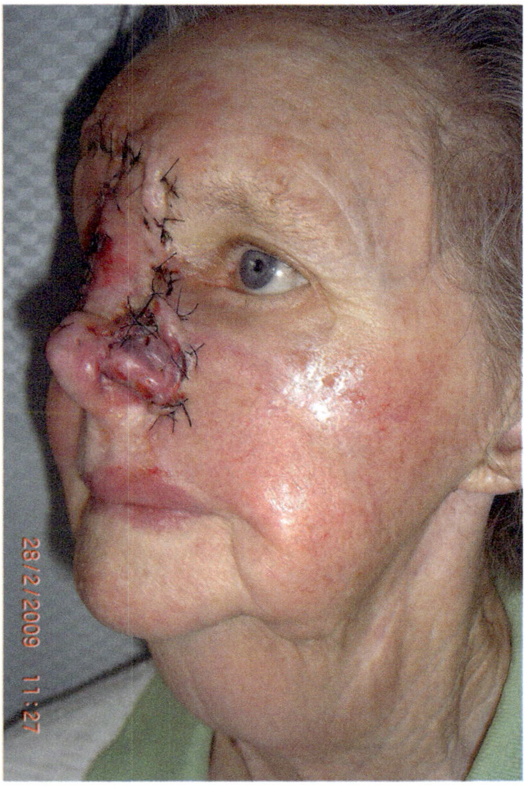

Fig. 2.408 Appearance at 8 days, with a full, successful graft

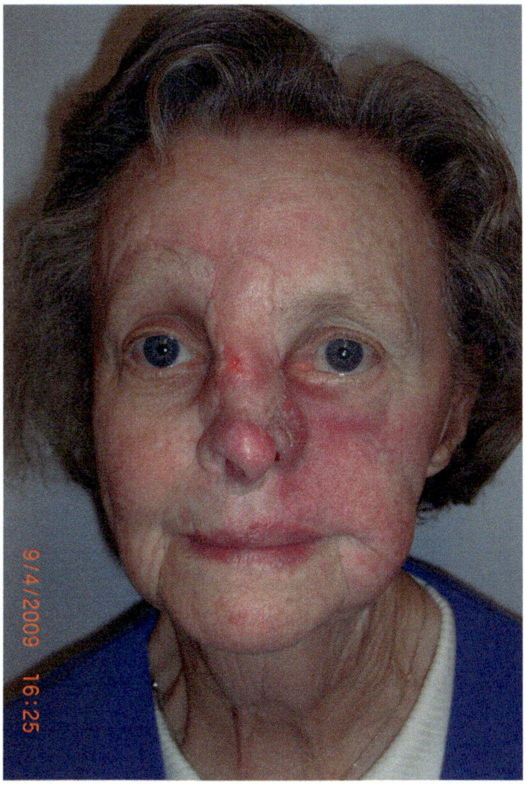

Fig. 2.409 The appearance at 3 months is shown, and the successful helix reconstruction can be attributed to the fenestrations in the composite graft—awaiting the correction of the ectropion of the L eye. The patient was extremely pleased with the outcome and could even form a smile, and this composite grafting technique using the ear certainly avoids multiple staged reconstructive manoeuvres

The PACES characteristics were all exemplified: pain-free, aesthetic, no vascular complications, economical in terms of time and sensory recovery with the resolution of oedema.

2.1.5 Cheek

The Keystone has universal applications in the closure of defects from the infraorbital region, the preauricular region and the bucco-mandibular alignment. The principles of direct closure, though possible in loose elderly skin, often leave lines of tension in the closure, and this is overcome by the Keystone, a single island flap, which bridges two surgical defects (the first defect originates from the flap, and the other defect is from the tumour excision). Simplistically, we have an umbrella of tissue, the Keystone, which opens to cover both sites, acting in the same manner as an open umbrella. I will not list the umpteen cases of cheek rotation flaps, V-Y island flaps and Mustarde's rotation flaps; nor will I quote Moncrief as a style of reconstruction. The rhombic flap, or Dufourmentel modification of the Limberg flap, creates angular designs with V-Y closures at various sites. The Keystone combines a lot of these designs with random subcutaneous pedicles, which are not defined. But the island apparently sympathectomises the tissues around the designs of the Keystone, which increases vascularity and creates the hyperaemic appearance, externally visualised by the red dot sign. The alignment of flaps around the dermatomes of the trigeminal design and the cervico-facial outlines constitutes the success of this reconstructive tool. The problem of using undermining to allow advancement in large wound closure is thus avoided because the tensional apposition—an edict of surgery that we have all experienced and respected—is now obsolete given that the hyperaemia is based on perforator circulation in this island concept and has no part in the subdermal plexus, except for input. The perforators lie in the 'stalk of the umbrella' that is used to cover the tissue defect thanks to random vascular support, not specific perforators. Microvascular free flap, radial forearm and even parascapular reconstruction almost necessitate performing secondary procedures to improve contour, bulk and volume because these three extremes seem to currently characterise microvascular reconstruction. However, if it is needed, it is needed, particularly to cover large bony defects. Yet according to our publications to date, the Keystone design is remarkable in its wide applications in reconstructive use.

2.1.5.1 Case 42—Melanoma in an Irradiated Field

Case 42 features melanoma in the R cheek in an irradiated field in a 62-year-old man. He had a history of cancer of the larynx treated with radiation. His lower neck skin necrosis was treated with a pectoralis-major reconstructive flap before the biopsy of the cheek lesion, which confirmed melanoma (Figs. 2.410, 2.411, 2.412, 2.413, 2.414 and 2.415).

In summary, the PACES charactristics of the Keystone were all exemplified in this island flap repair. An acceptable surgical repair in irradiated tissue, which is not a contraindication for Keystone applications as it is for other locoregional flaps. The islanding hypervascularises the tissue in spite of dermal and subdermal fibrous atrophy after radiation vasculitis.

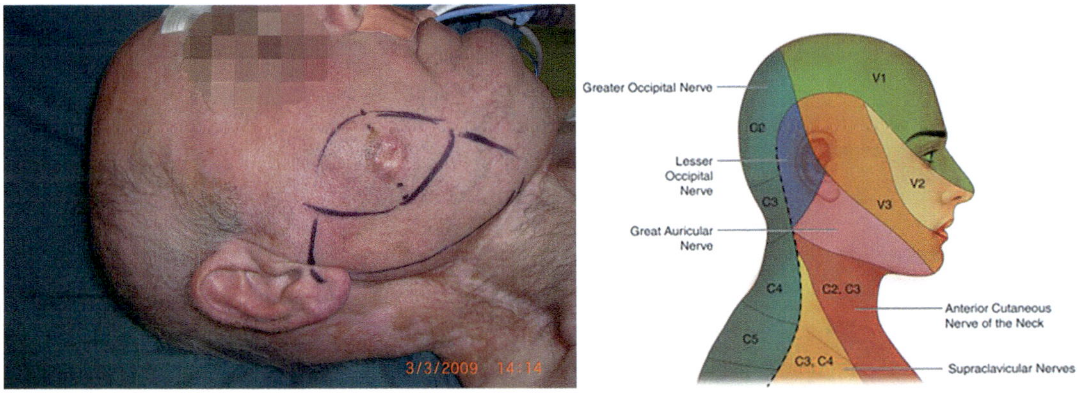

Fig. 2.410 This level II melanoma in an irradiated field doubled in size during the postoperative treatment of the lower cervical radio-necrosis, treated with a pectoralis-major flap. The dermatomal mark outs become the line of incision of the dermis and epidermis, ensuring that one-third deeply is attached with only partial undermining to facilitate the closure and vascular integrity of the defect. (Reprinted with permission from Atlas, *Reconstructive Technique in Melanoma Management* (p. 19), by Felix Behan, Springer Nature 2023)

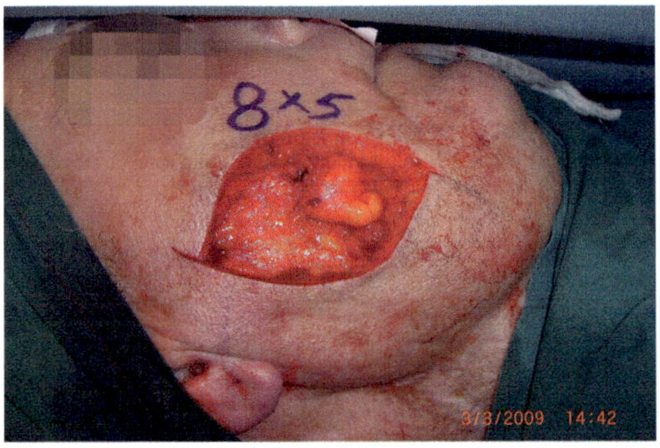

Fig. 2.411 The 8 × 5 cm defect and the buccal pad of fat are evident in the depths of the wound

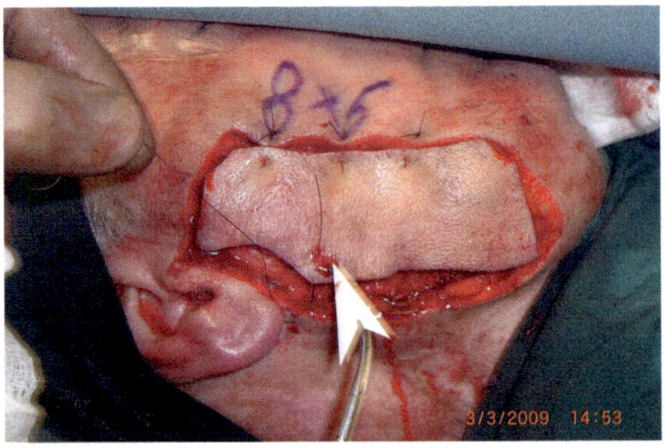

Fig. 2.412 The wound is closed under tension in this irradiated field, a Keystone characteristic reflecting that the hyperaemic reflex is evident in the posterior aspect of the Keystone (closer to a branch of the facial artery). The cyanotic superior margin indicates the possible vasculitis associated with radiation. The red dot sign is arrowed, confirming its hypervascularity, which ensures healing in this irradiated field—usually a contraindication for locoregional reconstruction

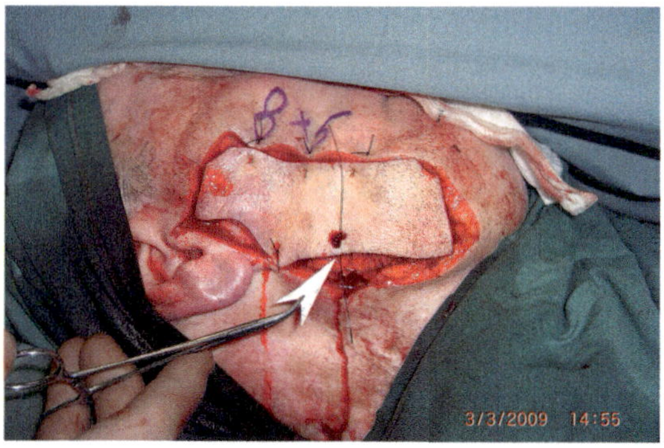

Fig. 2.413 The red dot sign in an irradiated field reflects the slight vascular impedance, and it borders on the cyanotic appearance

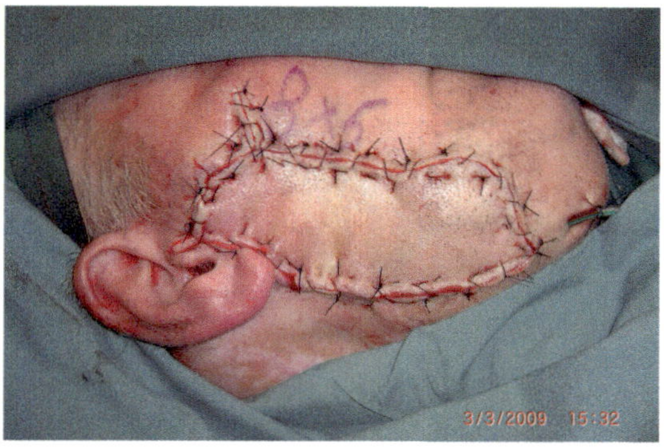

Fig. 2.414 Complete closure in a timeframe of 90 min with the standard three-phase suture technique is shown. The difference in vascular perfusion is evident, starting inferiorly and spreading up the flap

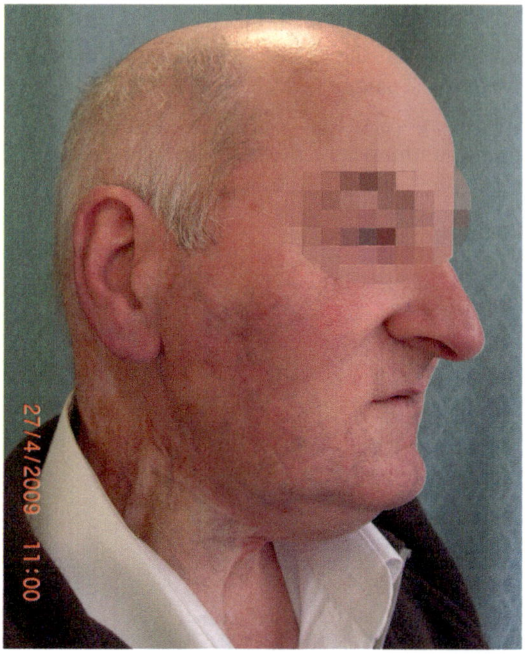

Fig. 2.415 Normal appearance at 6 weeks is shown, meeting the patient's satisfaction. The scar is indiscernible, reflecting the value of the three-phase single-layer nylon closure technique

2.1.5.2 Case 43—An Aesthetic Facial Closure Avoiding the Melon Slice Dip if the Wound Is Closed Directly (Figs. 2.416, 2.417, 2.418, 2.419, 2.420, 2.421, 2.422, 2.423, 2.424, 2.425 and 2.426)

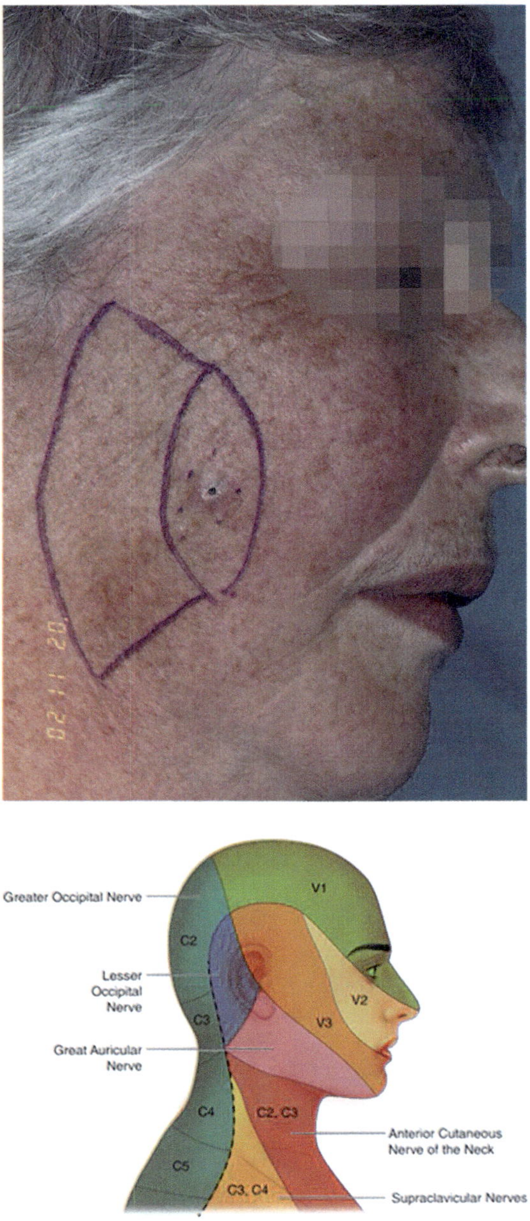

Fig. 2.416 Patient presents with the lesion marked out, and the Keystone repair indicates the preauricular line. The dermatomal mark outs become the line of incision of the dermis and epidermis, ensuring that one-third deeply is attached with only partial undermining to facilitate the closure and vascular integrity of the defect. (Reprinted with permission from Atlas, *Reconstructive Technique in Melanoma Management* (p. 19), by Felix Behan, Springer Nature 2023)

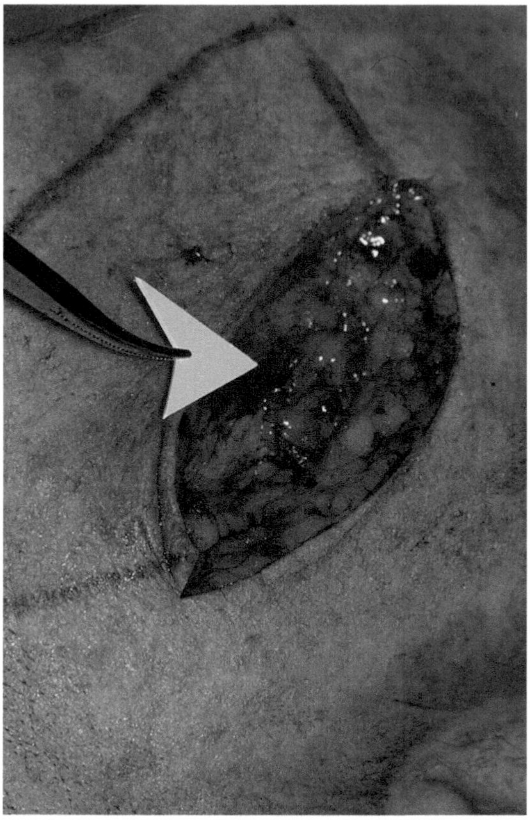

Fig. 2.417 Subdermal perforators originating from the facial artery

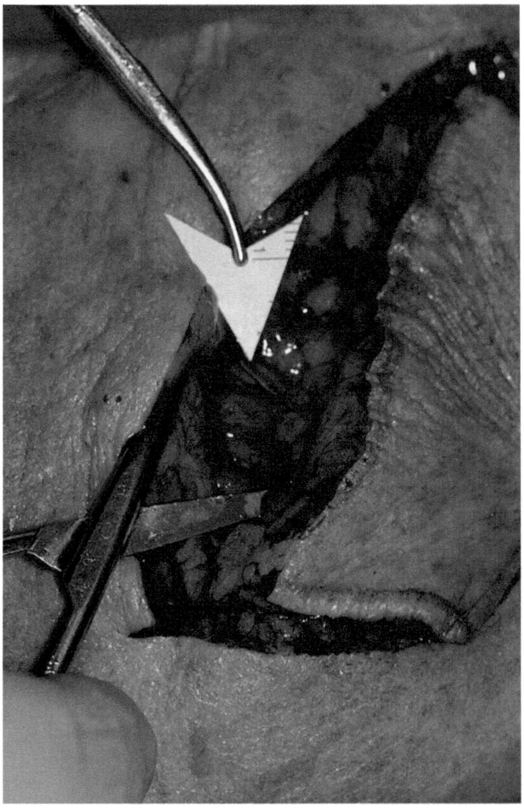

Fig. 2.418 The blunt dissection with scissors, displacing the flap into the defect

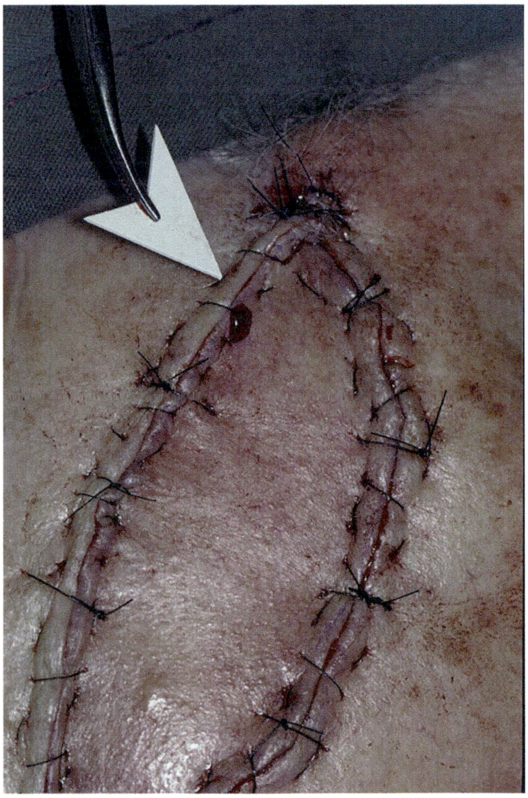

Fig. 2.419 Ongoing vascular indications show the vascular flare throughout, mainly in the superior part, and the red dot sign is a confirmation of the hyperaemia from the sympathetic principle

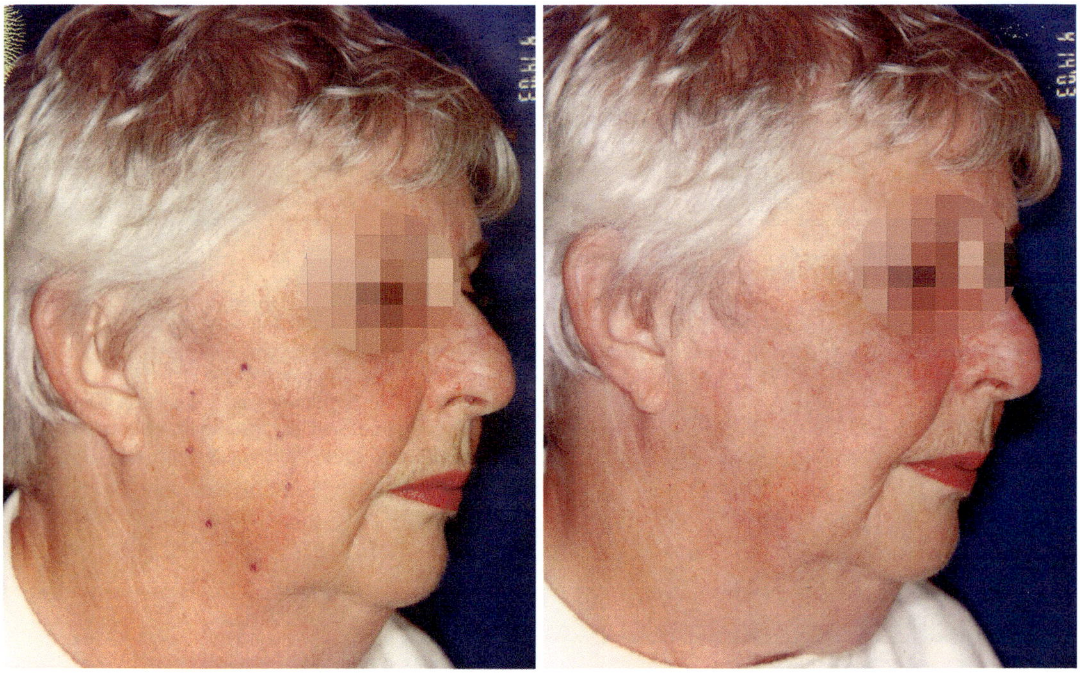

Fig. 2.420 The staged removal of the sutures is shown, and the outline is barely visible, using dots to highlight the flap insertion

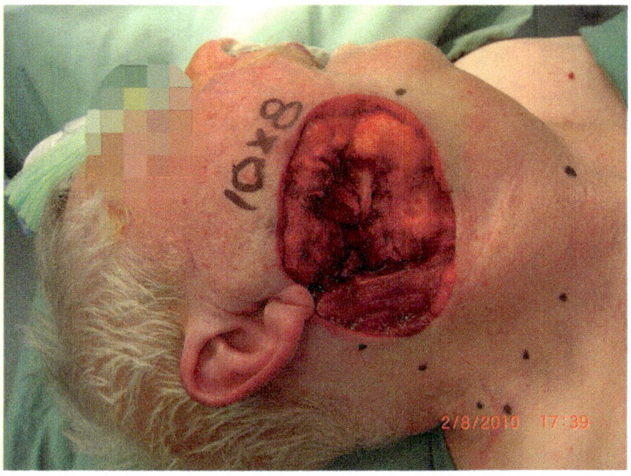

Fig. 2.421 Nodal secondaries in the upper echelon of cervical nodes—a 10 × 8 cm defect

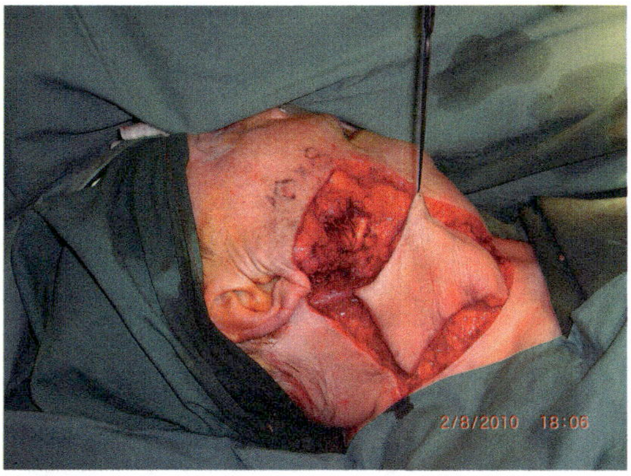

Fig. 2.422 The outline of the Keystone closure is shown, indicating that its deep attachments are in place. The dermatome outline is the mark of the incision for the Keystone

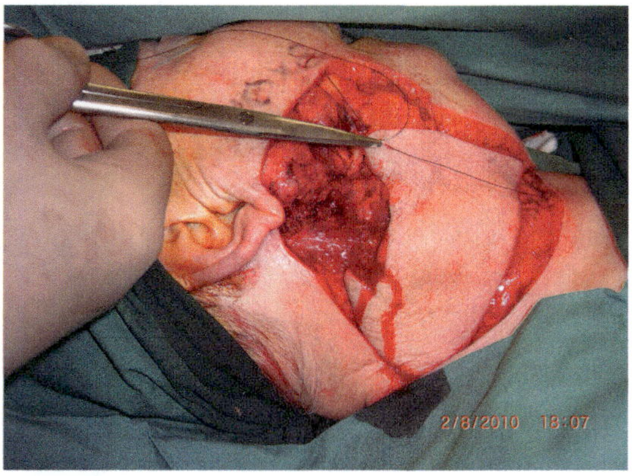

Fig. 2.423 Sequential closure with locking mattress sutures at the points of maximum tension

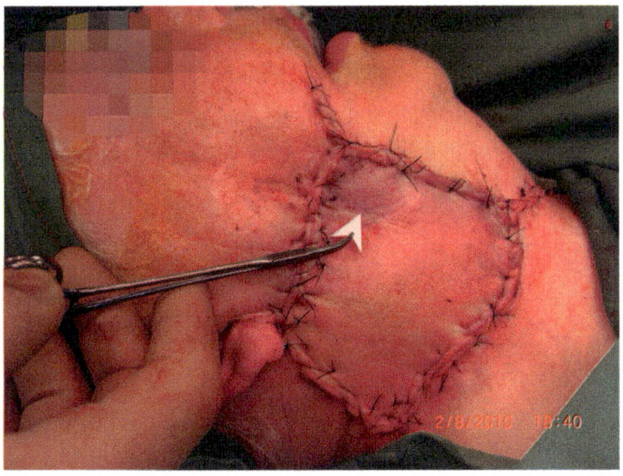

Fig. 2.424 On completion, showing that the hyperaemic phase is evident even under tension

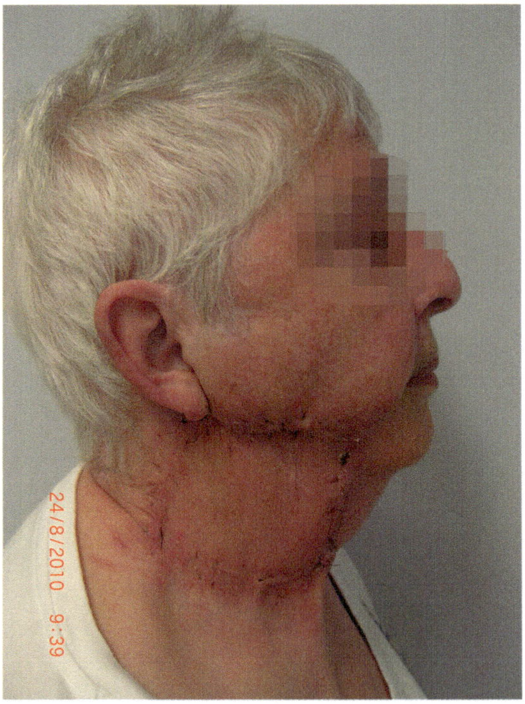

Fig. 2.425 The appearance at 3 weeks is shown with healing complete, and the maximum tension points of locking mattress sutures have been removed

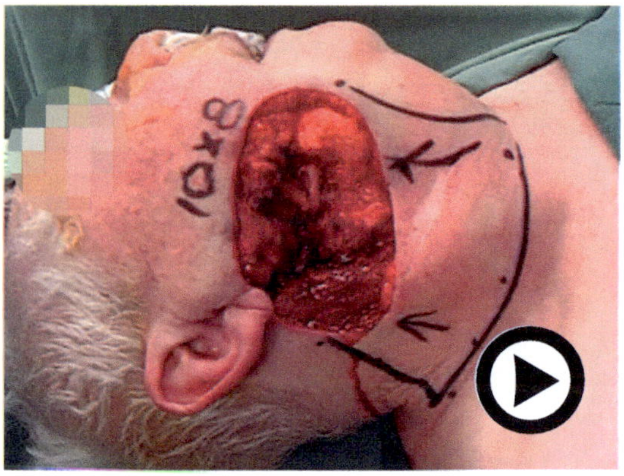

Fig. 2.426 Video 2.54 Keystone closure of a major parotid defect using lax neck tissue, another example of intrinsic expansion, not dissimilar to tailoring, where the tissue is fashioned to fill the defect (▶ https://doi.org/10.1007/000-k7k)

The PACES characteristics were all exemplified: pain-free, aesthetic, no vascular complications, economical in terms of time and sensory recovery with the resolution of oedema.

2.1.5.3 Case 44—Infraorbital Exposure of the Maxillary Sinus (Figs. 2.427, 2.428, 2.429, 2.430, 2.431 and 2.432)

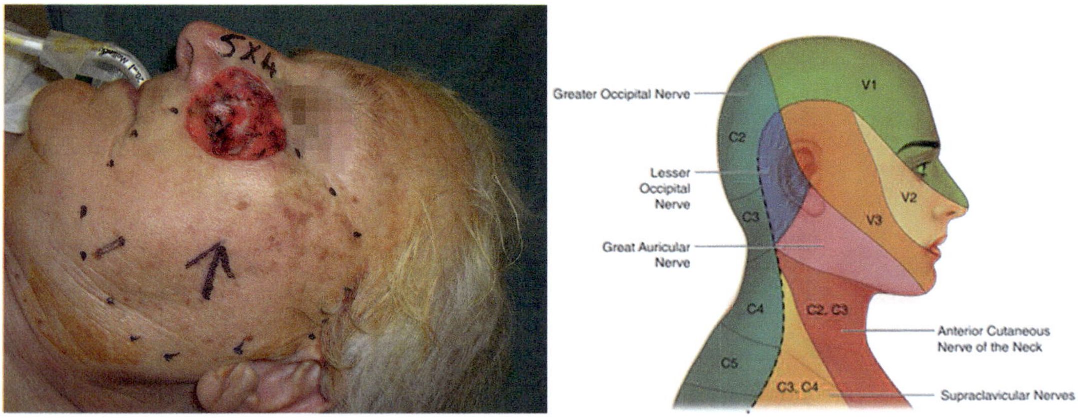

Fig. 2.427 The outline of the cheek Keystone in the vicinity of the V2 dermatome is shown, where the Keystone covers the 5 × 4 cm maxillary opening. The dermatomal mark outs become the line of incision of the dermis and epidermis, ensuring that one-third deeply is attached with only partial undermining to facilitate the closure and vascular integrity of the defect. (Reprinted with permission from Atlas, *Reconstructive Technique in Melanoma Management* (p. 19), by Felix Behan, Springer Nature 2023)

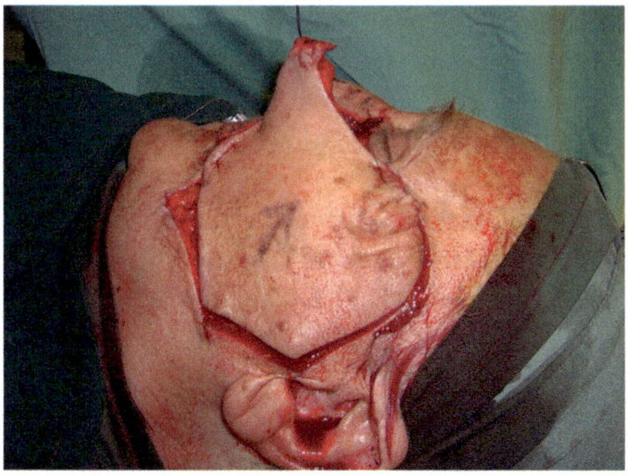

Fig. 2.428 The undermining with the point of the flap elevated is shown, and the V2 dermatome is surgically delineated to facilitate advancement and stretch to ensure closure

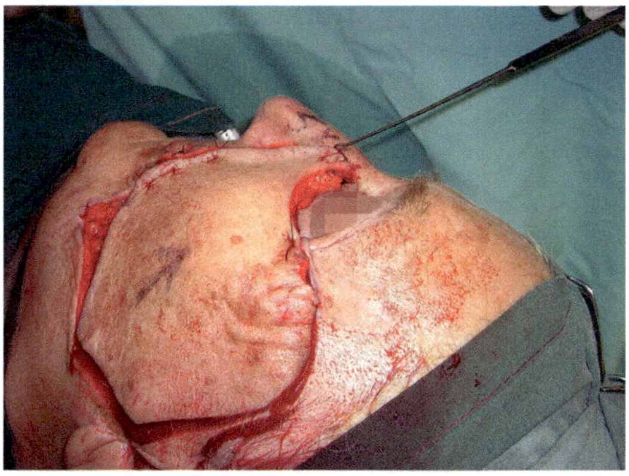

Fig. 2.429 Prior to insertion along the infraorbital margin without causing ectropion

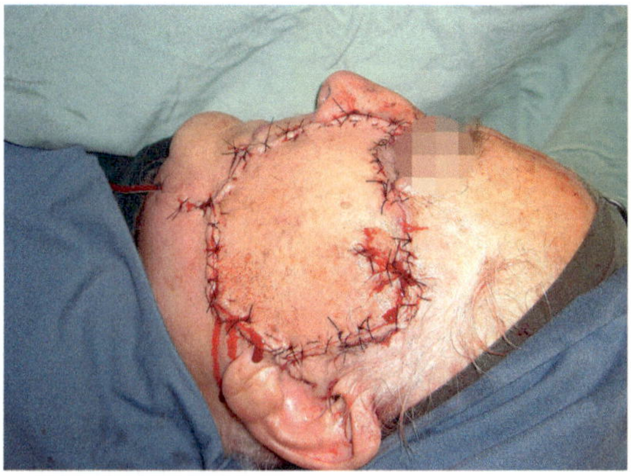

Fig. 2.430 Sequential suturing for closure is shown. The vascular flare is indicated along the inferior margin from branches of the facial artery, which are not defined—as long as it is pink, it is vascularised

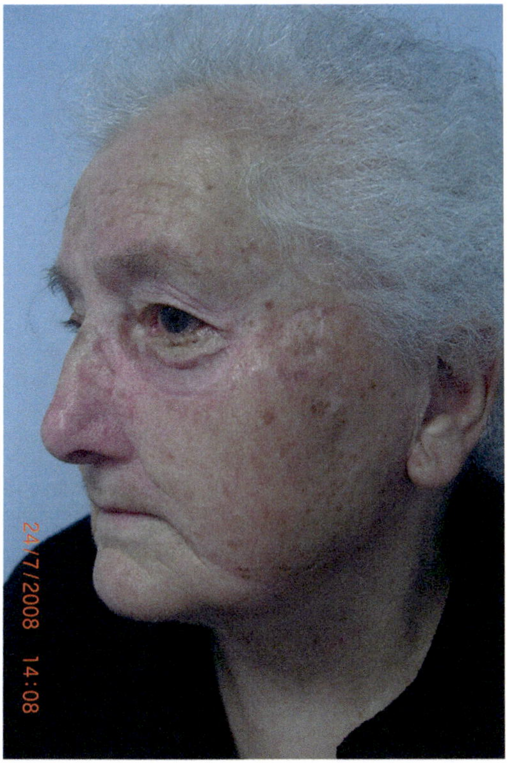

Fig. 2.431 The aesthetic outcome after the staged removal of sutures is shown, and the apical suture at the inner canthus is left in for 3 weeks

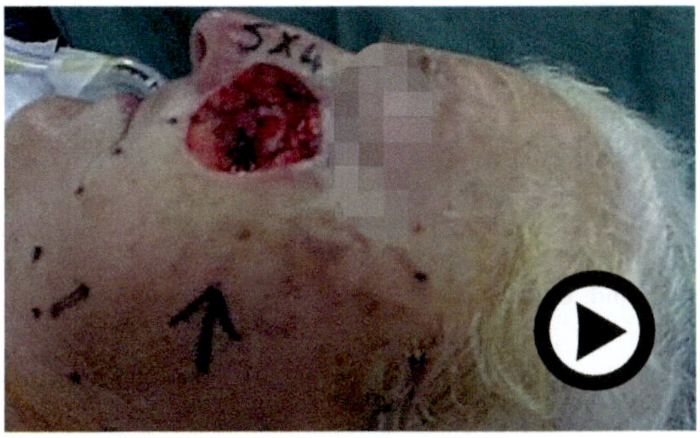

Fig. 2.432 Video 2.55 Planned operative reconstruction (▶ https://doi.org/10.1007/000-k7m)

The PACES characteristics were all exemplified: pain-free, aesthetic, no vascular complications, economical in terms of time and sensory recovery with the resolution of oedema.

2.1.5.4 Case 45—Another Nasolabial Lesion with the Potential for Causing Ectropion Pull

(Figs. 2.433, 2.434, 2.435, 2.436, 2.437, 2.438, 2.439, 2.440, 2.441 and 2.442)

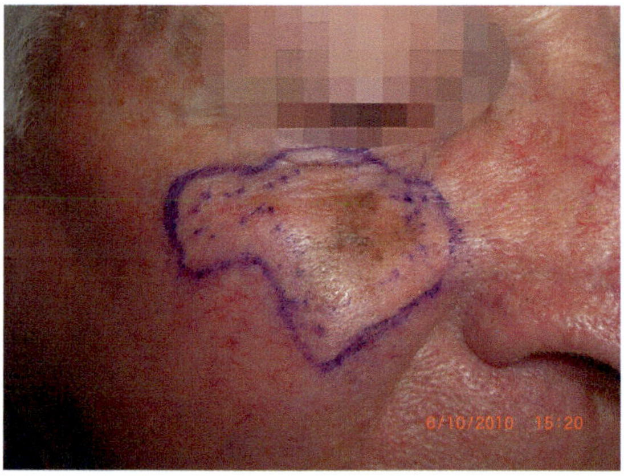

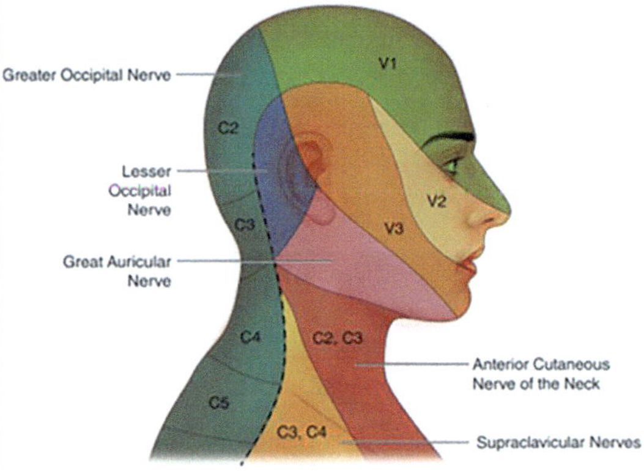

Fig. 2.433 The pigmented lesion is shown on presentation of level II melanoma. The dermatomal mark outs become the line of incision of the dermis and epidermis, ensuring that one-third deeply is attached with only partial undermining to facilitate the closure and vascular integrity of the defect. (Reprinted with permission from Atlas, *Reconstructive Technique in Melanoma Management* (p. 19), by Felix Behan, Springer Nature 2023)

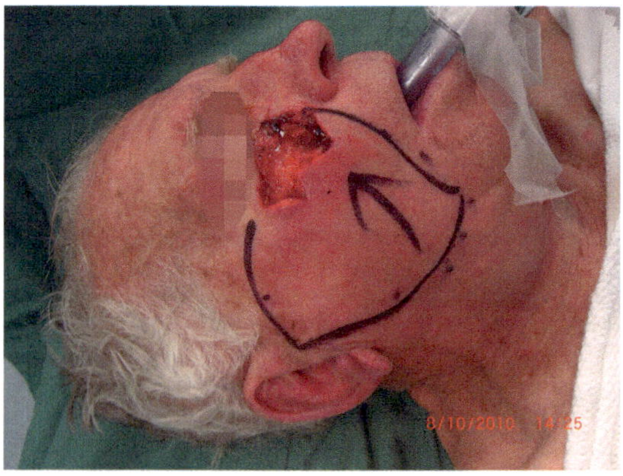

Fig. 2.434 The V2 dermatome is marked out to create the hypervascularity at the dermal-epidermal level on the basis of infraorbital V2 circulation, and the flap inserted into its definitive position to minimise ectropion

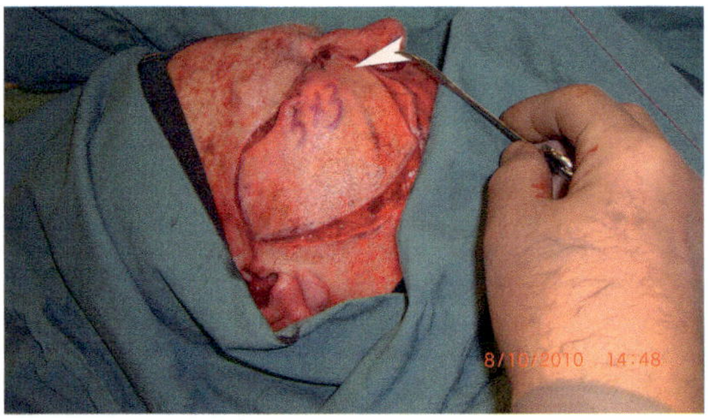

Fig. 2.435 Hypervascularity indicators and the vascular flare are evenly distributed, and the arrow indicates the red dot sign, consistent with perfusion to the tip, where the flap is fashioned to fill the defect, which is not dissimilar to tailoring and which thankfully reflects intrinsic expansion

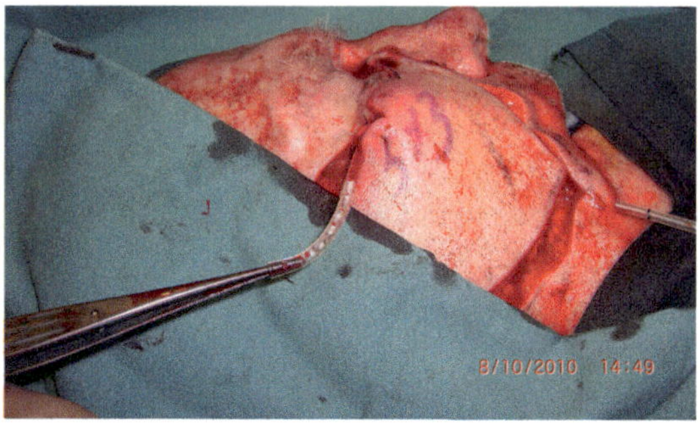

Fig. 2.436 Full V2 dermatome Keystone with a suction drainage support

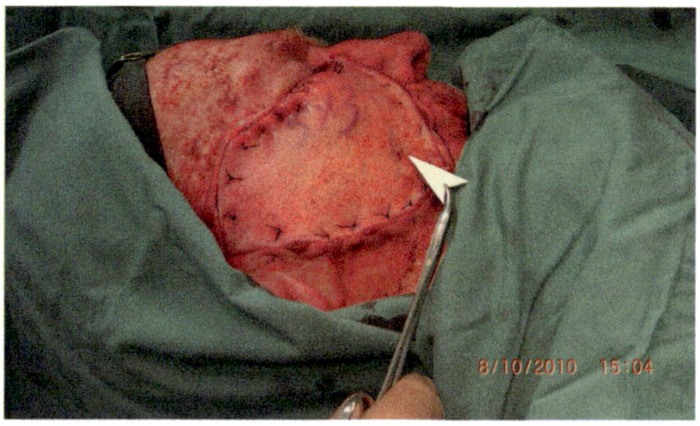

Fig. 2.437 the vascular flare is complete without defining perforators, and the red dot sign is dermal evidence of its complete perfusion

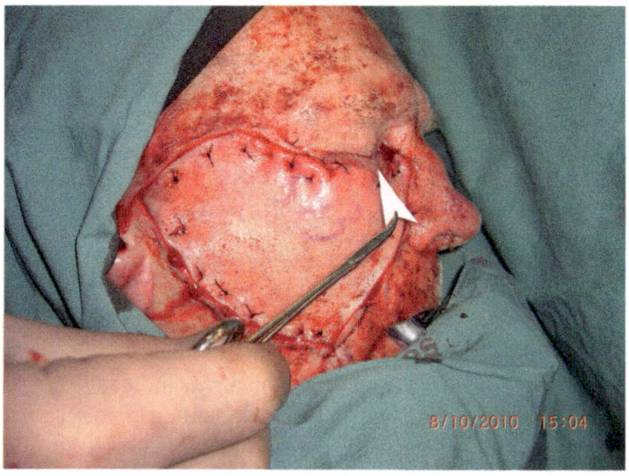

Fig. 2.438 The staged insertion of sutures

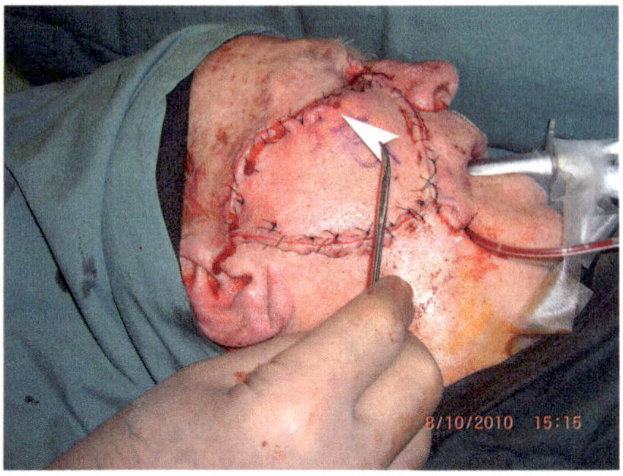

Fig. 2.439 The aesthetic appearance of wound closure with complete vascularity and the eversion of the suture margin, helping to achieve a good aesthetic closure

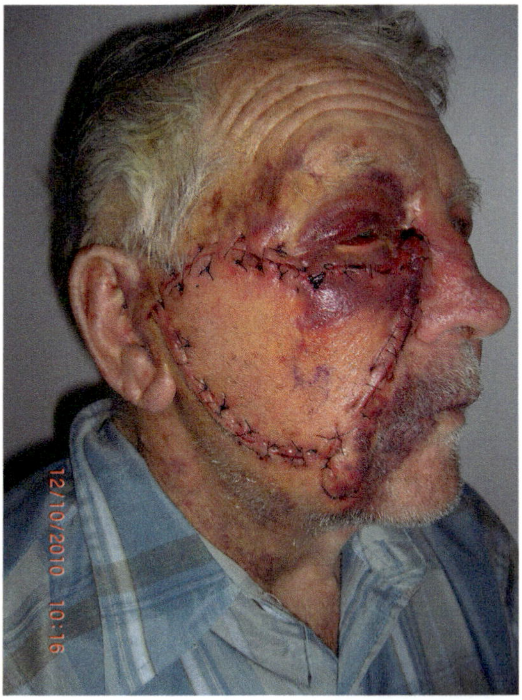

Fig. 2.440 Appearance at 4 days, requiring only eye toilets

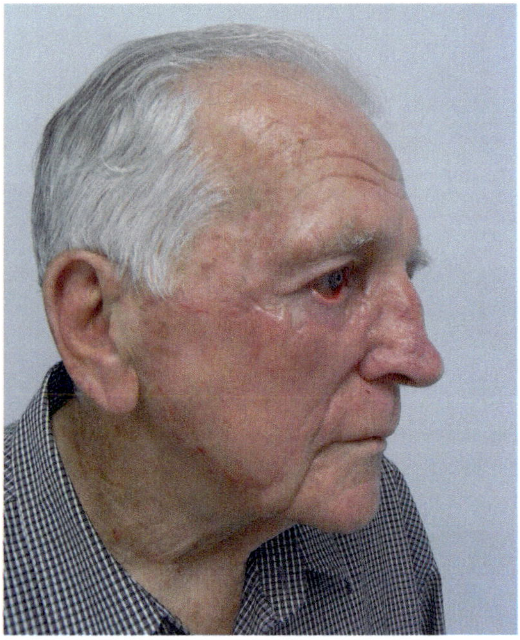

Fig. 2.441 The appearance at 2 months is shown, and the patient is extremely happy with the outcome

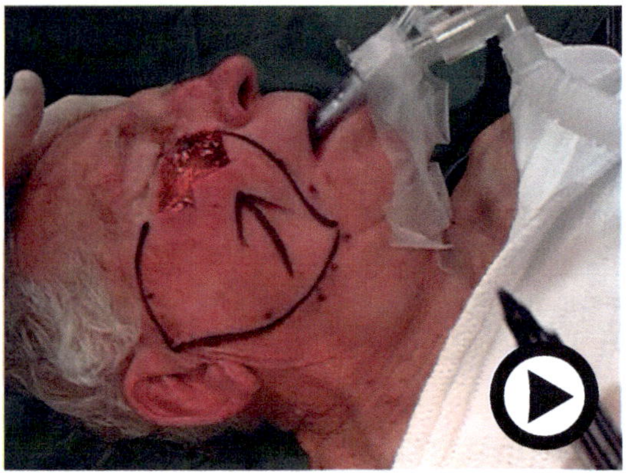

Fig. 2.442 Video 2.56 Planned operative reconstruction (▶ https://doi.org/10.1007/000-k7n)

The PACES characteristics were all exemplified: pain-free, aesthetic, no vascular complications, economical in terms of time and sensory recovery with the resolution of oedema.

2.1.5.5 Case 46—Recurrent Merkel Cell R Cheek

Case 46 shows another example of intrinsic expansion where the ageing tissue is supple enough to fill the defect like an example of tailoring, yet the delineations around the dermatomes with the fascial base support ensure its success (Figs. 2.443, 2.444, 2.445, 2.446, 2.447, 2.448, 2.449, 2.450, 2.451, 2.452, 2.453, 2.454, 2.455, 2.456, 2.457, 2.458, 2.459, 2.460 and 2.461).

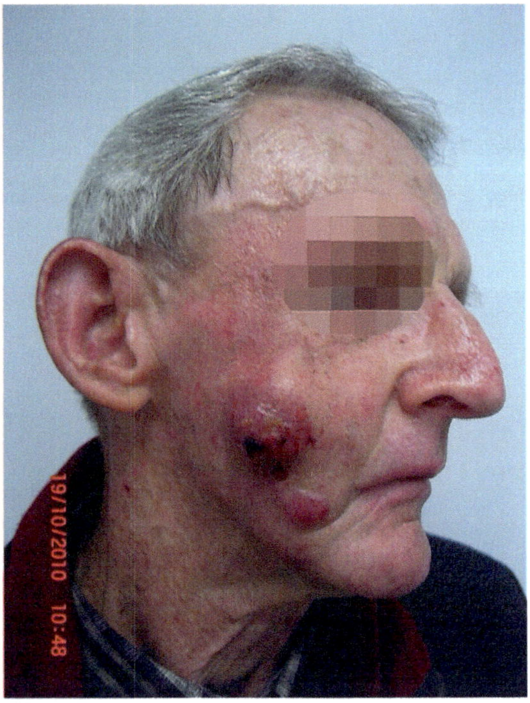

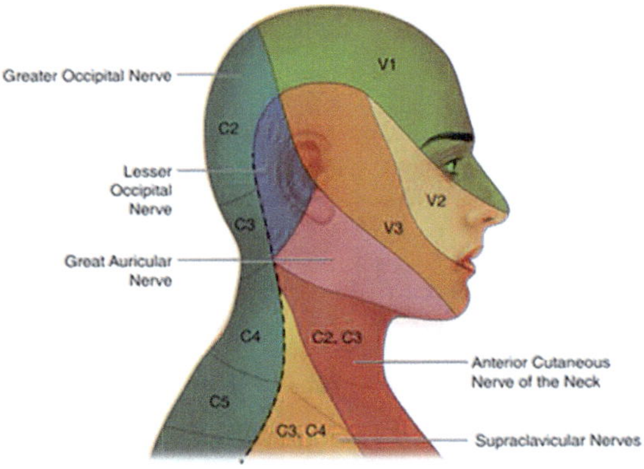

Fig. 2.443 Prior to excision. The dermatomal mark outs become the line of incision of the dermis and epidermis, ensuring that one-third deeply is attached with only partial undermining to facilitate the closure and vascular integrity of the defect. (Reprinted with permission from Atlas, *Reconstructive Technique in Melanoma Management* (p. 19), by Felix Behan, Springer Nature 2023)

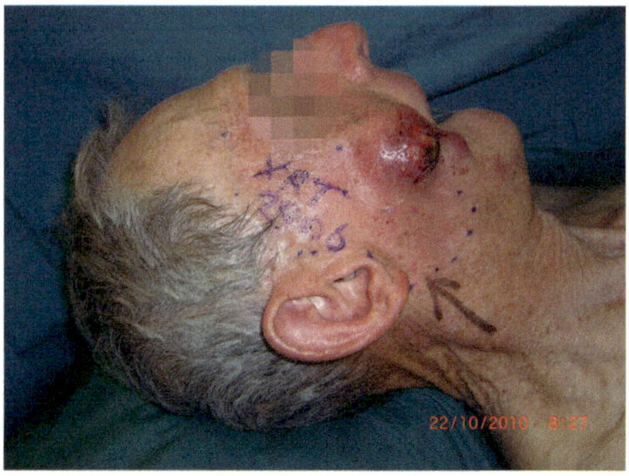

Fig. 2.444 The outline of the surgical margins for clearance

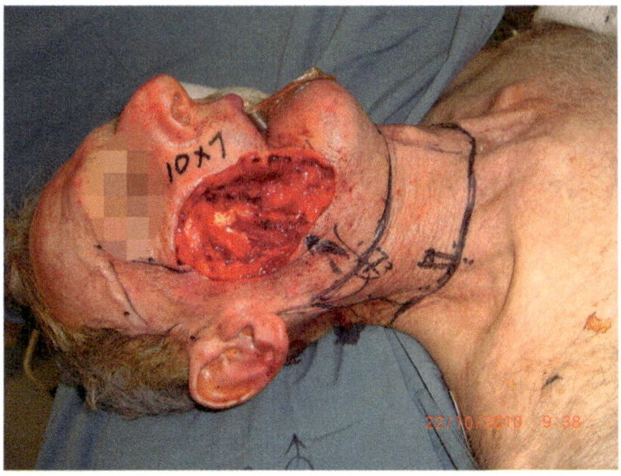

Fig. 2.446 Releasing incision in the R temple takes the tension off the wound

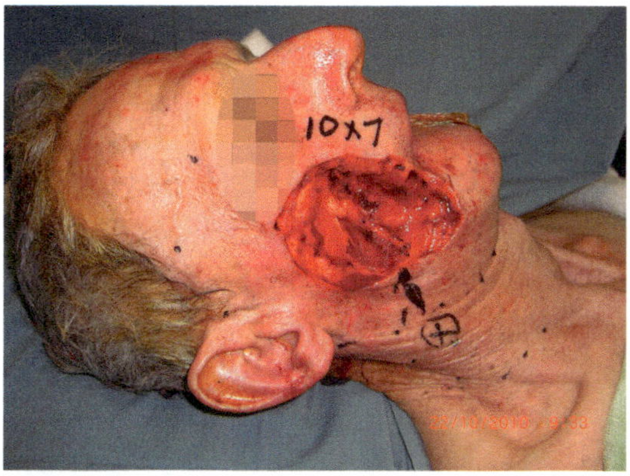

Fig. 2.445 The outline of the Keystone in the C2 dermatome

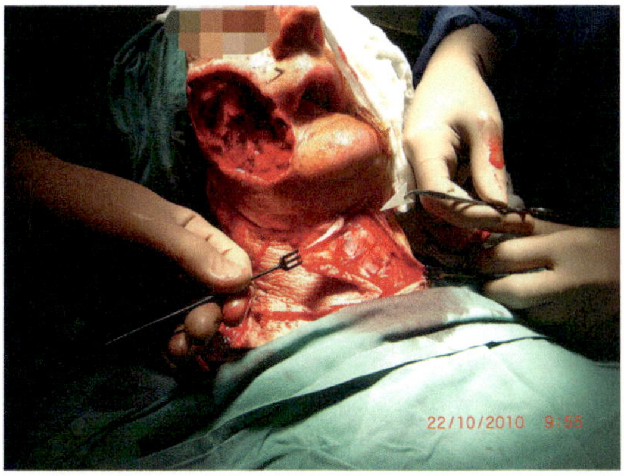

Fig. 2.447 The retraction of the flap in the neck is shown, and the white arrow indicates the upper perfusion

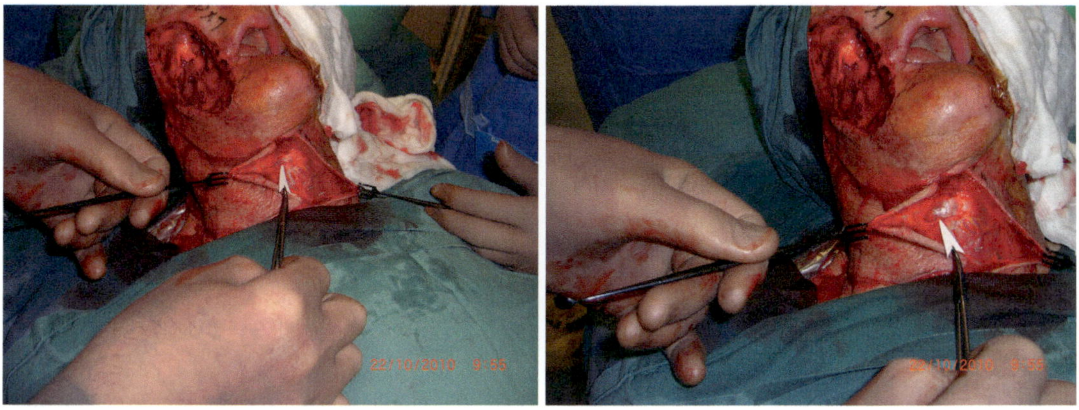

Fig. 2.448 Random perforators at the base of the cervical Keystone, which are closed with Weck clips, with the undermined part of the flap retracted at the cervical fascial level

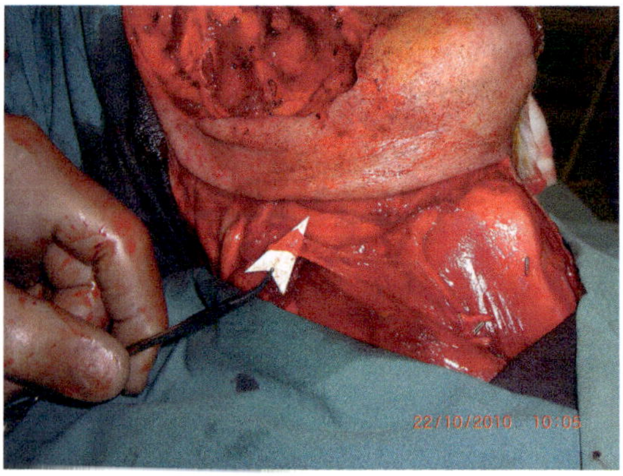

Fig. 2.449 Arrow highlighting the cervical fascia, which is the basis for the Keystone's success

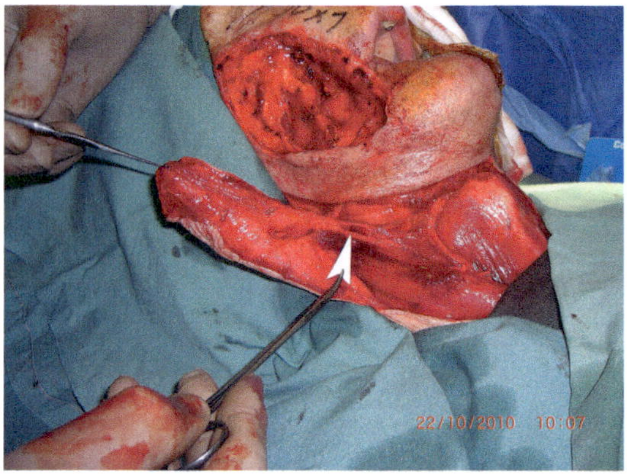

Fig. 2.450 More cervical fascia indications underneath the chin

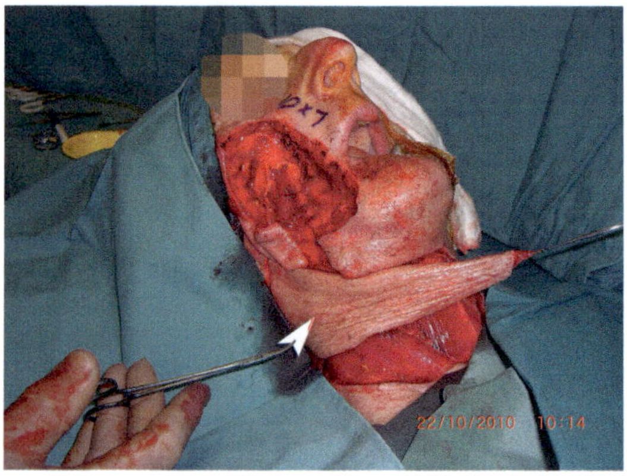

Fig. 2.451 The flap elevated and stretched before rotation and advancement into the nasolabial region to repair the facial defect. The cervical Keystone is inserted into this facial defect

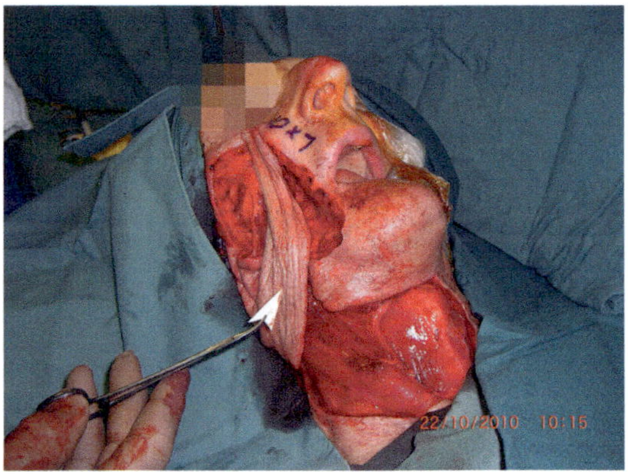

Fig. 2.452 Staged insertion is shown, and note the pink flare of the hypervascularity

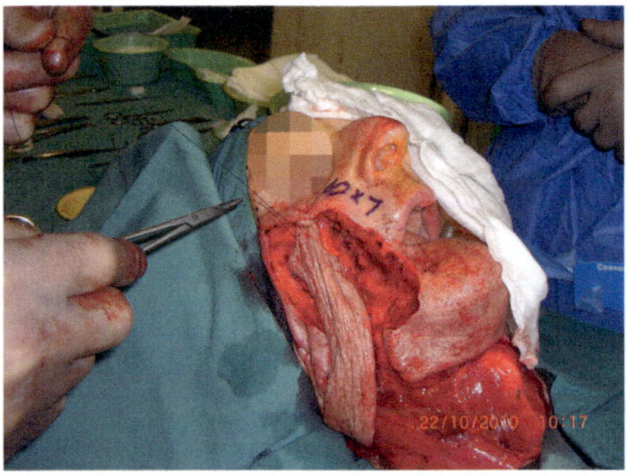

Fig. 2.453 Further closure sutures for the 10 × 7 cm defect, with the apical suture placed to avoid ectropion pull

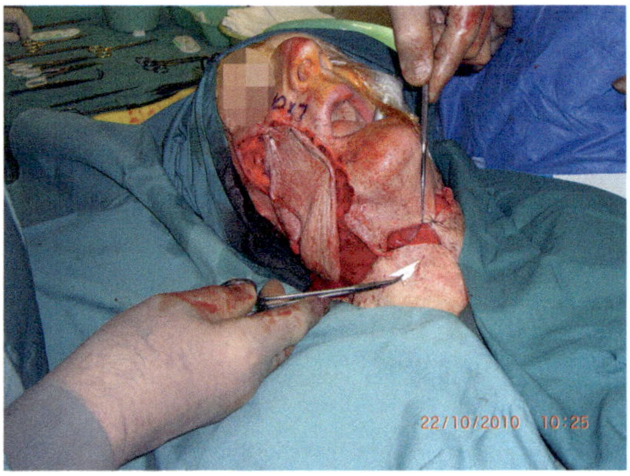

Fig. 2.454 Closure of the secondary defect with locking mattress sutures inserted for 3 weeks

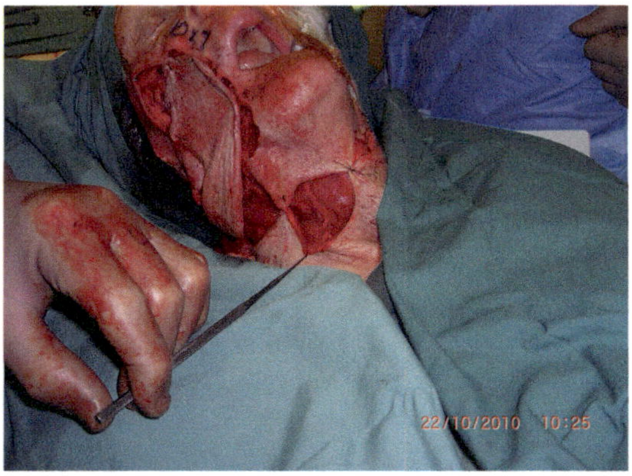

Fig. 2.455 The staged closure of the neck defect

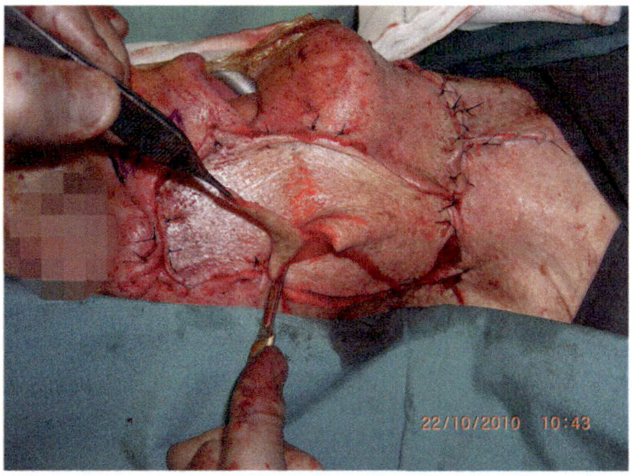

Fig. 2.456 The hypervascularity allows the excision of the dog ear, avoiding a secondary procedure for an aesthetic outcome

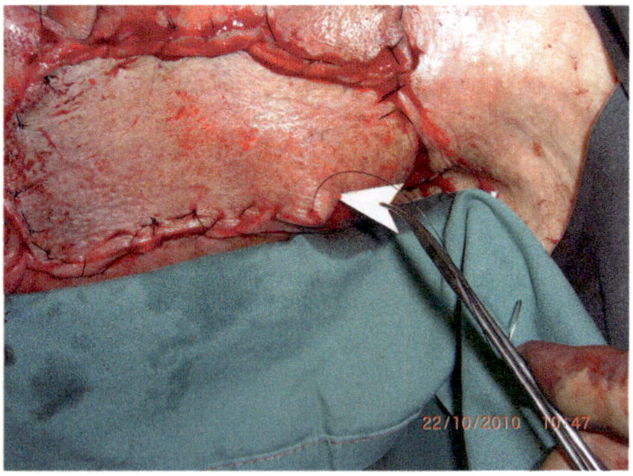

Fig. 2.457 Another dog ear trimmed because the flap rotation reveals the redundancy of tissue

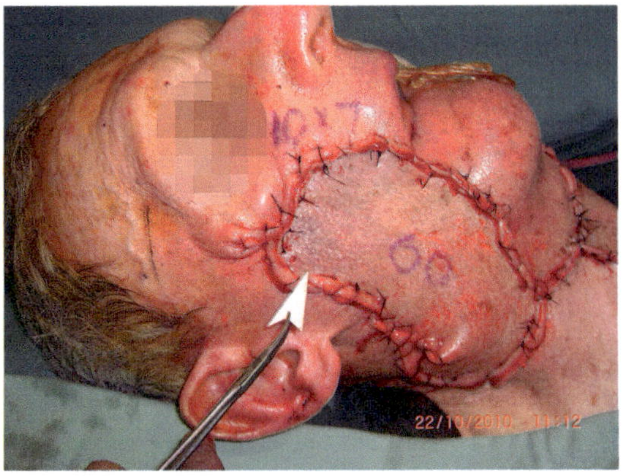

Fig. 2.458 The timeframe and the closure of 60 min are indicated. Free flap timeframe would take hours

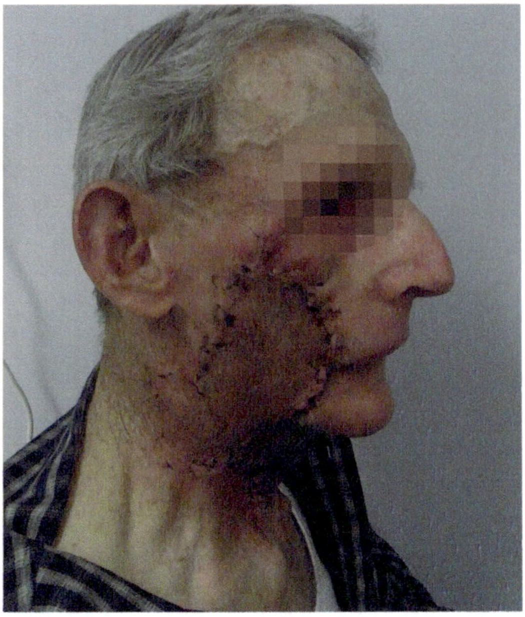

Fig. 2.459 Appearance at 3 weeks, showing no severe ectropion

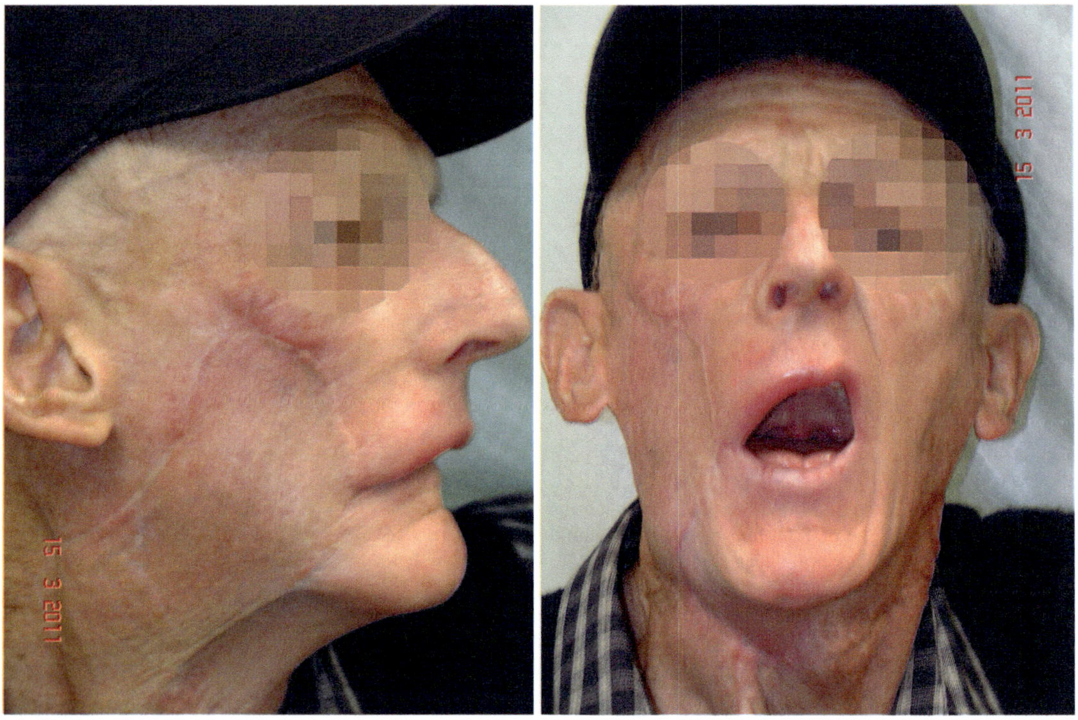

Fig. 2.460 The appearance at 5 months with just a mild facial neuropraxia of the buccal branch of the facial nerve, no doubt reflecting its initial pathology and proximity to the tumour growth, which is of no concern to the patient. It was skeletonised, but it was not resected, as was our policy with Prof. Andrew Sizeland, because it showed no involvement

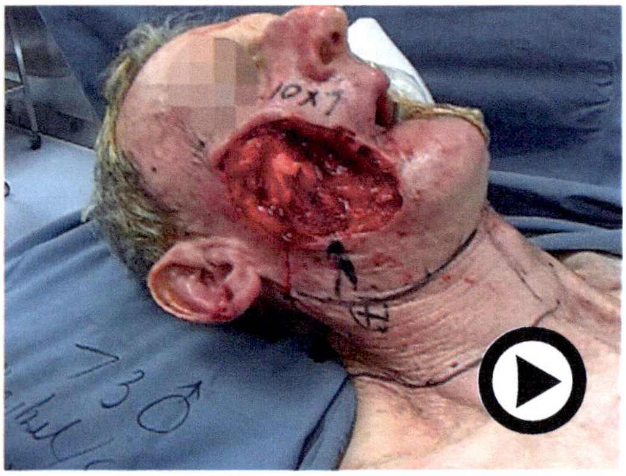

Fig. 2.461 Video 2.57 Planned operative reconstruction (▶ https://doi.org/10.1007/000-k7p)

The PACES characteristics were all exemplified: pain-free, aesthetic, no vascular complications, economical in terms of time and sensory recovery with the resolution of oedema.

2.1.5.6 Case 47—A Full-Cheek Defect from the Nasolabial Crease to the Preauricular Line

The repeat evidence of intrinsic expansion is once more illustrated, where the tissues are fashioned to fit the defect, relying on the integrity of the hypervascularity created by the Keystone concept, as detailed below (Figs. 2.462, 2.463, 2.464, 2.465, 2.466 and 2.467).

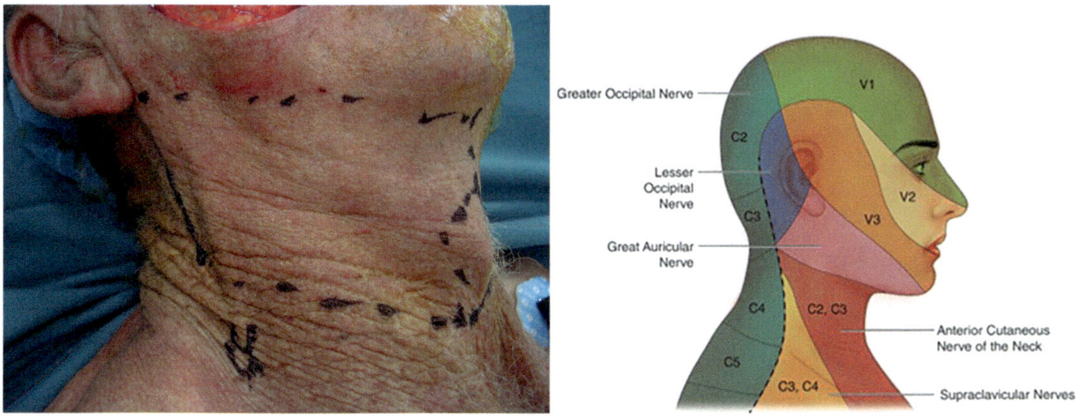

Fig. 2.462 The lines of the mark out are used to help hypervascularise the flap at the dermal-epidermal level, leaving the axis of rotation around the base of the sterno-mastoid attachment. The dermatomal mark outs become the line of incision of the dermis and epidermis, ensuring that one-third deeply is attached with only partial undermining to facilitate the closure and vascular integrity of the defect. (Reprinted with permission from Atlas, *Reconstructive Technique in Melanoma Management* (p. 19), by Felix Behan, Springer Nature 2023)

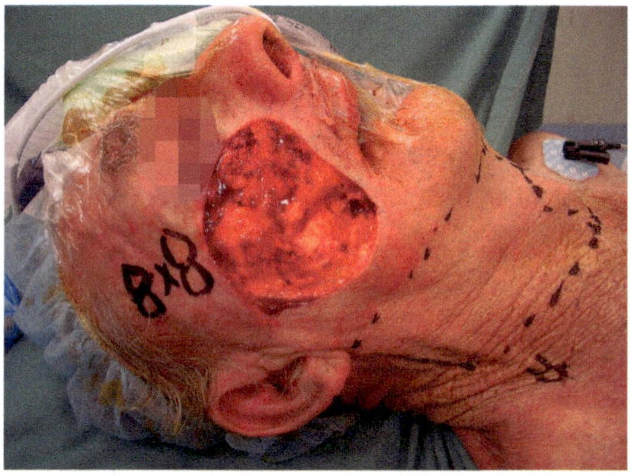

Fig. 2.463 The 8 × 8 cm defect is not insubstantial, and the Keystone supplies an aesthetic solution

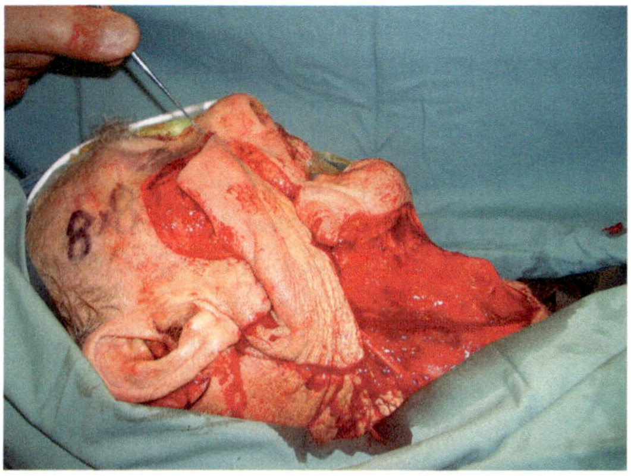

Fig. 2.465 The staged insertion before the neck is closed directly

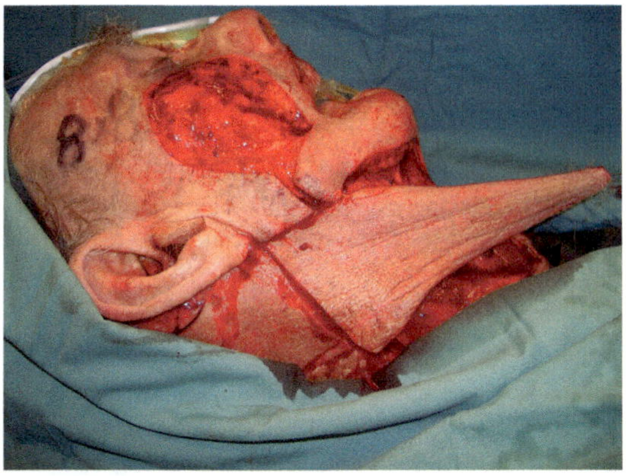

Fig. 2.464 The flap about to be inserted is shown, and note that the red dot sign confirms its vascular reliability. Size is not a contraindication for Keystone usefulness; the intrinsic expansion reflects this wide surgical application; and the flap is tailored to fill the defect aesthetically. The Keystone can be applied with all these variables by using a flap with wide reconstructive applications

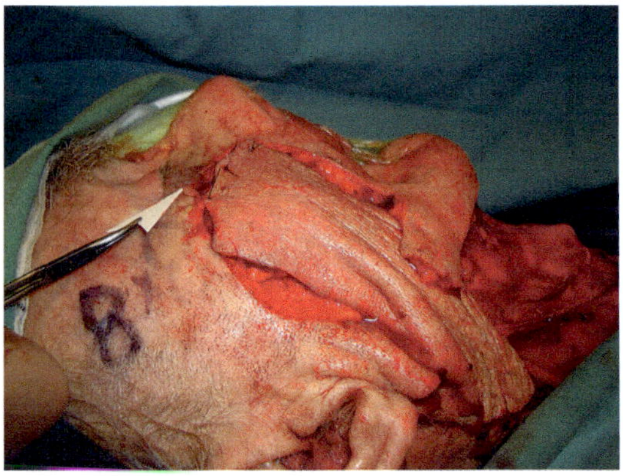

Fig. 2.466 The flap is inserted to avoid any ectropion pull

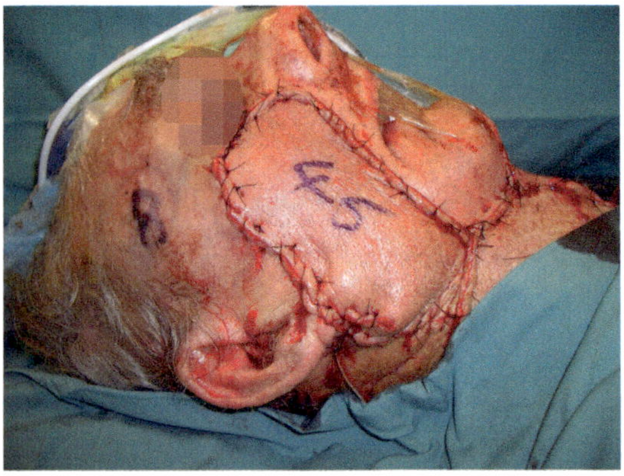

Fig. 2.467 The timeframe and the locking mattress tension suture in the neck must stay in for 3 weeks

The PACES characteristics were all exemplified: pain-free, aesthetic, no vascular complications, economical in terms of time and sensory recovery with the resolution of oedema.

2.1.5.7 Case 48—15 × 13 cm Large Size Is Rarely a Contraindication for Keystone Insertion

(Figs. 2.468, 2.469, 2.470, 2.471, 2.472 and 2.473)

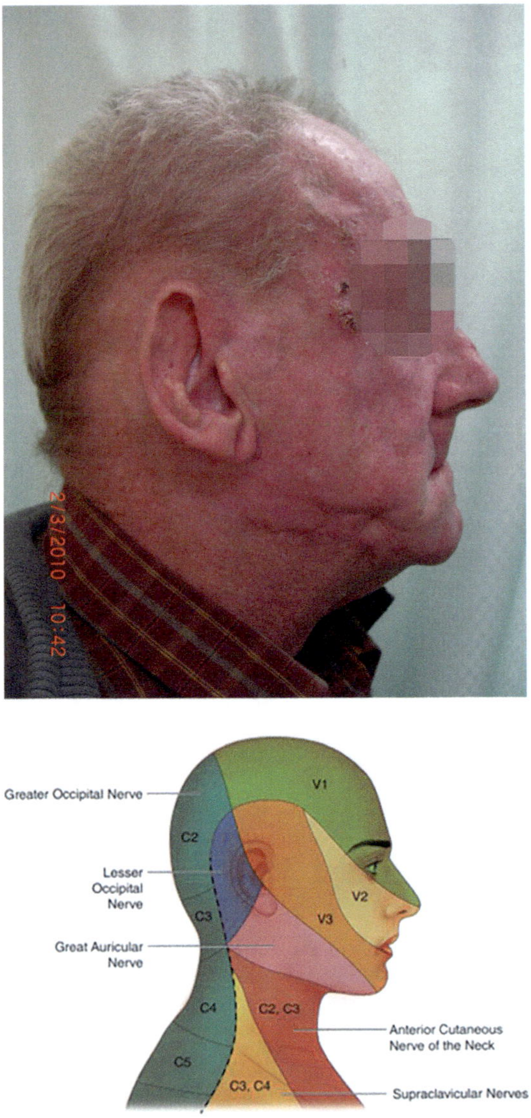

Fig. 2.468 Patient on presentation with SCCs of the cheek is shown. The dermatomal mark outs become the line of incision of the dermis and epidermis, ensuring that one-third deeply is attached with only partial undermining to facilitate the closure and vascular integrity of the defect. (Reprinted with permission from Atlas, *Reconstructive Technique in Melanoma Management* (p. 19), by Felix Behan, Springer Nature 2023)

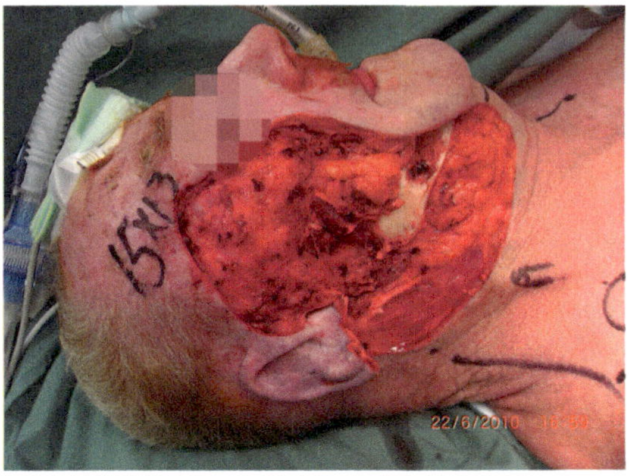

Fig. 2.469 The 15 × 13 cm defect and the mark out of the cervical Keystone

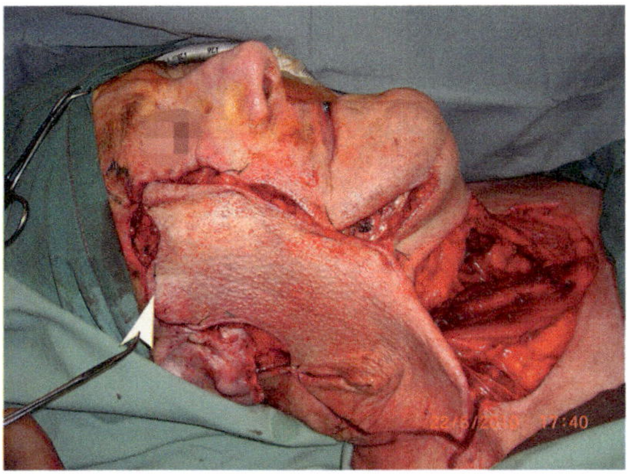

Fig. 2.470 Stages of the closure before the neck wound is closed directly under tension using locking mattress sutures

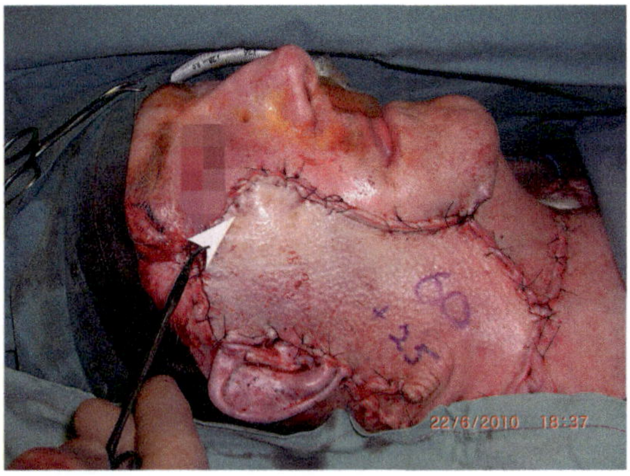

Fig. 2.471 Recovery of perfusion with the timeframes indicated (60 + 25), showing no vascular necrosis, and full vascular perfusion is reflected in its pink colour. This is an extensive defect, and the malleability of the Keystone is once more a reflection of its adaptability, enclosing surgical defects without reverting to alternative methods

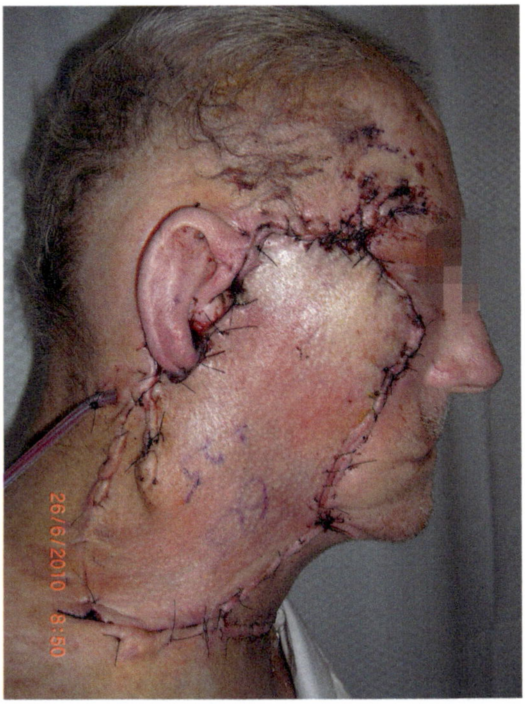

Fig. 2.472 Postoperative 4-day appearance with some slight vascular impedance

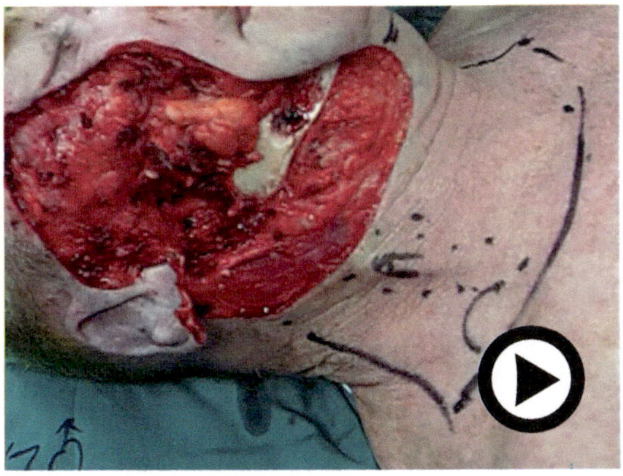

Fig. 2.473 Video 2.58 Planned operative reconstruction (▶ https://doi.org/10.1007/000-k7q)

The PACES characteristics were all exemplified: pain-free, aesthetic, no vascular complications, economical in terms of time and sensory recovery with the resolution of oedema.

2.1.5.8 Case 49—A 10 × 5 cm Cheek Defect Closed in 35 min (Figs. 2.474, 2.475, 2.476, 2.477, 2.478, 2.479, 2.480 and 2.481)

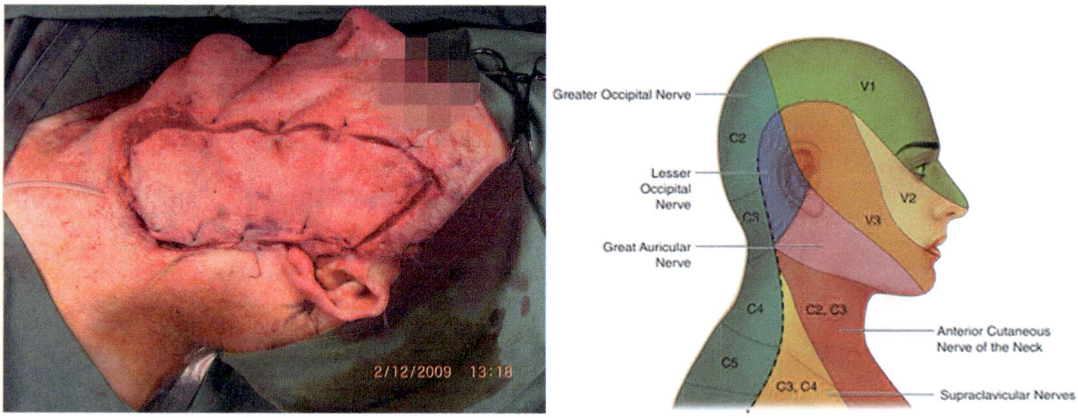

Fig. 2.474 The hypervascularisation is evident following the delineation after the dermatomal mark out, where the skin and epidermis are incised prior to direct closure after transfer. The dermatomal mark outs become the line of incision of the dermis and epidermis, ensuring that one-third deeply is attached with only partial undermining to facilitate the closure and vascular integrity of the defect. (Reprinted with permission from Atlas, *Reconstructive Technique in Melanoma Management* (p. 19), by Felix Behan, Springer Nature 2023)

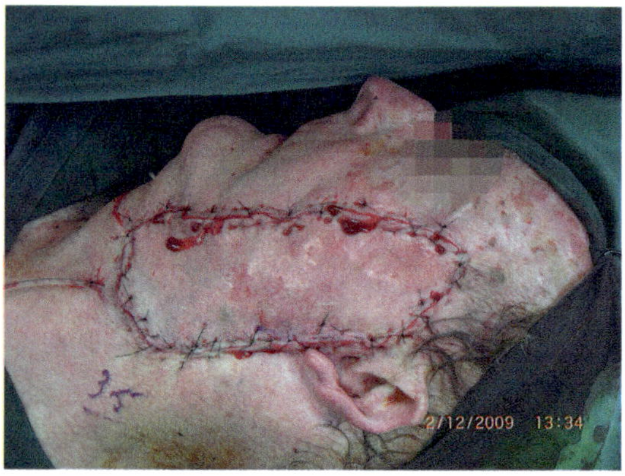

Fig. 2.475 Fully vascularised, hyperaemia is noted, and the red dot signs appear at the tension suture sites

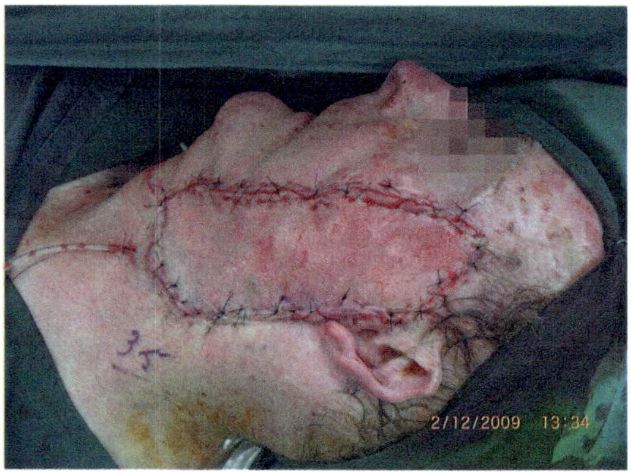

Fig. 2.476 On completion

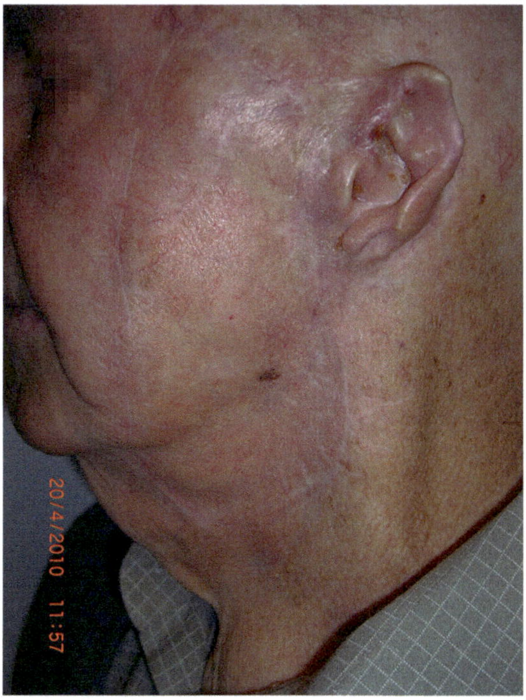

Fig. 2.477 Appearance at 4 months, with a totally contented patient

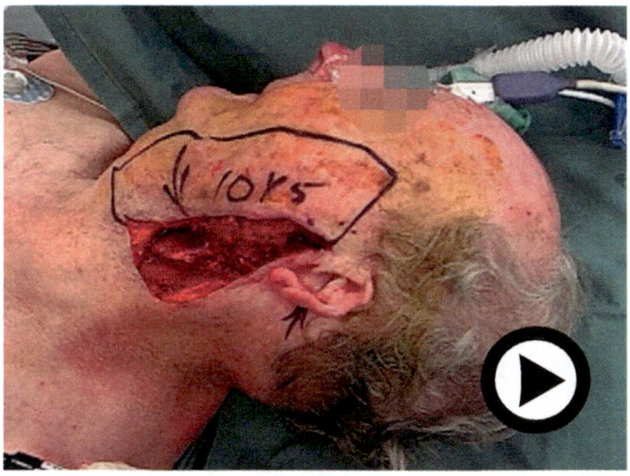

Fig. 2.478 Video 2.59 Planned operative reconstruction (▶ https://doi.org/10.1007/000-k7r)

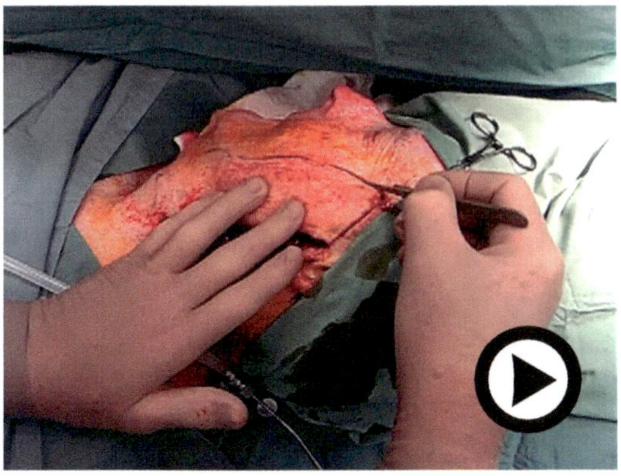

Fig. 2.479 Video 2.60 Islanding the Keystone flap via the division of the dermal-epidermal line (▶ https://doi.org/10.1007/000-k7s)

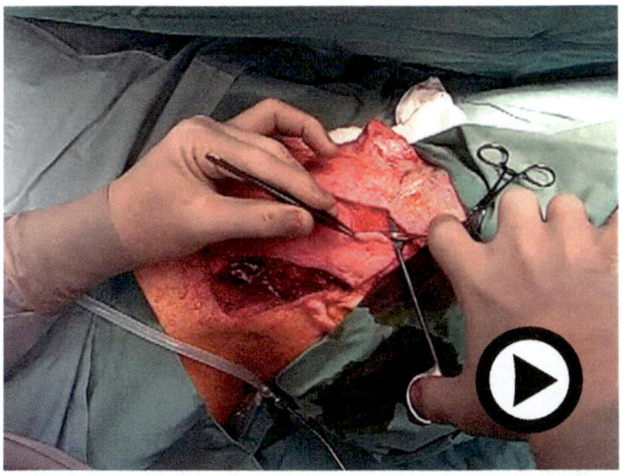

Fig. 2.480 Video 2.61 The blunt dissection technique is shown using scissors to separate the tissue planes to allow it to fit. There is minimal sharp dissection, whereas the blunt dissection retains any incontinuity from the microperforators without division, thus preserving its intact circulation. Note the hyperaemic flare preserving the vascular continuity (▶ https://doi.org/10.1007/000-k7t)

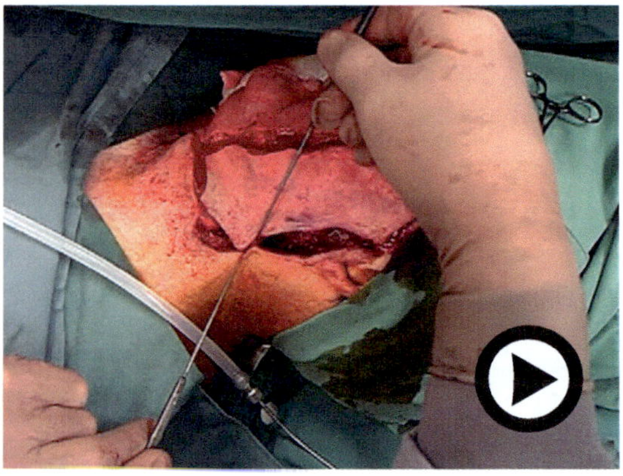

Fig. 2.481 Video 2.62 Approximating the insertion of the Keystone into the defect to minimise lines of tension (▶ https://doi.org/10.1007/000-k7v)

The PACES characteristics were all exemplified: pain-free, aesthetic, no vascular complications, economical in terms of time and sensory recovery with the resolution of oedema.

2.1.5.9 Case 50—Nodular SCC on the Jawline

Case 50 is another example of the adaptability of the Keystone regardless of the site or size, but the designs demonstrate that the repairs can be successfully completed when based on embryological principles (Figs. 2.482, 2.483, 2.484, 2.485, 2.486, 2.487, 2.488, 2.489, 2.490, 2.491, 2.492, 2.493, 2.494, 2.495, 2.496, 2.497, 2.498, 2.499, 2.500, 2.501, 2.502 and 2.503).

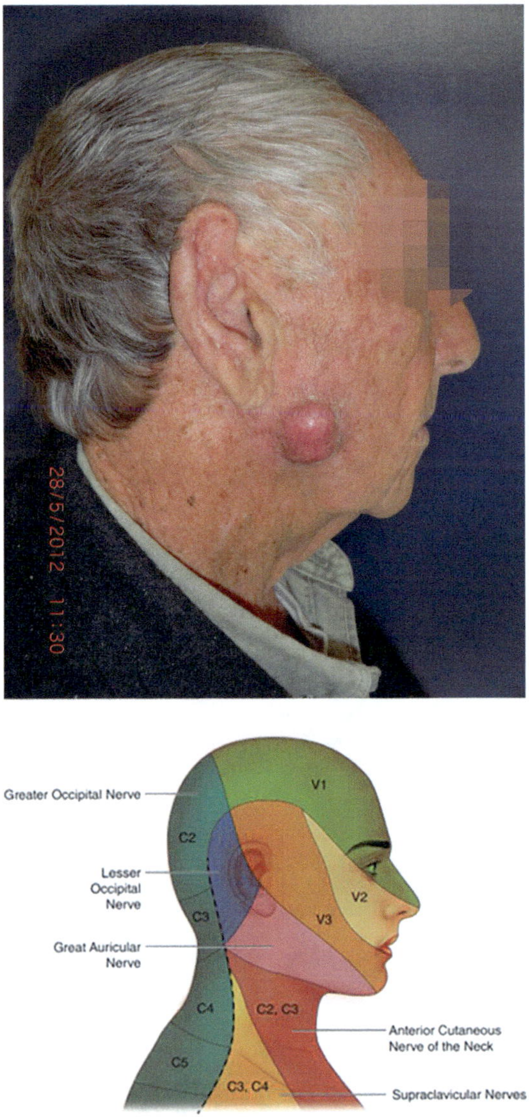

Fig. 2.482 The patient presents with SCC along the line of the mandible below the parotid. The dermatomal mark outs become the line of incision of the dermis and epidermis, ensuring that one-third deeply is attached with only partial undermining to facilitate the closure and vascular integrity of the defect. (Reprinted with permission from Atlas, *Reconstructive Technique in Melanoma Management* (p. 19), by Felix Behan, Springer Nature 2023)

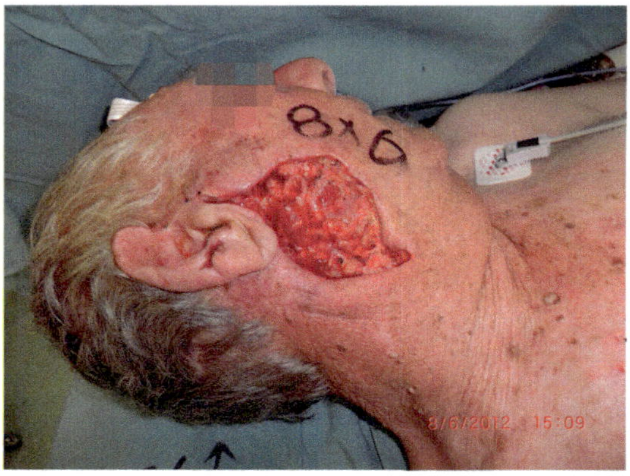

Fig. 2.483 The 8 × 6 cm clinical defect

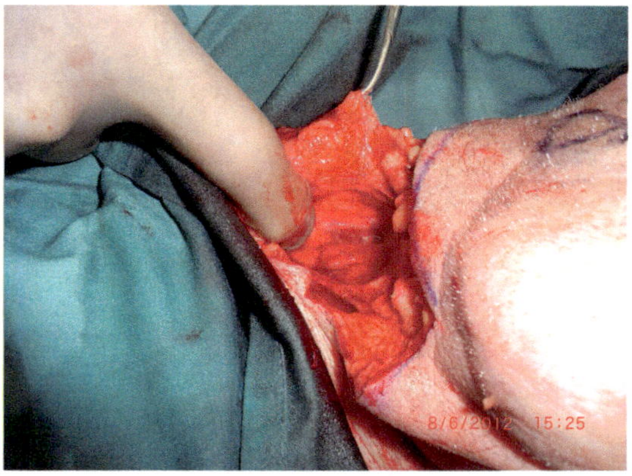

Fig. 2.484 The site of the perforators at the limits of the sternomastoid base

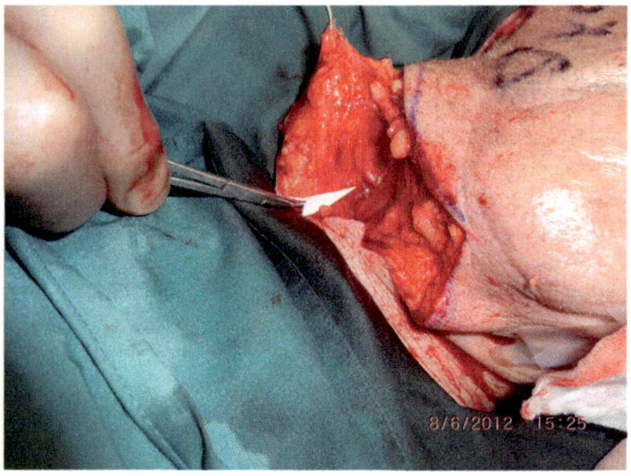

Fig. 2.485 Prior to haemostasis with the Weck clip

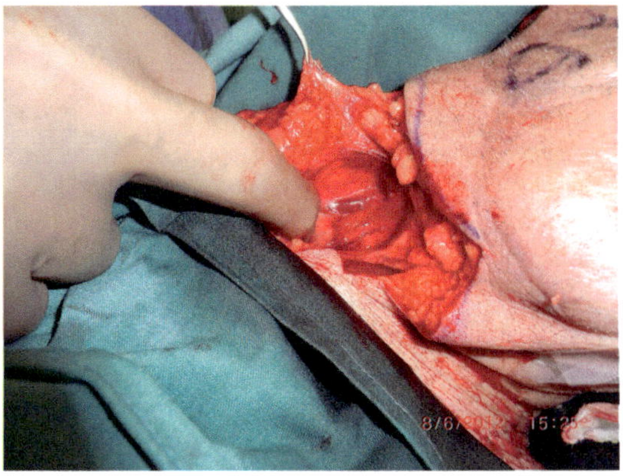

Fig. 2.486 Various perforators at the base of the sterno-mastoid protected by the cervical fascia

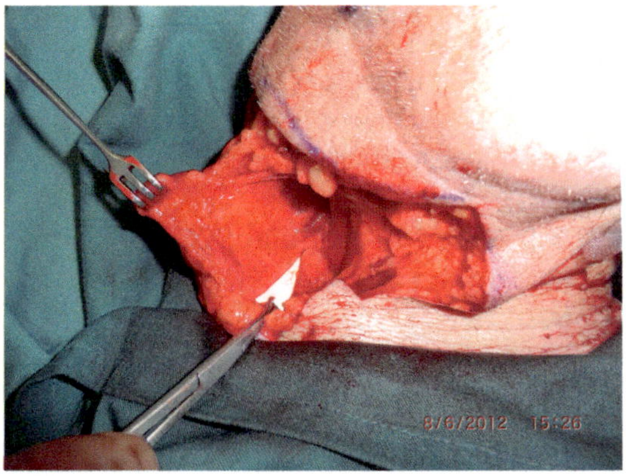

Fig. 2.487 Arrow showing the intact cervical fascia

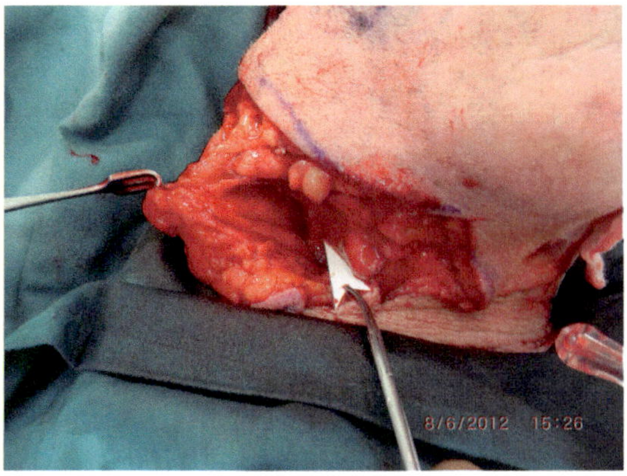

Fig. 2.488 Arrow indicating various structures in the neck dissection, such as the vagus nerve

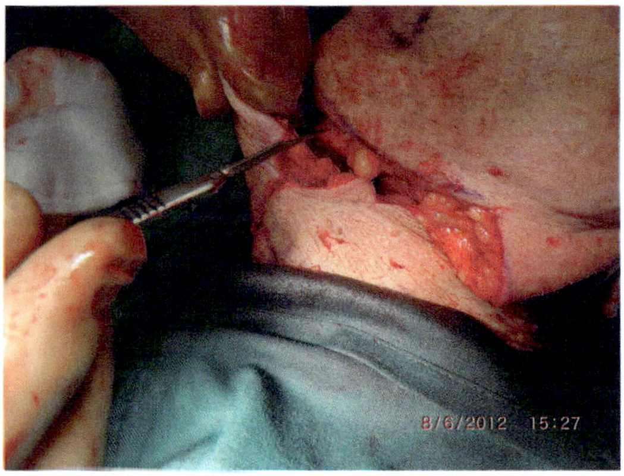

Fig. 2.489 The reliability of the vascular perfusion allows the trimming of dog ears in the acute phase

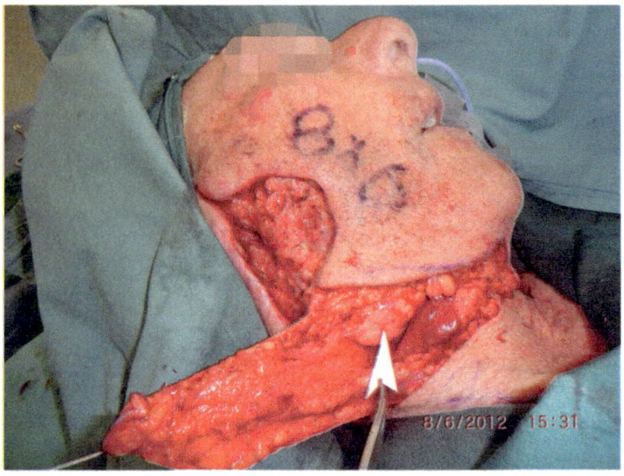

Fig. 2.490 Skirting over the submandibular gland with the intact cervical fascia in the Keystone

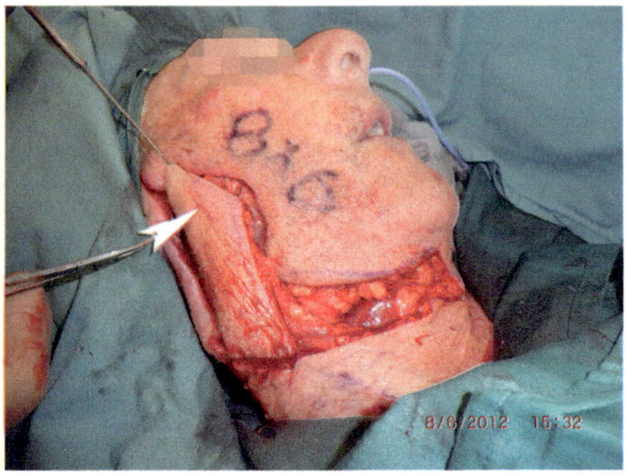

Fig. 2.491 Prior to insertion before the neck closure is done with locking mattress sutures

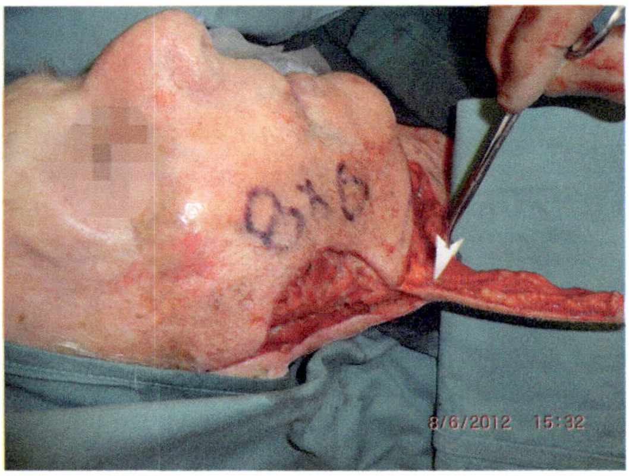

Fig. 2.492 Arrow indicating perfusional dynamics

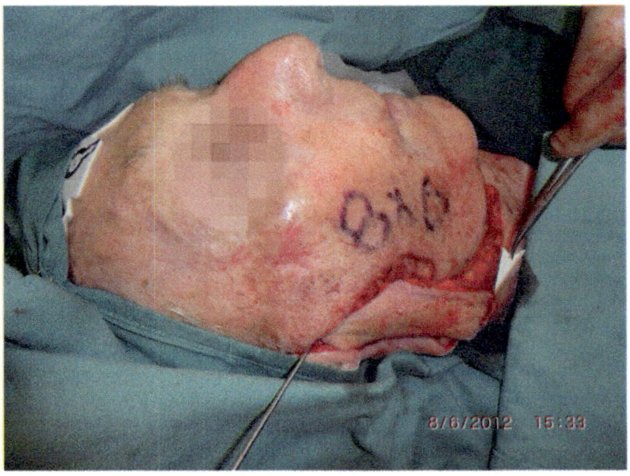

Fig. 2.493 Prior to closure

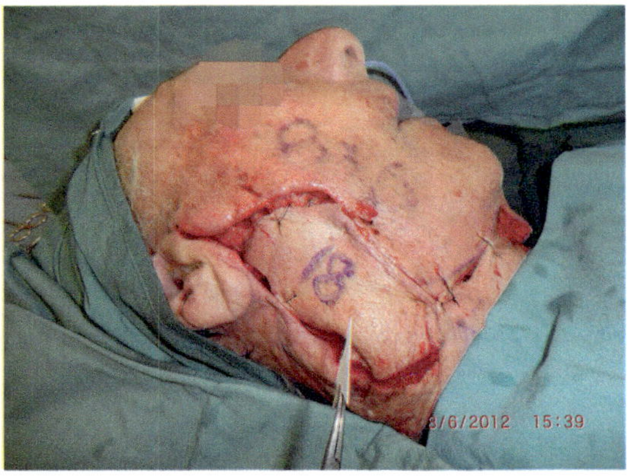

Fig. 2.494 18 min, as timestamped

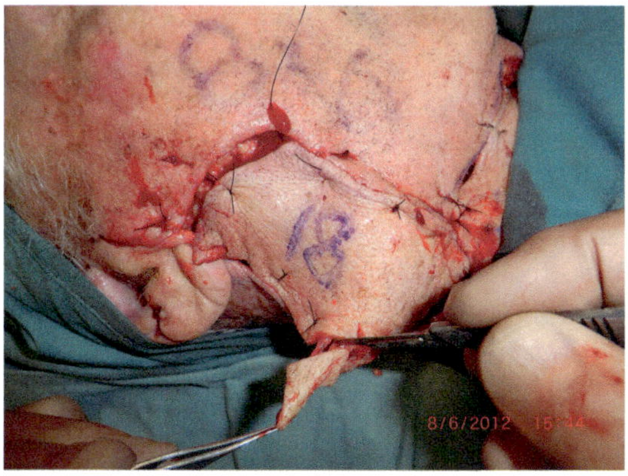

Fig. 2.495 Trimming the dog ear in the acute phase to avoid any readmission for aesthetic scar revision

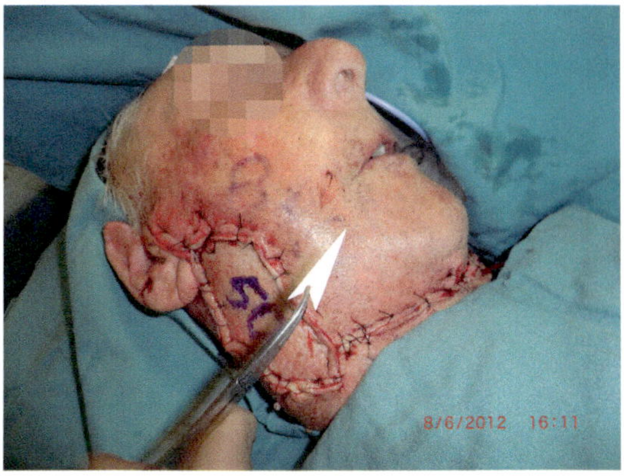

Fig. 2.498 Vascular perfusion is complete in spite of tensional closure

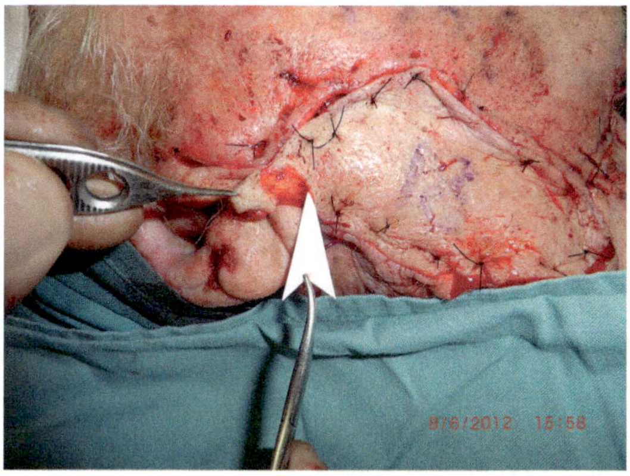

Fig. 2.496 A robust flow in the subdermal plexus

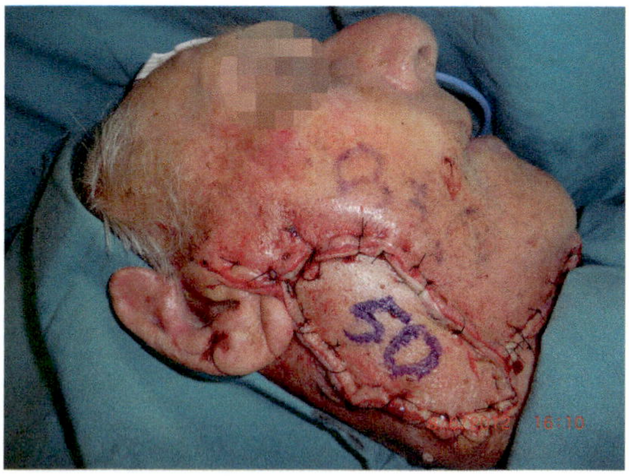

Fig. 2.497 Timeframe of 50 min for an 8 × 6 cm defect

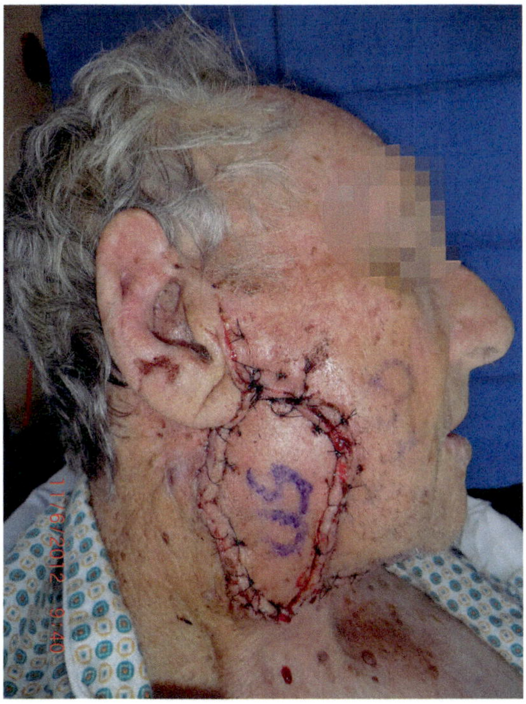

Fig. 2.499 Appearance at 3 days

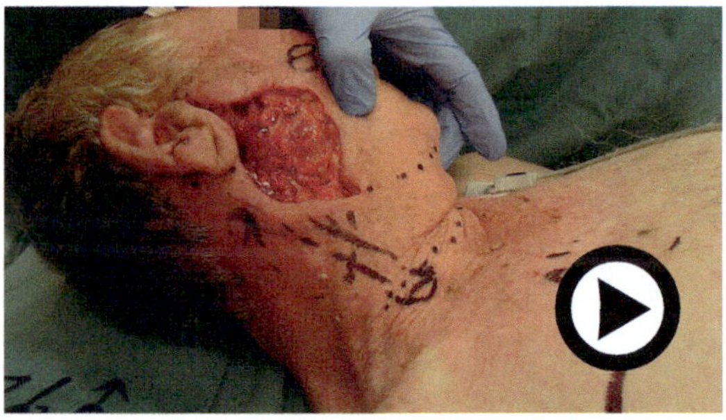

Fig. 2.500 Video 2.63 The details of raising a cervico-submental Keystone for a parotid defect and marking out the external jugular vein to preserve its continuity (▶ https://doi.org/10.1007/000-k7w)

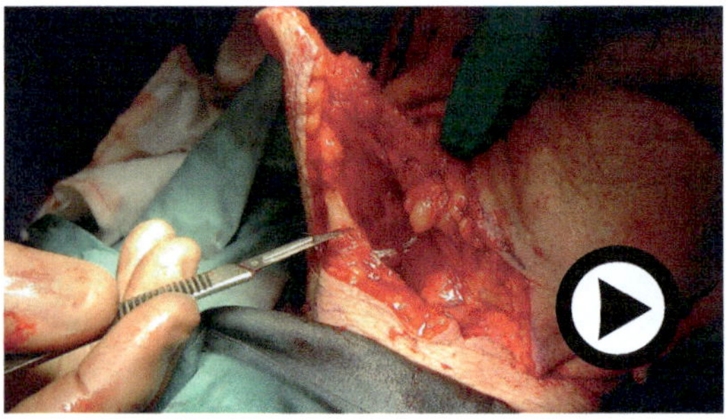

Fig. 2.501 Video 2.64 The fascial layer and the retained circulation support for the Keystone design (▶ https://doi.org/10.1007/000-k7x)

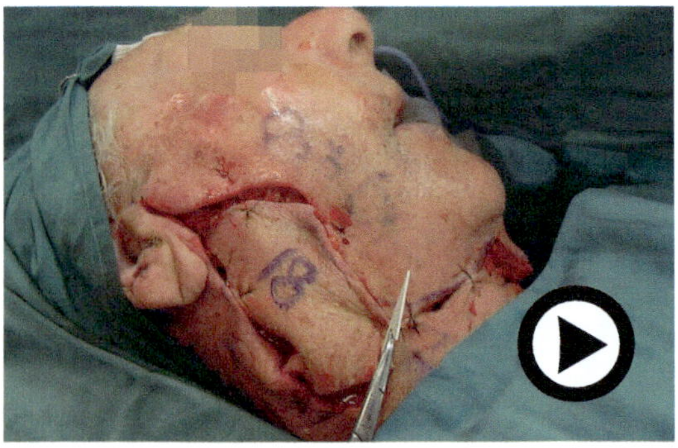

Fig. 2.502 Video 2.65 Indicating the timeframe and the stages in wound closure (▶ https://doi.org/10.1007/000-k7y)

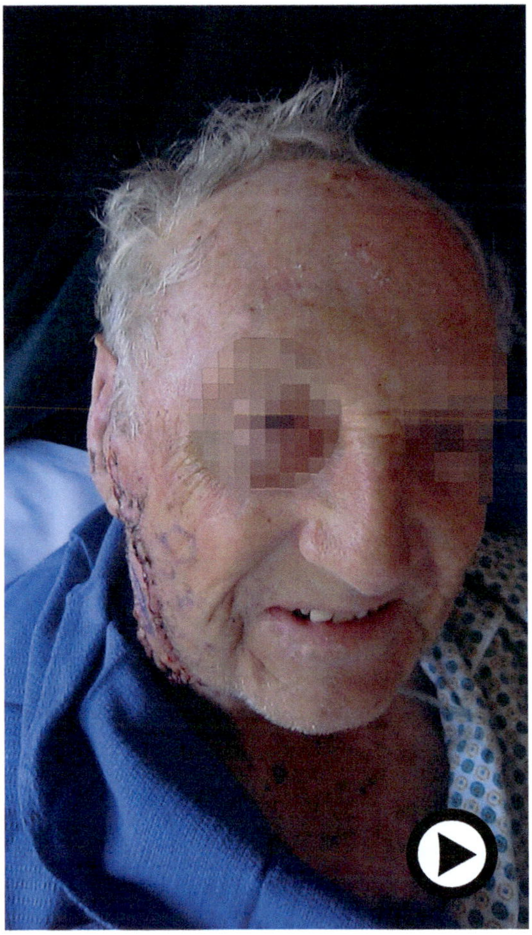

Fig. 2.503 Video 2.66 Patient's postoperative response, indicating his satisfaction in this pain-free stage of the repair (▶ https://doi.org/10.1007/000-k7z)

The PACES characteristics were all exemplified: pain-free, aesthetic, no vascular complications, economical in terms of time and sensory recovery with the resolution of oedema.

2.1.5.10 Case 51—Incomplete SCC Removal for Re-excision (Figs. 2.504, 2.505, 2.506, 2.507, 2.508, 2.509, 2.510, 2.511, 2.512, 2.513, 2.514, 2.515 and 2.516)

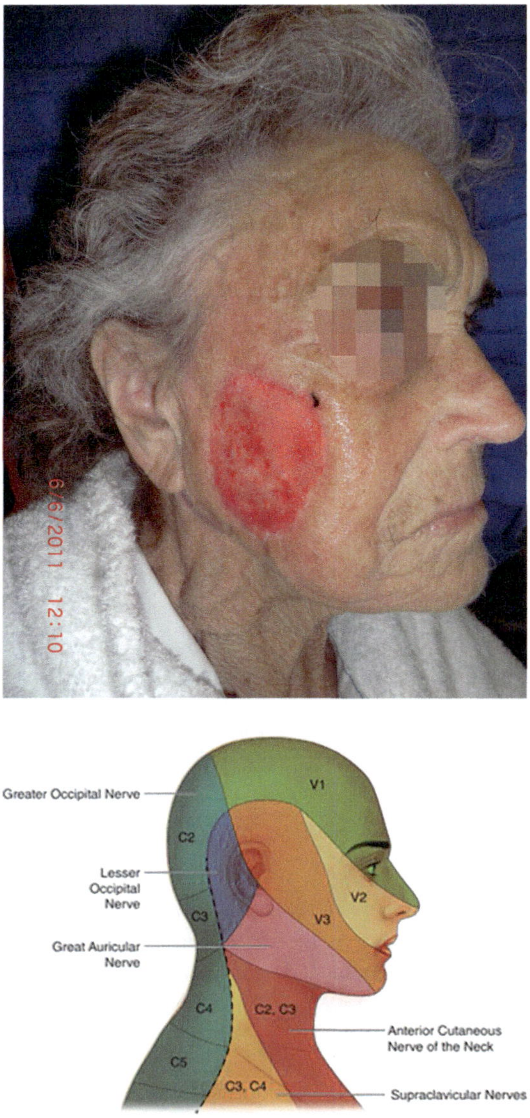

Fig. 2.504 The 7 × 5 cm excision is closed via a cervico-submental Keystone. The dermatomal mark outs become the line of incision of the dermis and epidermis, ensuring that one-third deeply is attached with only partial undermining to facilitate the closure and vascular integrity of the defect. (Reprinted with permission from Atlas, *Reconstructive Technique in Melanoma Management* (p. 19), by Felix Behan, Springer Nature 2023)

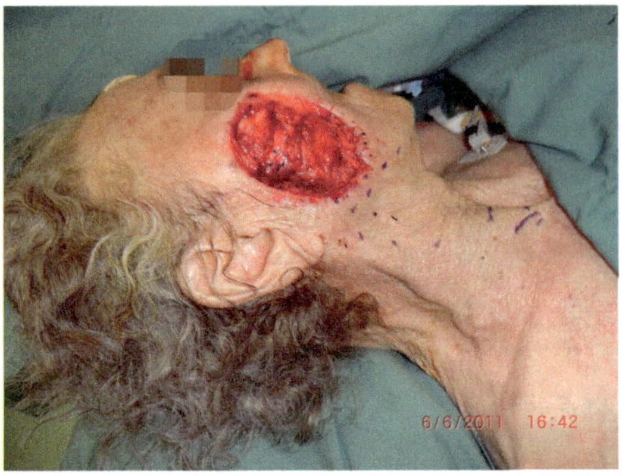

Fig. 2.505 The cervico-submental mark out

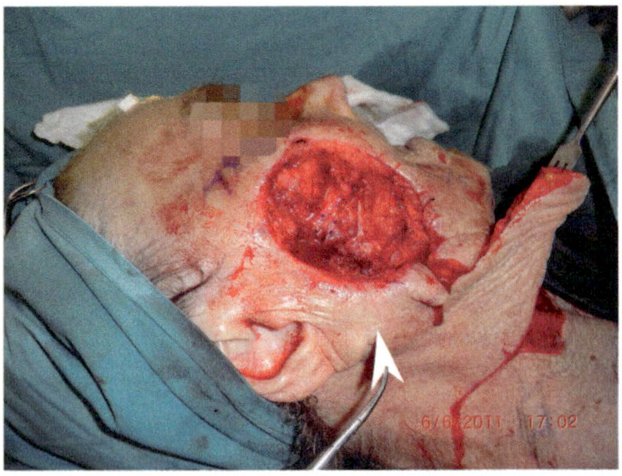

Fig. 2.506 Raising the flap with the cervical fascial base

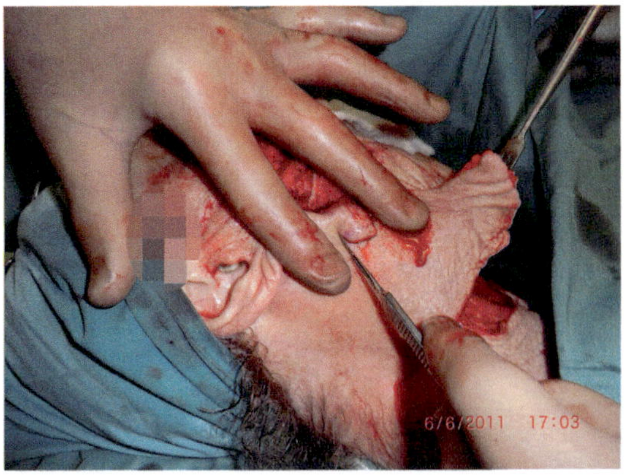

Fig. 2.507 Trimming the dog ear in the acute phase as a consequence of the hypervascularity in the dermal-epidermal layer—avoiding a revisional procedure

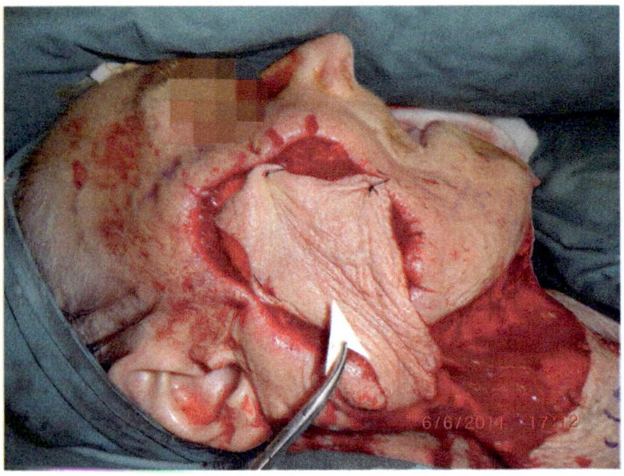

Fig. 2.508 Inserting locking mattress sutures at key points

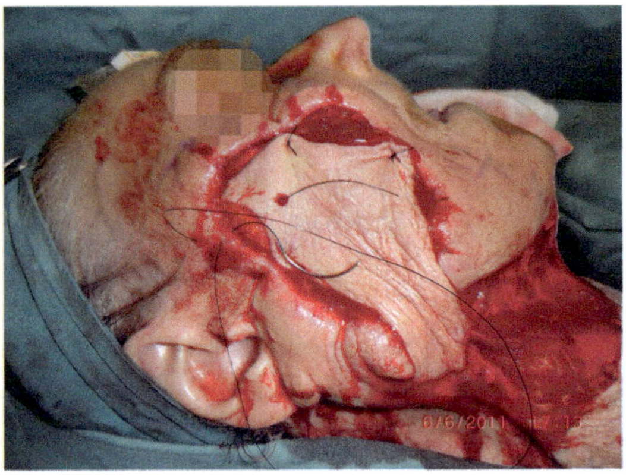

Fig. 2.509 Red dot sign indicating hypervascularity at the suture point

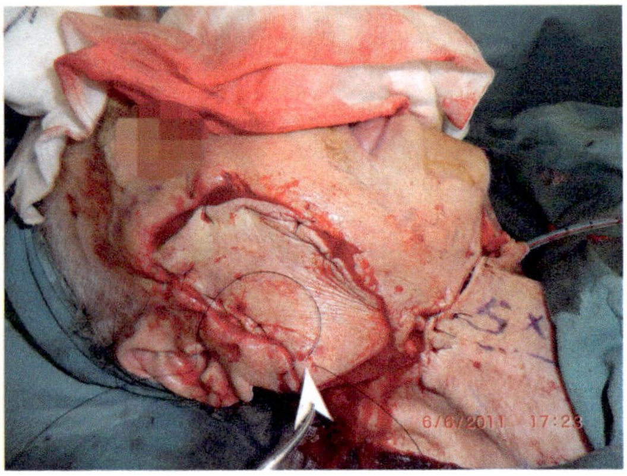

Fig. 2.510 Progress insertion

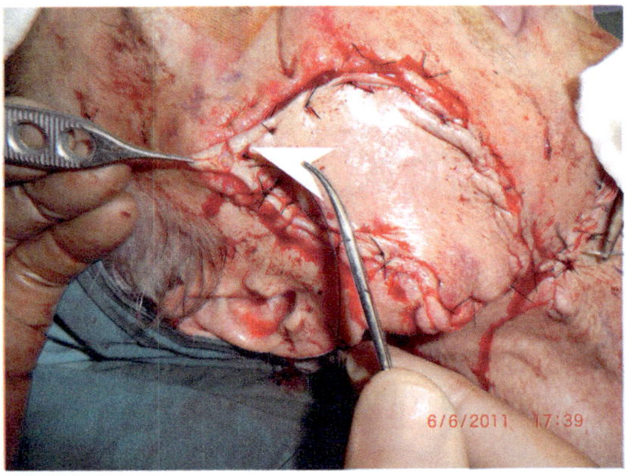

Fig. 2.511 The red dot sign at the apex

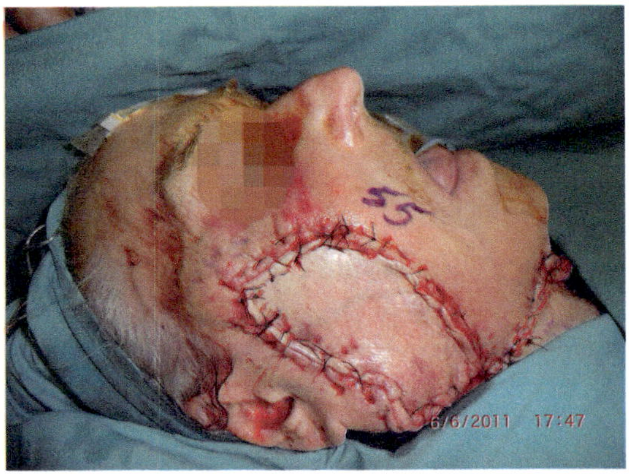

Fig. 2.512 The 7 × 5 cm defect closed in 55 min

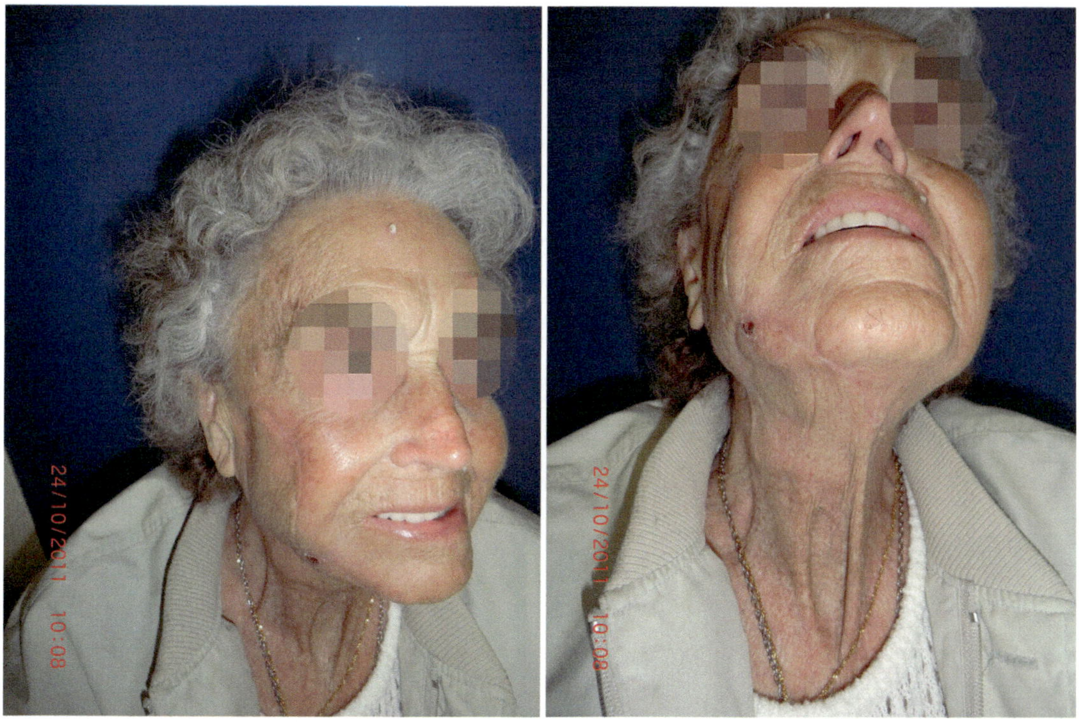

Fig. 2.513 Appearance at 4 months—aesthetically acceptable and patient pleased

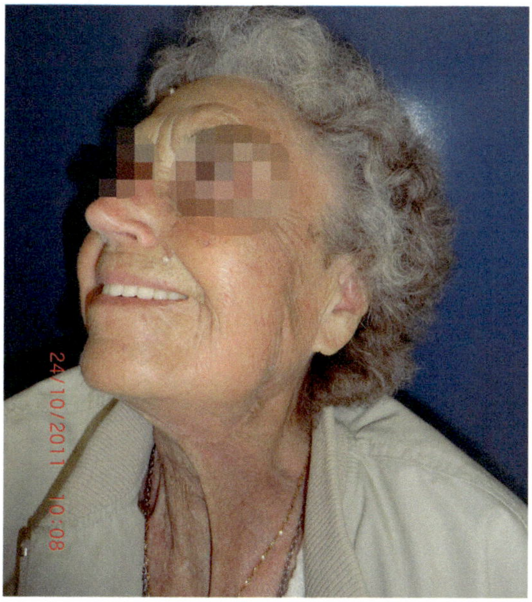

Fig. 2.514 Patient's smile, indicating her satisfaction

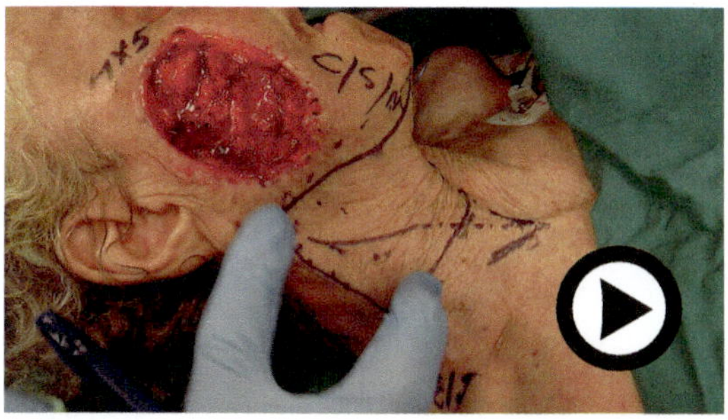

Fig. 2.515 Video 2.67 The mark out of the cervico-submentalKeystoneflap(▶https://doi.org/10.1007/000-k80)

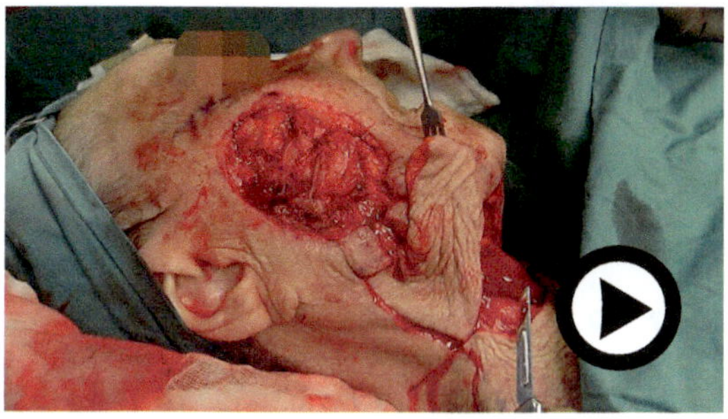

Fig. 2.516 Video 2.68 How the island flap is created on the basis of perforators through the sternomastoid (▶ https://doi.org/10.1007/000-k81)

The PACES characteristics were all exemplified: pain-free, aesthetic, no vascular complications, economical in terms of time and sensory recovery with the resolution of oedema.

2.1.5.11 Case 52—7 × 3 cm Parotid Mass (Figs. 2.517, 2.518 and 2.519)

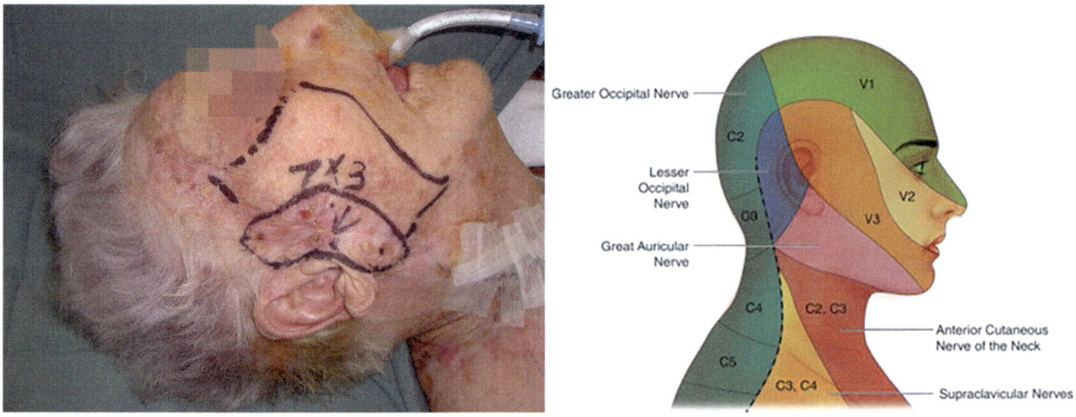

Fig. 2.517 The Keystone mark out down the nasolabial line and along the jawline is used to close the 7 × 3 cm defect. The dermatomal mark outs become the line of incision of the dermis and epidermis, ensuring that one-third deeply is attached with only partial undermining to facilitate the closure and vascular integrity of the defect. (Reprinted with permission from Atlas, *Reconstructive Technique in Melanoma Management* (p. 19), by Felix Behan, Springer Nature 2023)

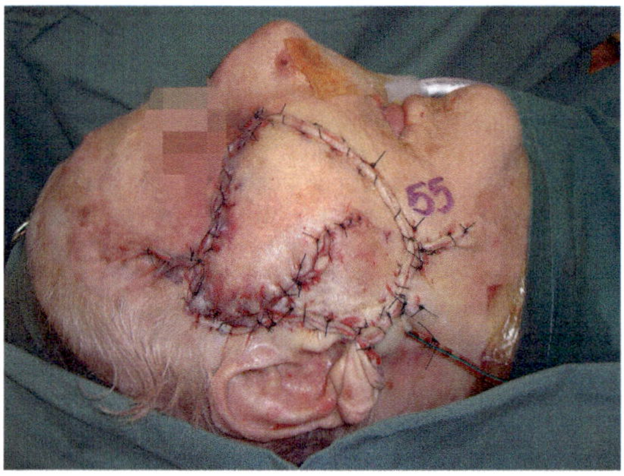

Fig. 2.518 The Keystone closure after the neck clearance in 55 min

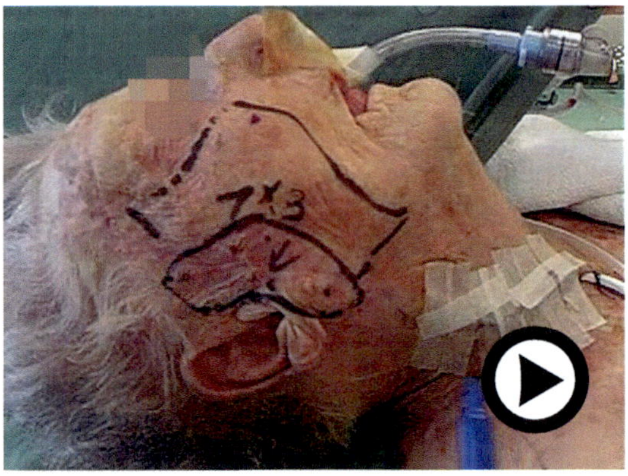

Fig. 2.519 Video 2.69 The mark out and the planned reconstruction (▶ https://doi.org/10.1007/000-k82)

2.1.5.12 Case 53—SCC at the Ear Lobule

Large defects of the parotid are particularly suitable for Keystone reconstruction, which relies particularly on their ease of use and shorter duration of operating time (Figs. 2.520, 2.521, 2.522, 2.523, 2.524, 2.525, 2.526, 2.527, 2.528, 2.529, 2.530, 2.531, 2.532, 2.533, 2.534, 2.535 and 2.536).

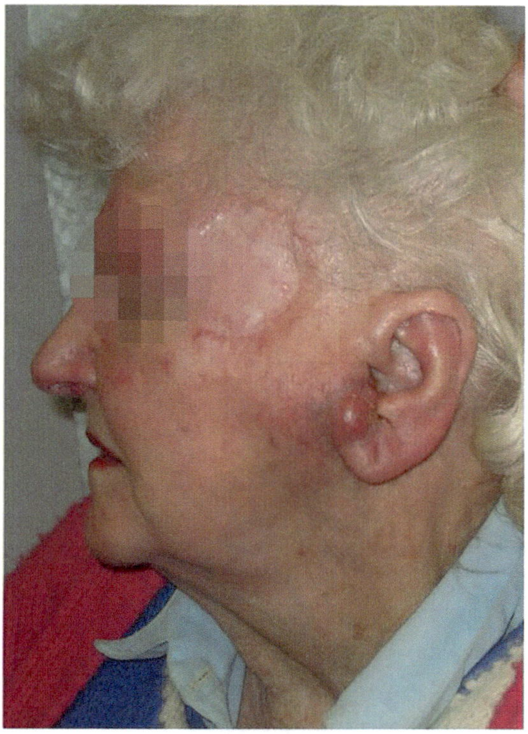

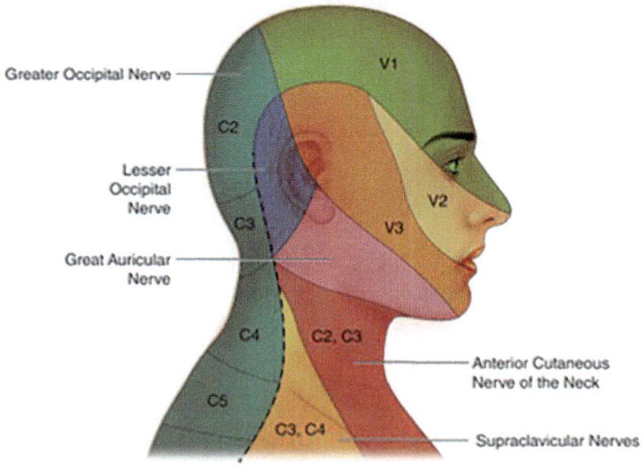

Fig. 2.520 On presentation, where the dermatomal mark outs become the line of incision of the dermis and epidermis, ensuring that one-third deeply is attached with only partial undermining to facilitate the closure and vascular integrity of the defect. (Reprinted with permission from Atlas, *Reconstructive Technique in Melanoma Management* (p. 19), by Felix Behan, Springer Nature 2023)

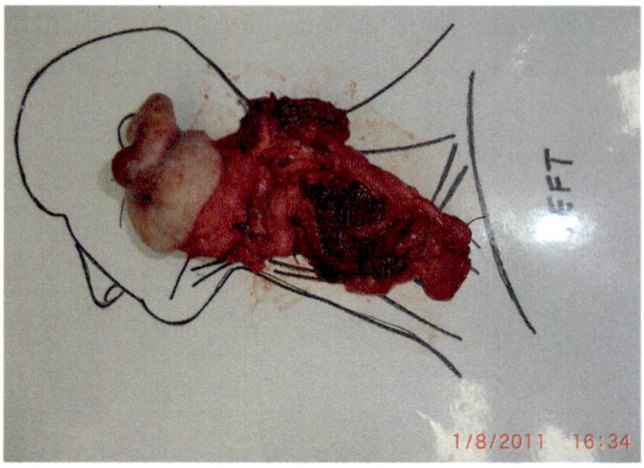

Fig. 2.521 The pathology specimen

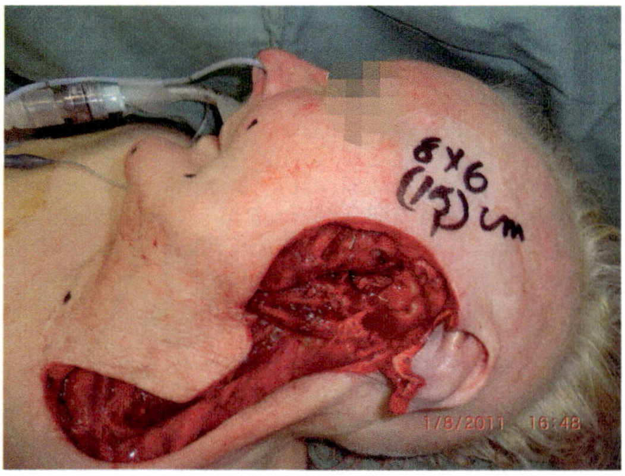

Fig. 2.522 The problem is an SCC of the temple, having been previously grafted over the parotid. Secondary dissemination into the parotid echelon of nodes (the Australian disease) with parotidectomy and clearance of level II, III, IV and V nodes, with gross undermining creating a ~8 × 6 × 15 cm defect including the neck dissection defect. The Keystone mark out creates hypervascularity to ease the closure of the neck dissection

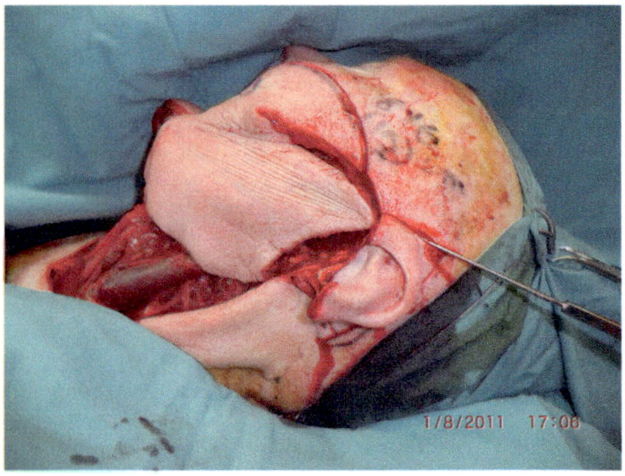

Fig. 2.523 Closure with the cervical Keystone up to the level of the zygomatic arch down to cover the internal jugular vein along the supraclavicular incision

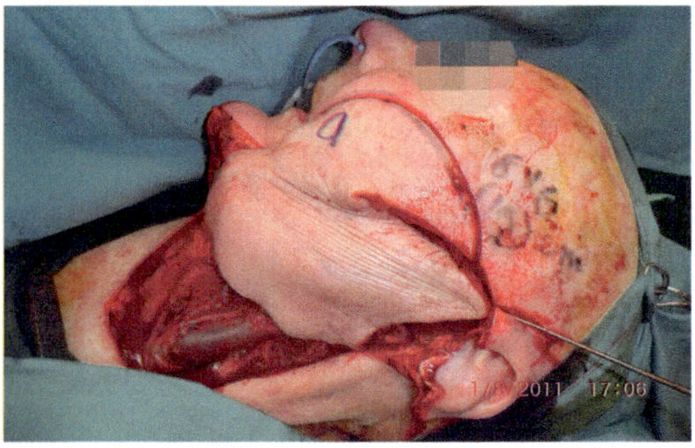

Fig. 2.524 The solution is direct closure, which would cause vascular problems. The cyanotic ear is hypervascularised by outlying the periphery through the Keystone island flap principle (KIFP). The neck flaps are similarly hypervascularised by creating an island around the periphery with 30% attachment to the deeper tissues (see video). This establishes the hypervascularity as a means of avoiding any potential tissue necrosis. This feature of hypervascularity, a Keystone characteristic, facilitates closure while avoiding necrosis. Creating the omega variant facilitates closure

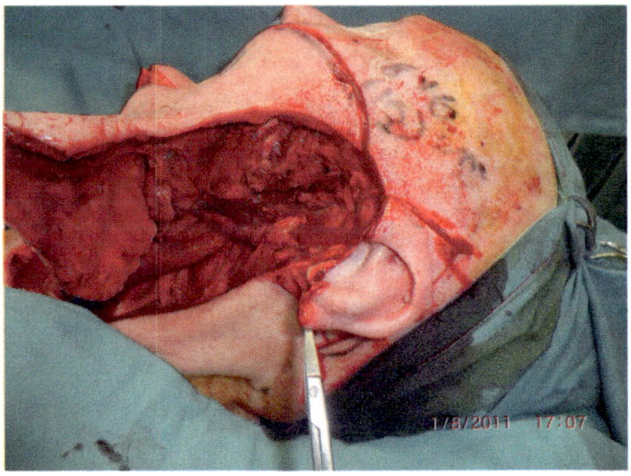

Fig. 2.525 The lax neck tissue hypervascularised with the Keystone mark out is interdigitated over the parotid, and the rest of the wounds are closed directly

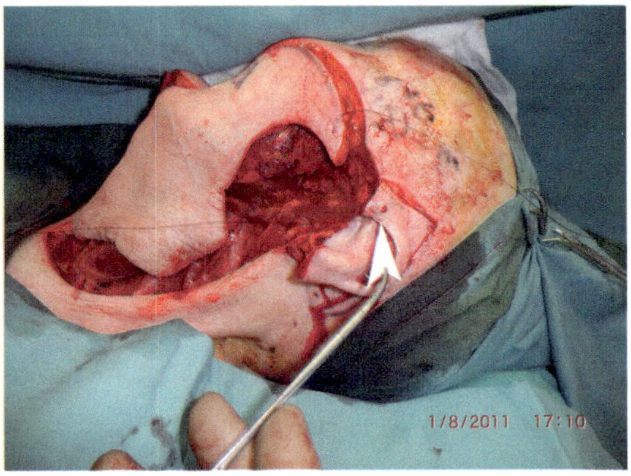

Fig. 2.526 Another red dot sign confirming its hypervascularity and therefore an indicator that necrosis is not anticipated

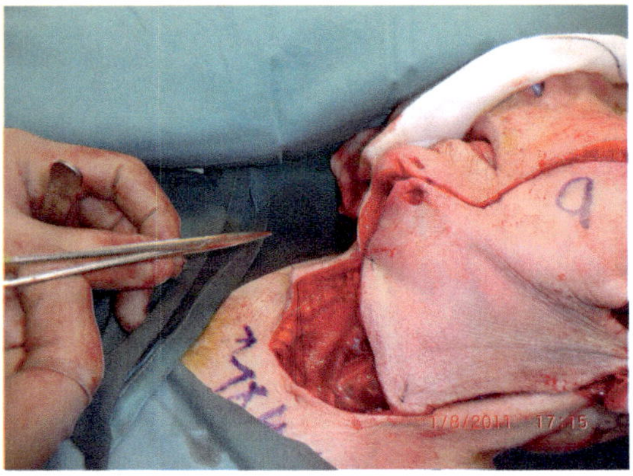

Fig. 2.527 The staged insertion of the Keystone is shown; the red dot signs are noted; and this hypervascularisation phase removes any anxiety about poor perfusion, which is rewarding

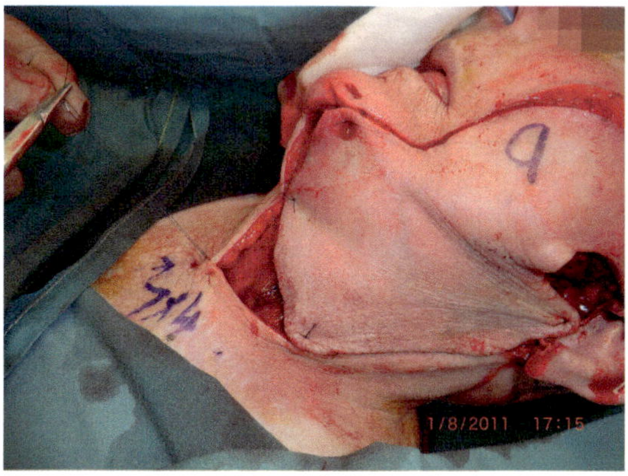

Fig. 2.528 Sequential stages of the closure using locking mattress sutures as a single layer

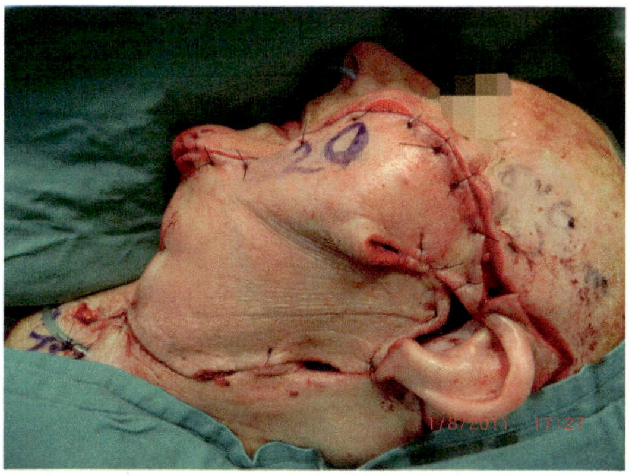

Fig. 2.529 Closure in 20 min and the dog ear about to be trimmed because of its reliable hypervascularity

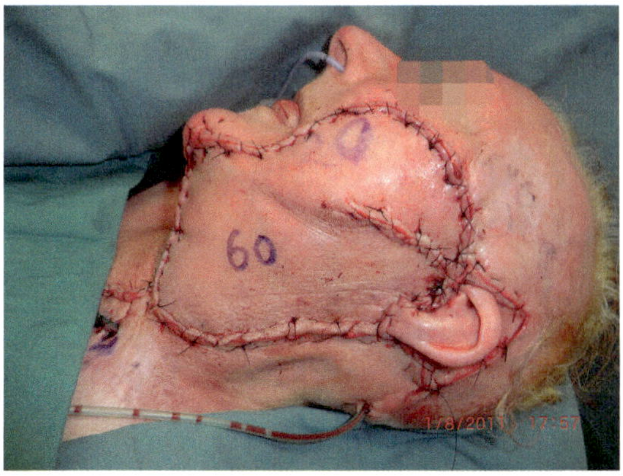

Fig. 2.530 The procedure is completed in 20 min with a double drainage system. Importantly, the island in the Keystone hypervascularises the tissues to promote healing and minimise necrotic changes when closed under tension. If this flap had not been islanded, the consequences would have been untoward

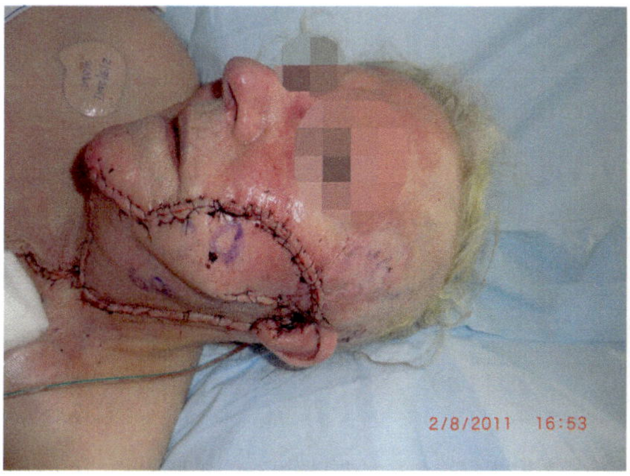

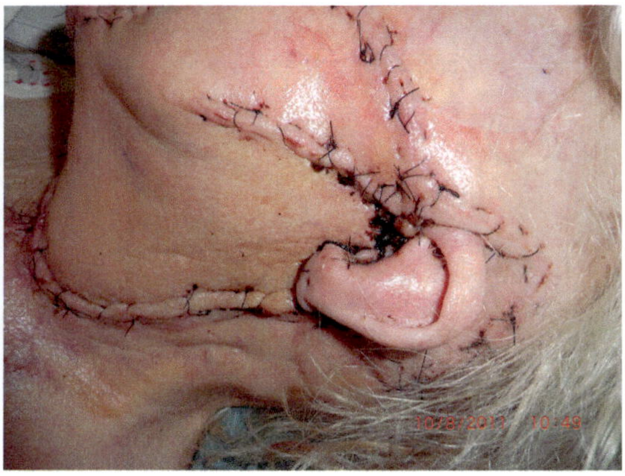

Fig. 2.531 Postoperative appearance at 1 day, showing no vascular impedance, a rewarding sign thanks to the hypervascularity

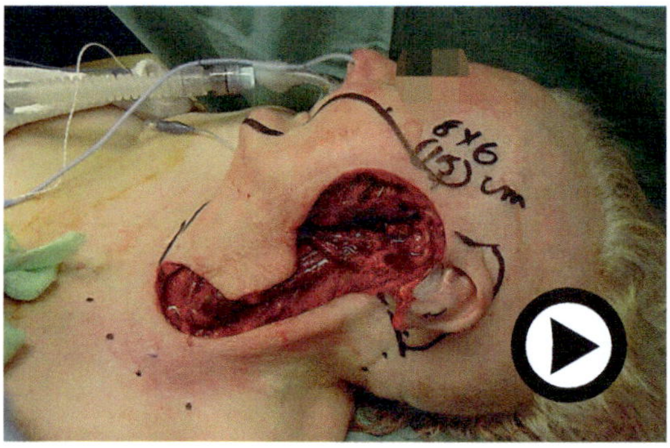

Fig. 2.532 Video 2.70 The mark out along the V2 dermatome before division, then insertion for a 8 × 6 cm defect (▶ https://doi.org/10.1007/000-k83)

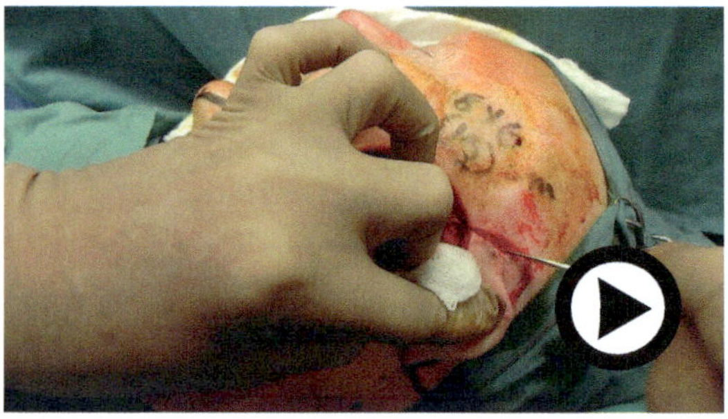

Fig. 2.533 Video 2.71 Islanding the ear to create a field of hypervascularity, reflecting Keystone principles (▶ https://doi.org/10.1007/000-k84)

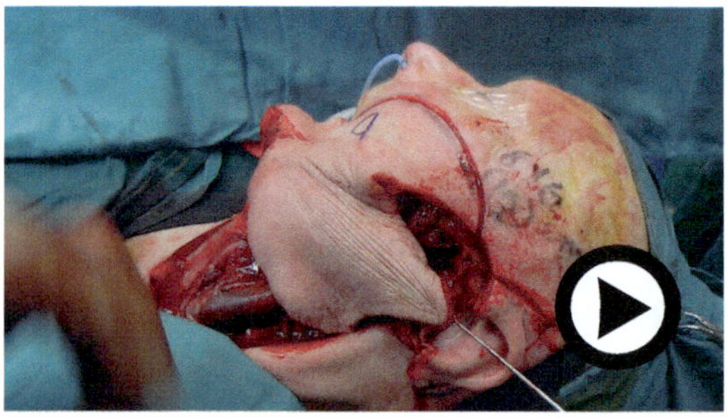

Fig. 2.534 Video 2.72 The inferior Keystone limits of closing the defect is shown. Note the increase in hypervascularity phase now evident in the ear remnant (▶ https://doi.org/10.1007/000-k85)

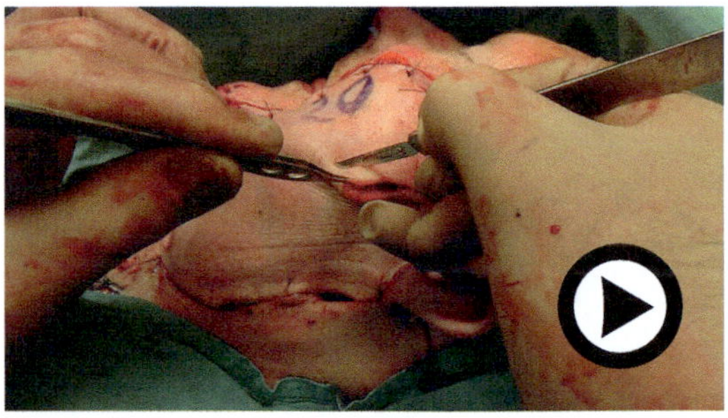

Fig. 2.535 Video 2.73 Removing the dog ear while avoiding a second stage scar revisional procedure (▶ https://doi.org/10.1007/000-k86)

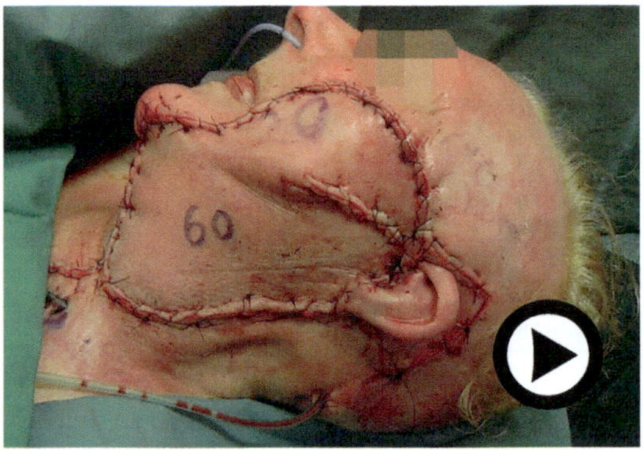

Fig. 2.536 Video 2.74 The 60 min timeframe (▶ https://doi.org/10.1007/000-k87)

The PACES characteristics were all exemplified: pain-free, aesthetic, no vascular complications, economical in terms of time and sensory recovery with the resolution of oedema.

2.1.5.13 Case 54—Melanoma over the Parotid with Neck Clearance

Cause 54 is a good example of intrinsic expansion, where the flap is tailored to fit the defect with V-Y points of closure under tension (Figs. 2.537, 2.538, 2.539, 2.540 and 2.541)

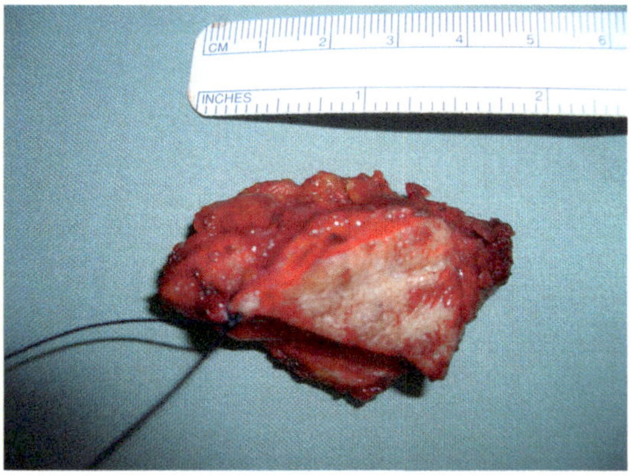

Fig. 2.537 The 5 × 3 cm pathology specimen including the neck gland

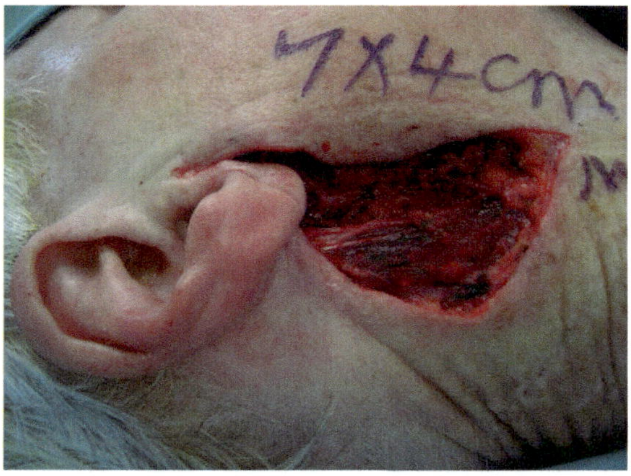

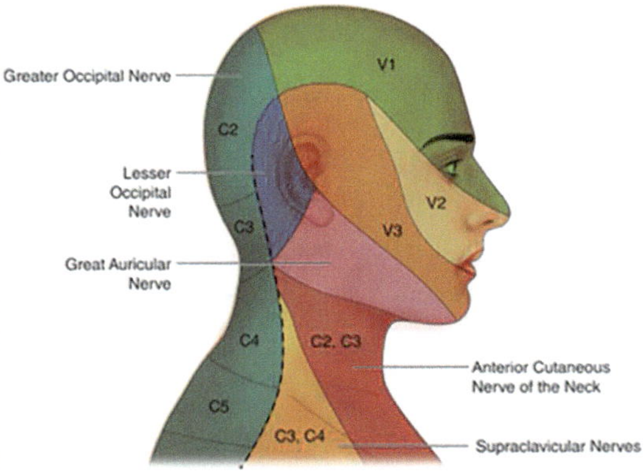

Fig. 2.538 The surgical defect before closure with a cheek Keystone is shown. The dermatomal mark outs become the line of incision of the dermis and epidermis, ensuring that one-third deeply is attached with only partial undermining to facilitate the closure and vascular integrity of the defect. (Reprinted with permission from Atlas, *Reconstructive Technique in Melanoma Management* (p. 19), by Felix Behan, Springer Nature 2023)

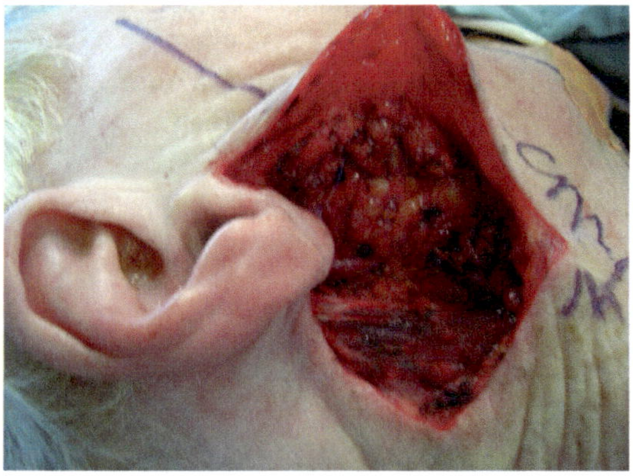

Fig. 2.539 Along the nasolabial line and along the jaw

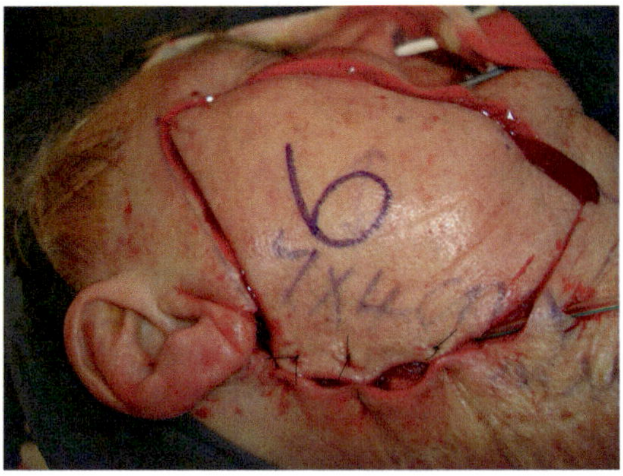

Fig. 2.540 The 7 × 4 cm defect closed in 6 min with drainage

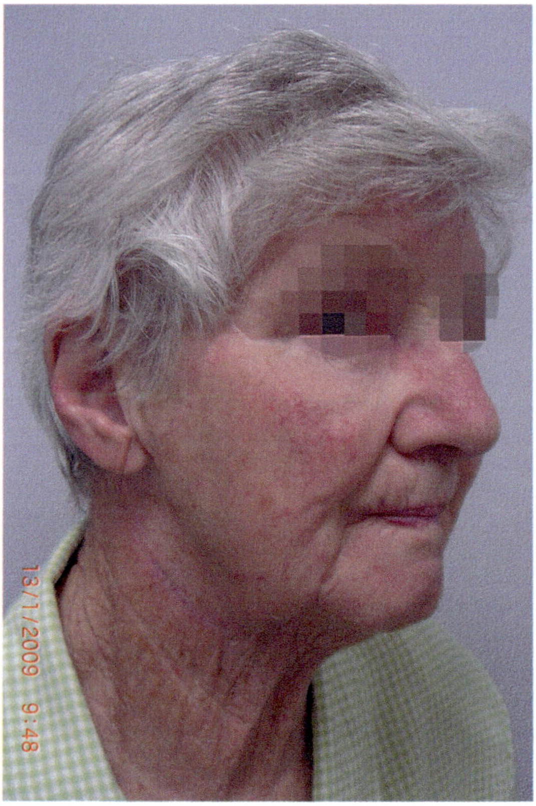

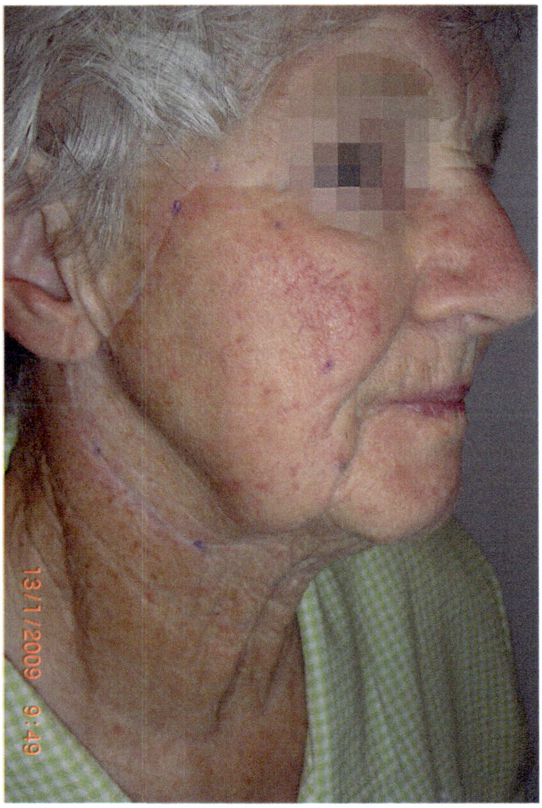

Fig. 2.541 The patient is pleased with her postoperative appearance. No signs of the major surgical incision appear, and the dotted outline emphasises the perfect skin apposition for the surgical defect with the standard three-phase single-layer nylon suture technique, which puts the dermal and epidermal areas into perfect alignment

The PACES characteristics were all exemplified: pain-free, aesthetic, no vascular complications, economical in terms of time and sensory recovery with the resolution of oedema.

2.1.5.14 Case 55—SCC L Cheek with Incomplete Removal and Inappropriately Covered with a Flap Needed for Repeat Excisions for Clearance (× 5)

The Keystone provides a solution for a major aesthetic problem, where two-thirds of the cheek were invovled with recurrent SCC previously treated with other forms of surgery and flaps. The Keystone was a single unit solution to the problem thanks to its intrinsic expansion (Figs. 2.542, 2.543, 2.544, 2.545, 2.546, 2.547 and 2.548).

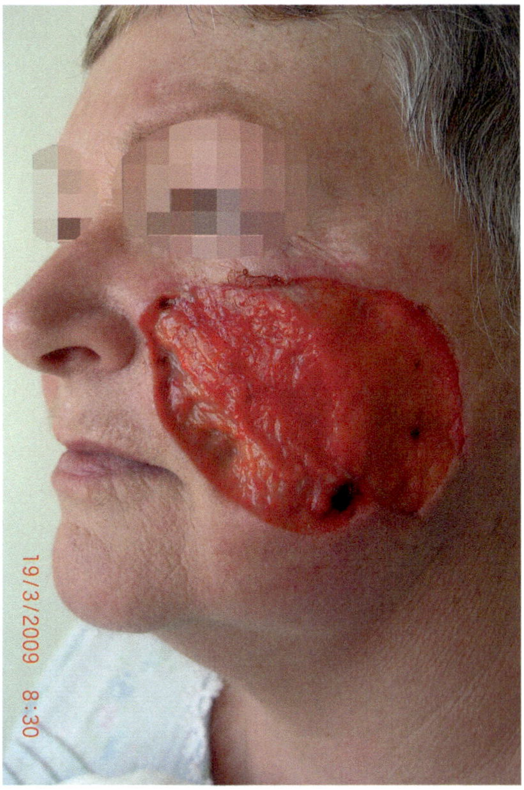

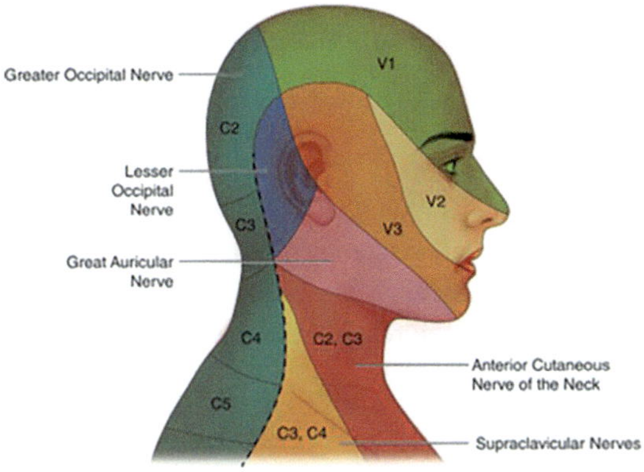

Fig. 2.542 The 8 × 5 cm cheek defect has important aesthetic implications for closure. The dermatomal mark outs become the line of incision of the dermis and epidermis, ensuring that one-third deeply is attached with only partial undermining to facilitate the closure and vascular integrity of the defect. (Reprinted with permission from Atlas, *Reconstructive Technique in Melanoma Management* (p. 19), by Felix Behan, Springer Nature 2023)

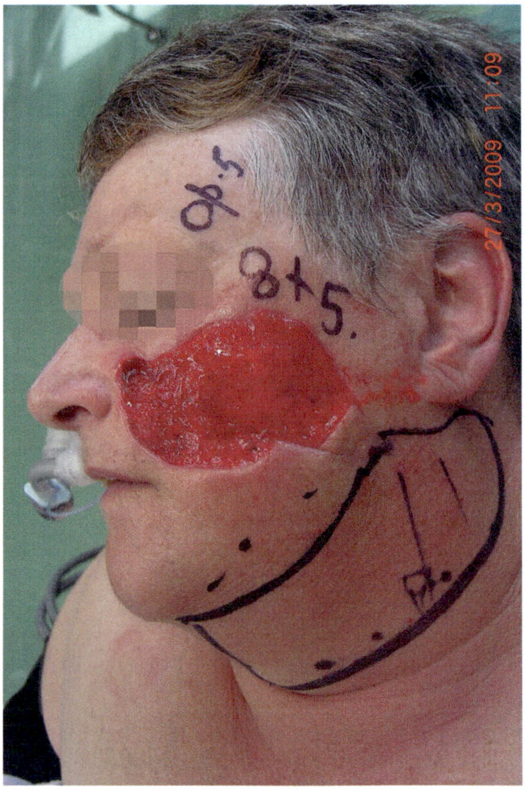

Fig. 2.543 The mark out of the Keystone of the cervico-submental design with the axis of rotation near the sterno-mastoid attachment, which is the area for the microperforators

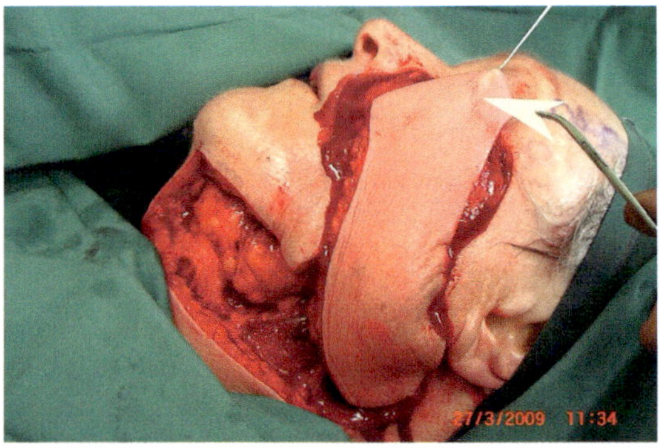

Fig. 2.544 Staged insertion where the arrow indicates the hypervascularity phase, based on the axis of rotation

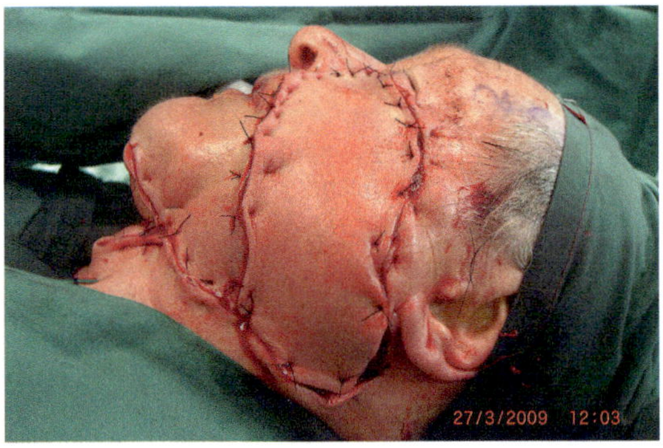

Fig. 2.545 An almost complete insertion is shown, and the insertion is arranged to avoid any ectropion pull of the L eye

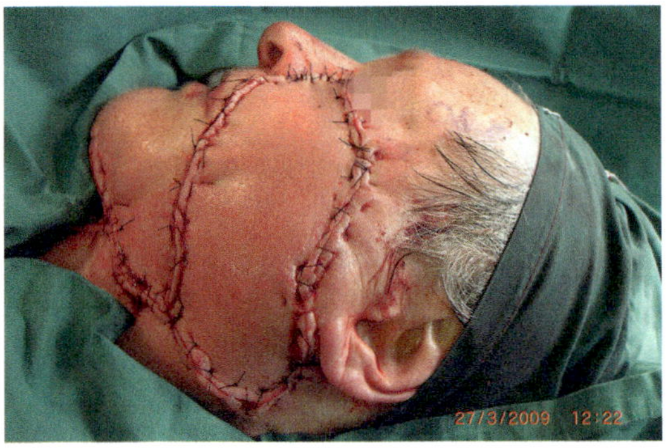

Fig. 2.546 The neck wound is closed directly with the standard three-phase suture technique

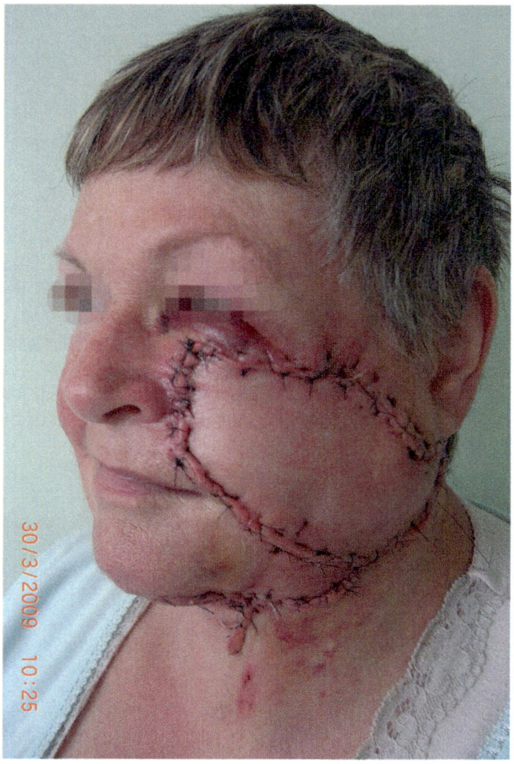

Fig. 2.547 The appearance at 3 days is shown, and the submental closure is not visible

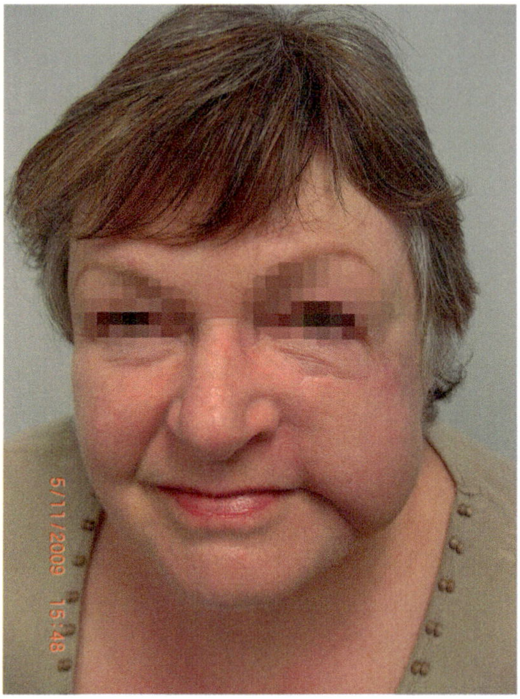

Fig. 2.548 The appearance at 8 months is shown, and the patient was able to resume her duties as a lord mayor, causing her no embarrassment at council meetings

The PACES characteristics were all exemplified: pain-free, aesthetic, no vascular complications, economical in terms of time and sensory recovery with the resolution of oedema.

2.1.5.15 Case 56—A Parotid Mass with Cheek Keystone After Bone Marrow Transplant and Acute Myeloid Leukaemia in Remission (Figs. 2.549, 2.550, 2.551, 2.552, 2.553, 2.554, 2.555, 2.556, 2.557, 2.558 and 2.559)

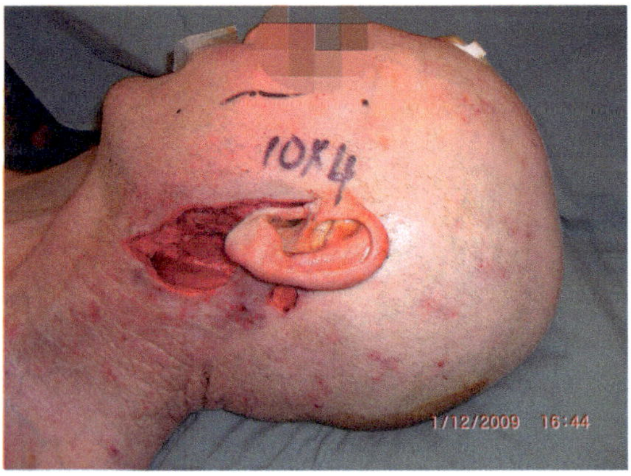

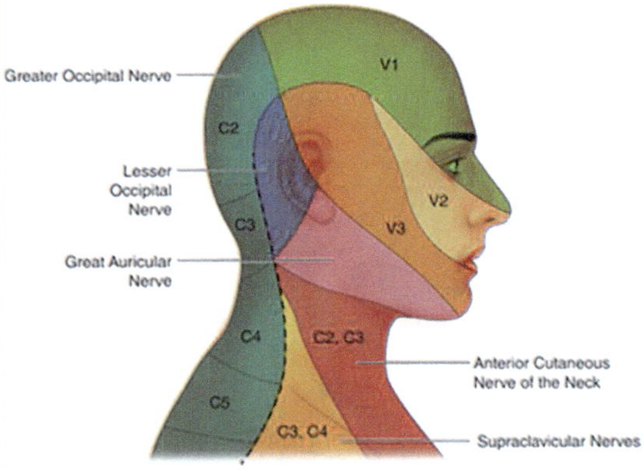

Fig. 2.549 The 10 × 4 cm surgical defect with a preauricular SCC spreading to the parotid node is shown. The dermatomal mark outs become the line of incision of the dermis and epidermis, ensuring that one-third deeply is attached with only partial undermining to facilitate the closure and vascular integrity of the defect. (Reprinted with permission from Atlas, *Reconstructive Technique in Melanoma Management* (p. 19), by Felix Behan, Springer Nature 2023)

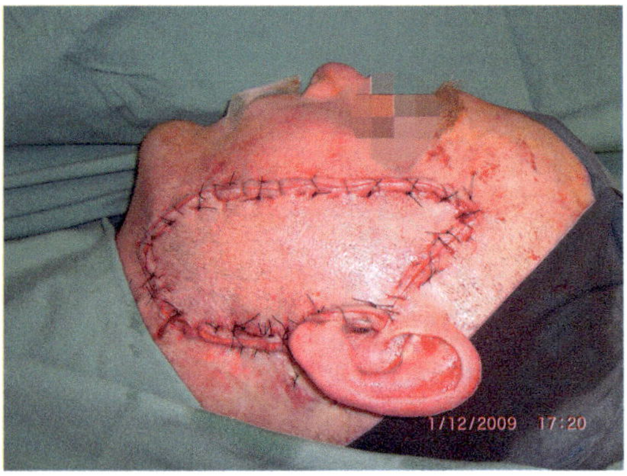

Fig. 2.550 Closure in 45 min in spite of his comorbidities

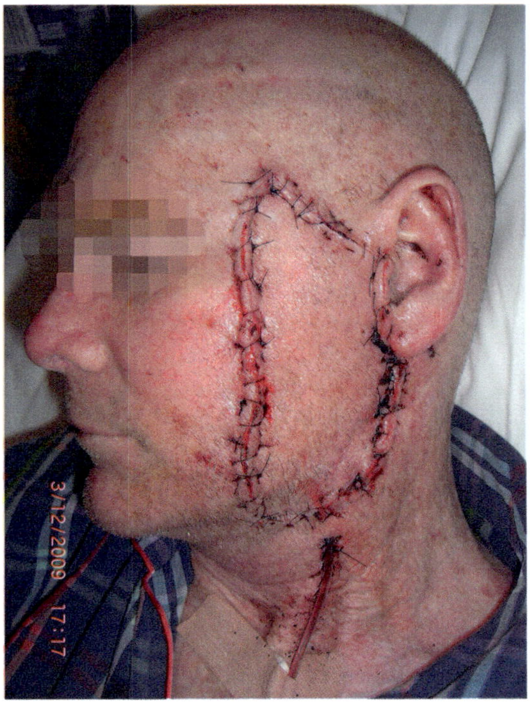

Fig. 2.551 Appearance at 2 days

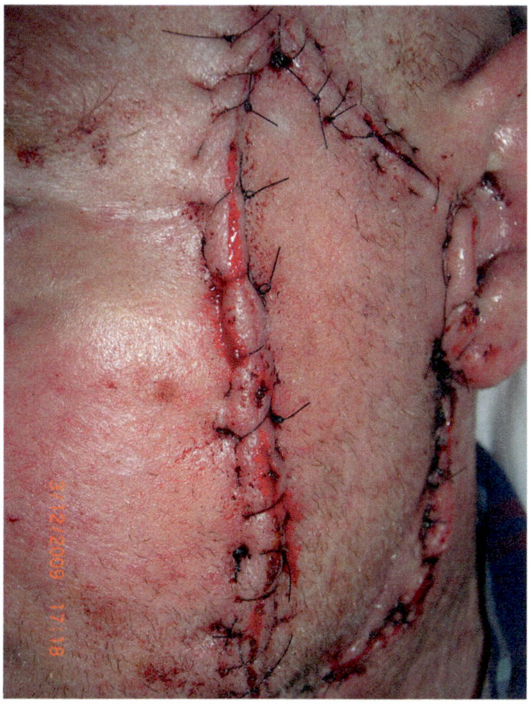

Fig. 2.552 The hypervascularity is a factor causing extra ooze along the wound margin

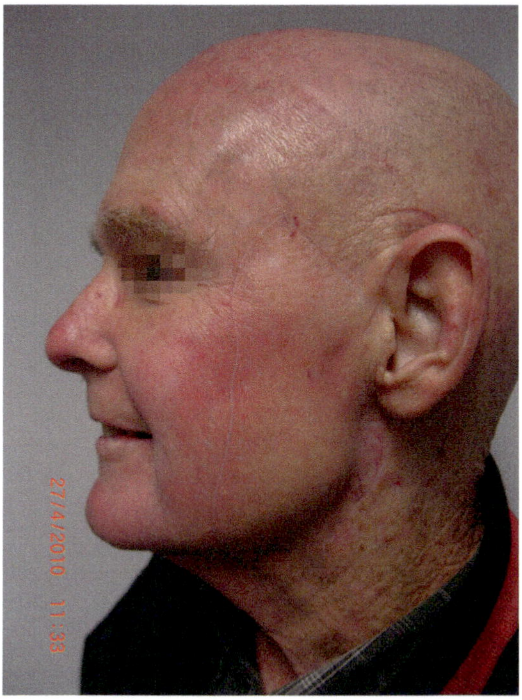

Fig. 2.554 The patient is very pleased with his aesthetic outcome—note the smile

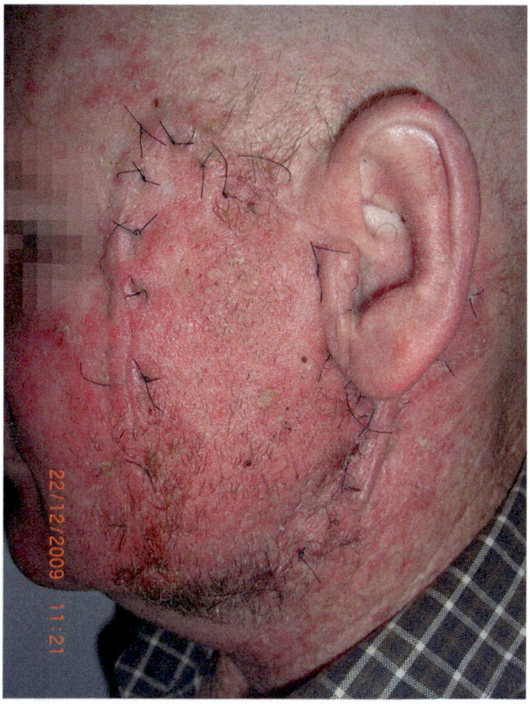

Fig. 2.553 Appearance at 2 weeks

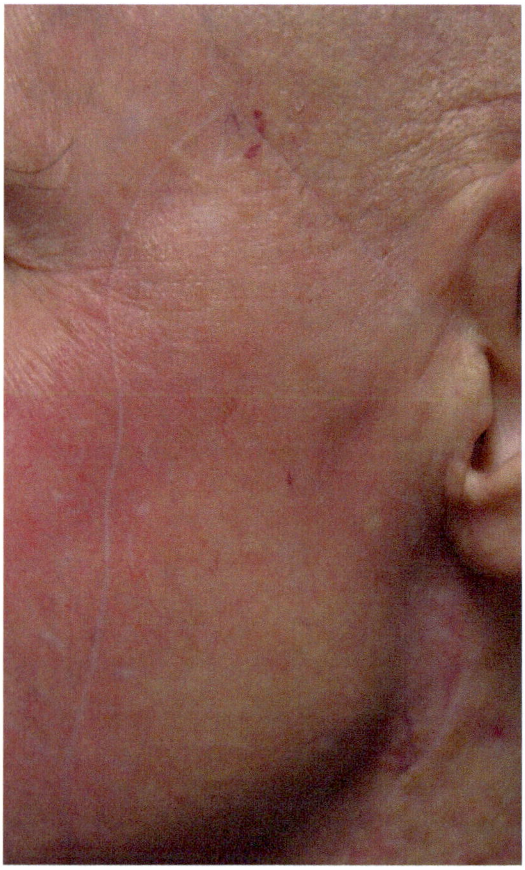

Fig. 2.555 The surgical margin and the standard three-phase suture technique produce this result because the dermis and epidermis are aligned accurately

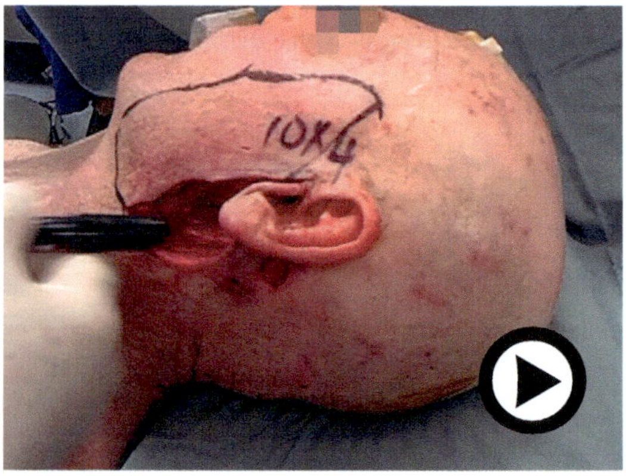

Fig. 2.556 Video 2.75 The staged reconstruction of the cheek Keystone over the parotid (▶ https://doi.org/10.1007/000-k88)

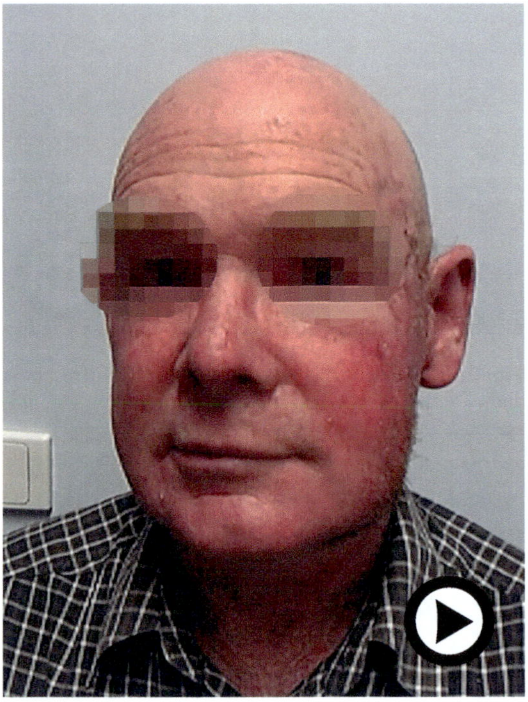

Fig. 2.557 Video 2.76 The patient's clinical history—comorbidities that did not cause any Keystone complication (▶ https://doi.org/10.1007/000-k89)

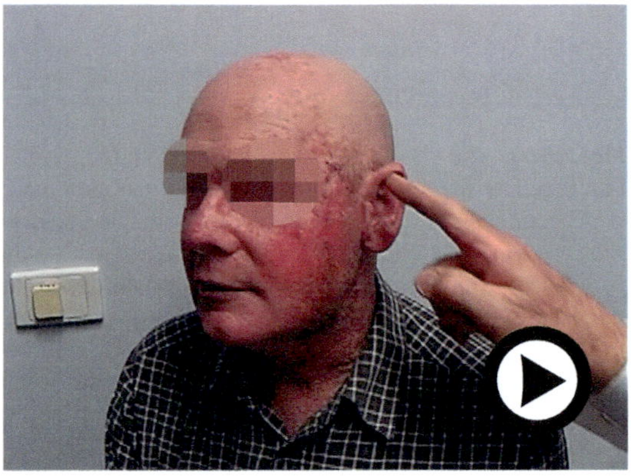

Fig. 2.558 Video 2.77 The healed wound with no evidence of necrosis (▶ https://doi.org/10.1007/000-k8a)

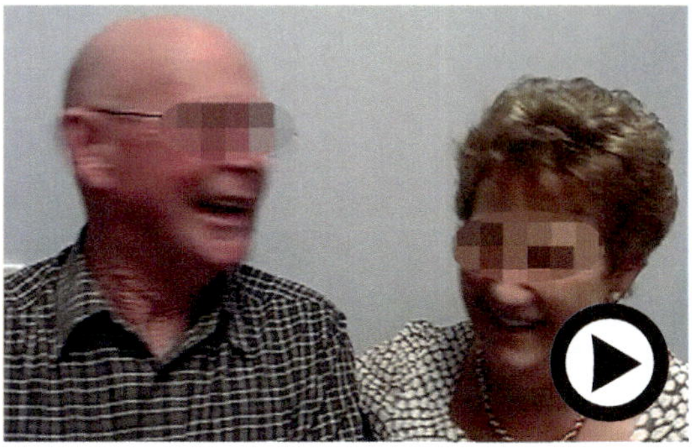

Fig. 2.559 Video 2.78 The family's positive response and satisfaction with the surgical outcome (▶ https://doi.org/10.1007/000-k8b)

The PACES characteristics were all exemplified: pain-free, aesthetic, no vascular complications, economical in terms of time and sensory recovery with the resolution of oedema.

2.1.5.16 Case 57—A Total-Cheek Melanoma from the Nasolabial Region to the Preauricular Groove, Creating an 8 × 6 cm Surgical Defect and a Lesion of the Glabella Crease (Figs. 2.560, 2.561, 2.562, 2.563, 2.564, 2.565, 2.566, 2.567 and 2.568)

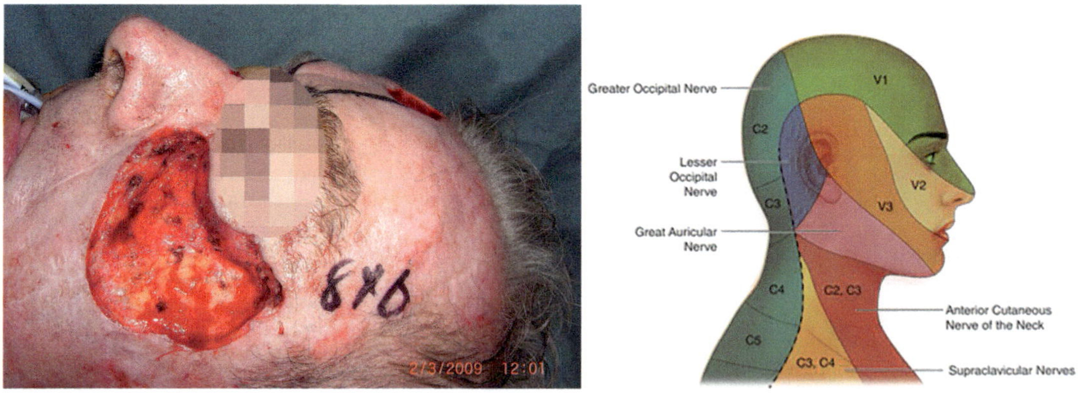

Fig. 2.560 The 8 × 6 cm surgical defect from the nasolabial region to the temple is shown. The dermatomal mark outs become the line of incision of the dermis and epidermis, ensuring that one-third deeply is attached with only partial undermining to facilitate the closure and vascular integrity of the defect. (Reprinted with permission from Atlas, *Reconstructive Technique in Melanoma Management* (p. 19), by Felix Behan, Springer Nature 2023)

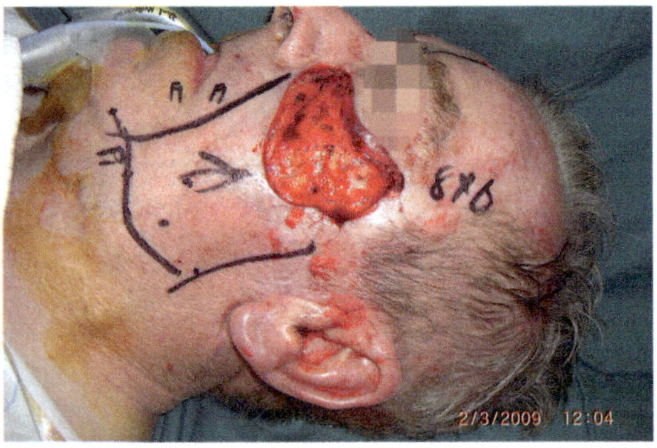

Fig. 2.561 The Keystone mark out plan using loose neck tissue for upward advancement based on supraclavicular perforators

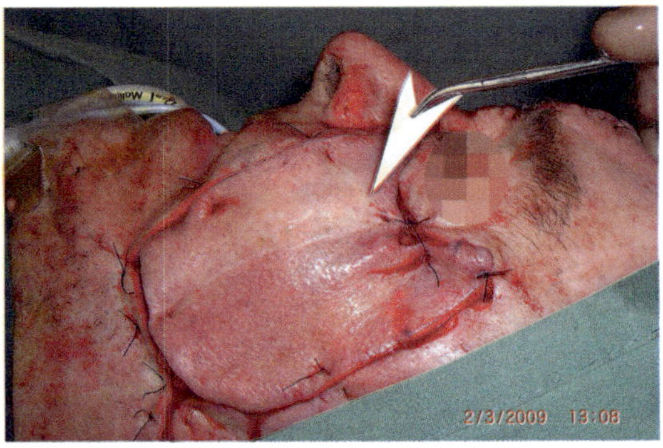

Fig. 2.564 Further stages in the closure of the cheek defect, which are followed to avoid ectropion pull by advancing the flap laterally

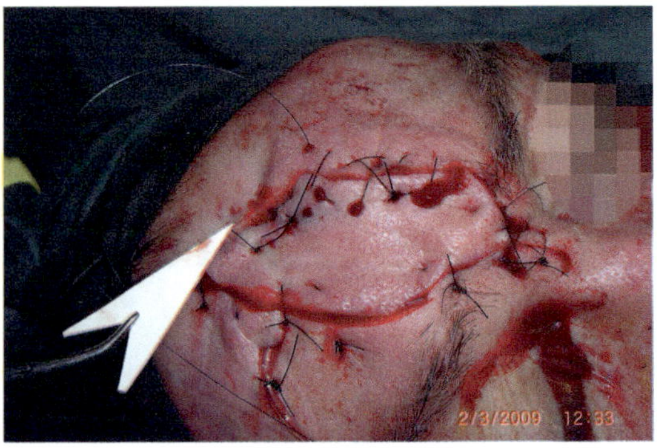

Fig. 2.562 The hypervascularity indicates the reliability of the flap closure of the glabella Keystone, contributing to safe closure even under tension

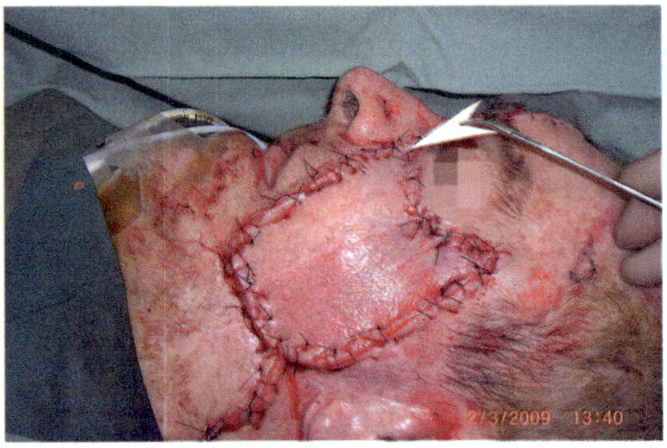

Fig. 2.565 The hypervascularity—an indicator of success

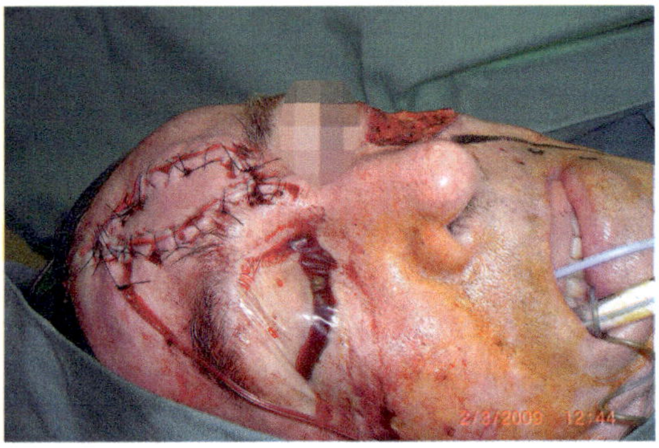

Fig. 2.563 Hypervascularity indicating the reliability of the glabellar Keystone

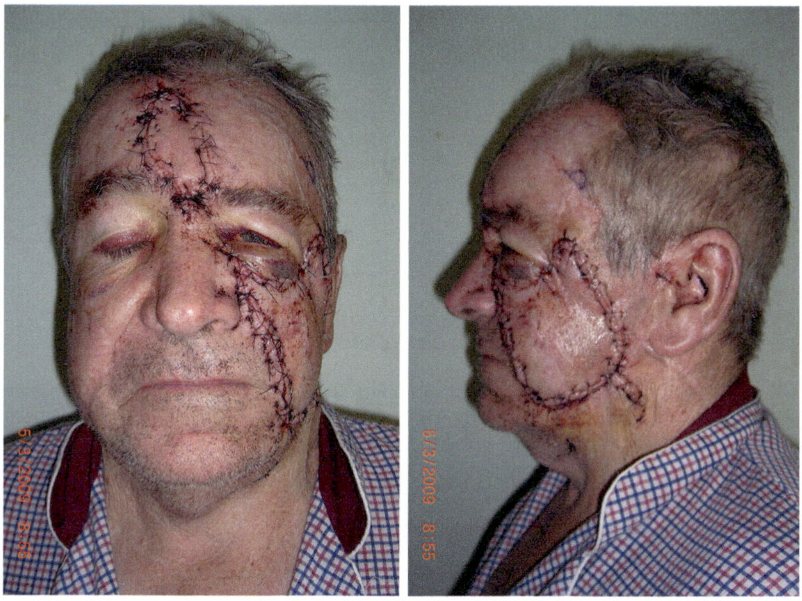

Fig. 2.566 Appearance at 3 days

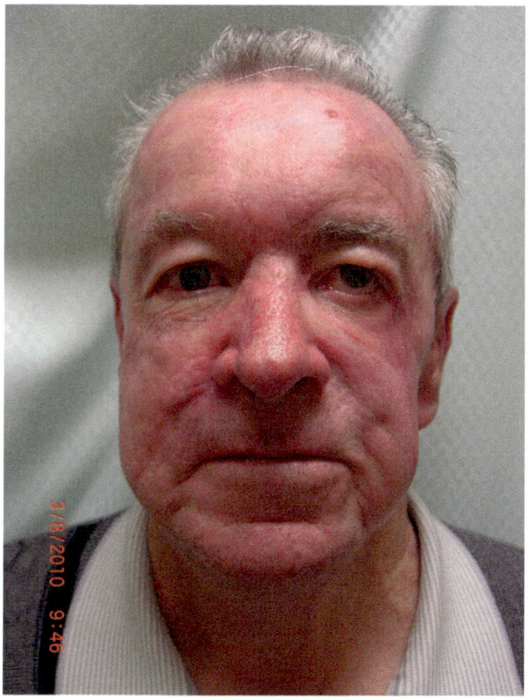

Fig. 2.567 The appearance at 15 months is shown, as timestamped on image, and the patient is extremely satisfied, with no recurrence and a good aesthetic outcome

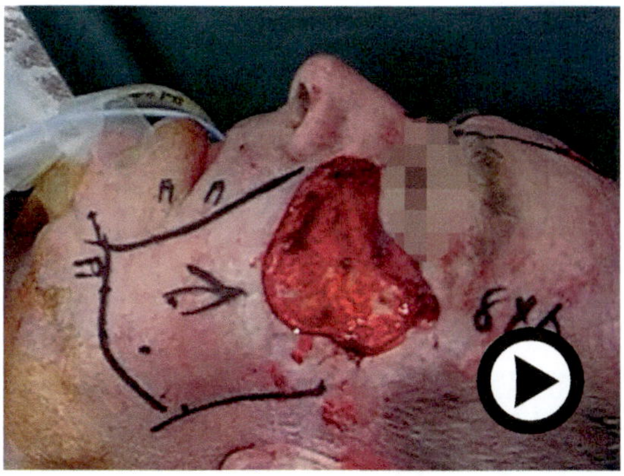

Fig. 2.568 Video 2.79 The Keystone reconstruction technique used on the cheek defect (▶ https://doi.org/10.1007/000-k8c)

The PACES characteristics were all exemplified: pain-free, aesthetic, no vascular complications, economical in terms of time and sensory recovery with the resolution of oedema.

2.1.6 Neck

The Keystone application in neck reconstruction becomes a bonus thanks to its simplicity, avoiding free flap reconstruction on many occasions. The line of the clavicular perforators above and the intercostal perforators below and posterior are the random sources of neurovascular axes that do not revert to angiographic investigations, which is a cost-saving exercise. Most cutaneous eruptions are associated with metastatic deposits, and often there is severe undermining of the flaps for oncological access. The assortment of cases shows the applications of the Keystone when its characteristics are evident from a clinical perspective. The undermining of the first case is part of the secondary dissemination, which means that the Keystone, using the advantage of loose neck skin, becomes **hypervascularised by creating an island** with deep attachment and perforators dotted along the clavicle. Leaving one-third deep attachment is the source of its vascular integrity. It does not preclude closing under tension with suction drainage intact.

The melanoma on the nape of the neck is closed by using a similar random perforator design along the margin of the T1 and T2 intercostal circulation, which is randomly placed, but the island, reflecting Keystone characteristics, allows adequate closure under tension.

The neck closure over the mastoid region following nodal excision is evident in this series. One outstanding comment is warranted: These facial tissues are hypervascularised. A dermal-epidermal incision along the V2 dermatome creates a sympathectomy effect, which ensures rapid healing without evident necrosis, even under tension.

2.1.6.1 Case 58—Infraclavicular Keystone for Closing a Defect of the Anterior Neck Following a Neck Dissection

Case 58 features a recurrent melanoma of the L neck in the supraclavicular region part of the neck, with clearance levels I–IV in an 80-year-old man who has a history of cerebrovascular accident (CVA). His comorbidities indicate that time on the theatre table is of the essence. (Figs. 2.569, 2.570, 2.571, 2.572, 2.573, 2.574, 2.575 and 2.576).

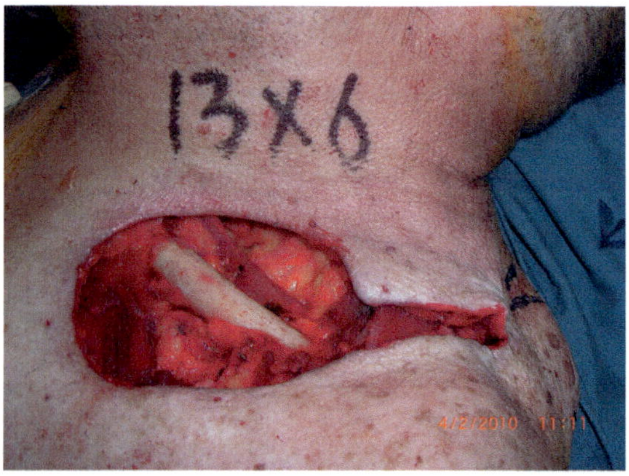

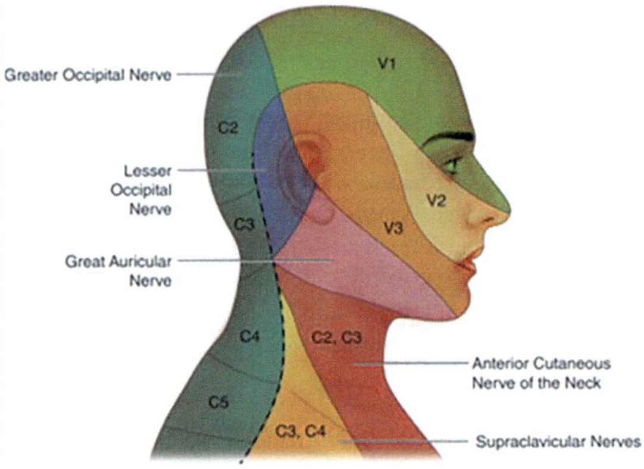

Fig. 2.569 The 13 × 6 cm oncological defect following nodal clearances of levels I–IV is shown. The exposed clavicle is not a contraindication for Keystone applications. The posterior extension of the wound is used merely to facilitate the clearance of level IV nodes. The dermatomal mark outs become the line of incision of the dermis and epidermis, ensuring that one-third deeply is attached with only partial undermining to facilitate the closure and vascular integrity of the defect. (Reprinted with permission from Atlas, *Reconstructive Technique in Melanoma Management* (p. 19), by Felix Behan, Springer Nature 2023)

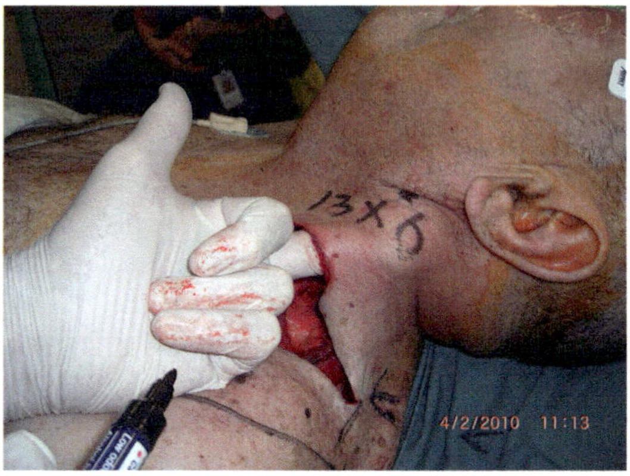

Fig. 2.570 The limits of undermining the flaps to achieve oncological nodal clearance is indicated by the L middle finger, which reaches the L mastoid. This is not a contra-indication for flap closure, because it is hypervascularised with the Keystone design, and the aesthetic outcome and the intrinsic expansion are valid contributors to its success

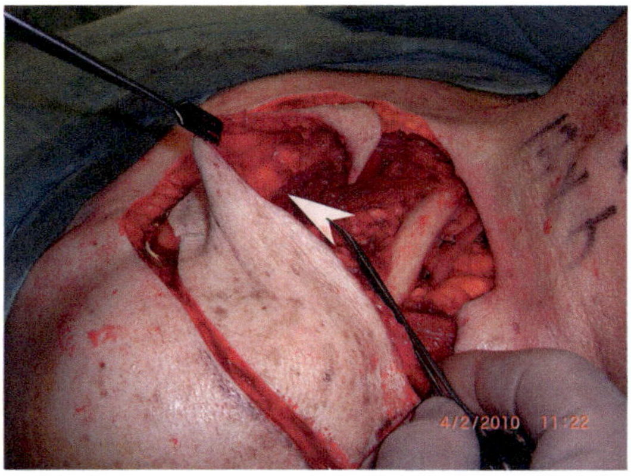

Fig. 2.571 The undermining of the inferior limits of the defect is indicated by the arrow in the vicinity of the intercostal sternal perforators, which have not been dissected intentionally. The Keystone design reflects intrinsic expansion almost like an umbrella effect, where a small tissue expanse can cover a wide surgical defect thanks to the looseness of the surrounding tissues. The facial lining supports this reconstructive principle

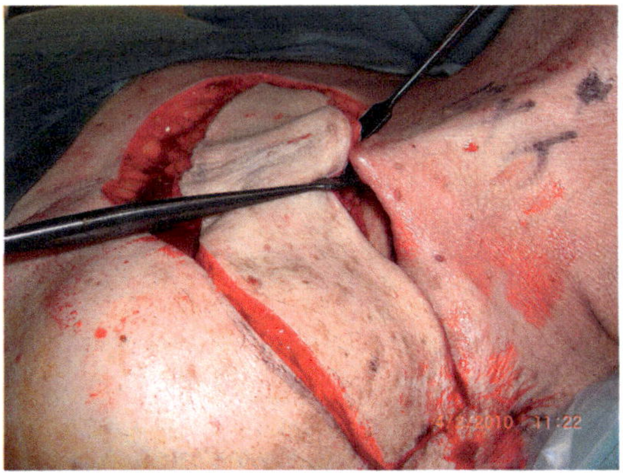

Fig. 2.572 The design mark out of the Keystone for neck closure

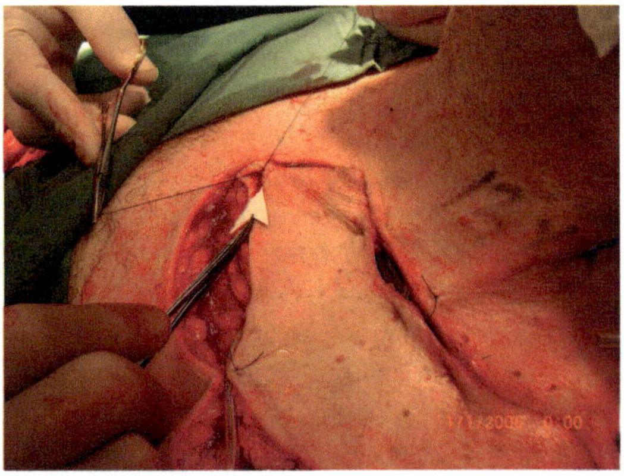

Fig. 2.573 Progress in wound closure using the three-phase single-layer nylon suture technique is shown. The arrow points to the hyperaemia along the medial side of the flap, indicating the major contribution from the intercostal perforators

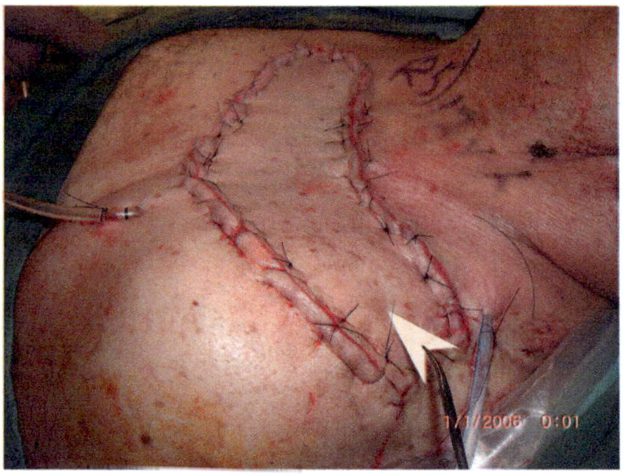

Fig. 2.574 Wound closure after 60 min is shown. Redivac installation and the hyperaemic flow without any lines of tension and potential necrosis have been overcome by the suprafascial and infrafascial support of this Keystone because random clavicular perforators have reverted to the intrinsic expansion of the looser tissues in elderly patients

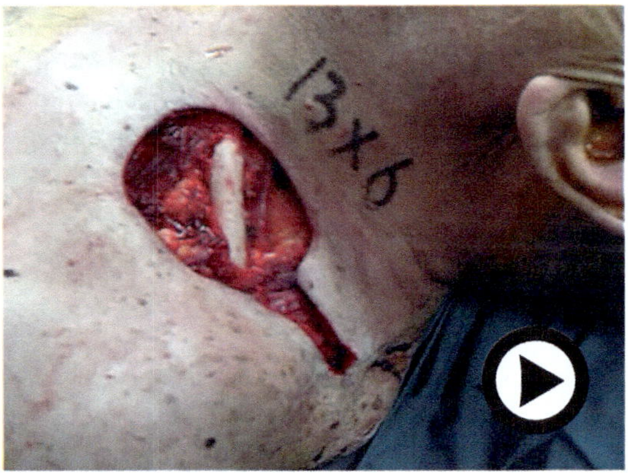

Fig. 2.576 Video 2.80 The planned Keystone reconstruction of the supraclavicular defect based on infraclavicular perforators (▶ https://doi.org/10.1007/000-k8d)

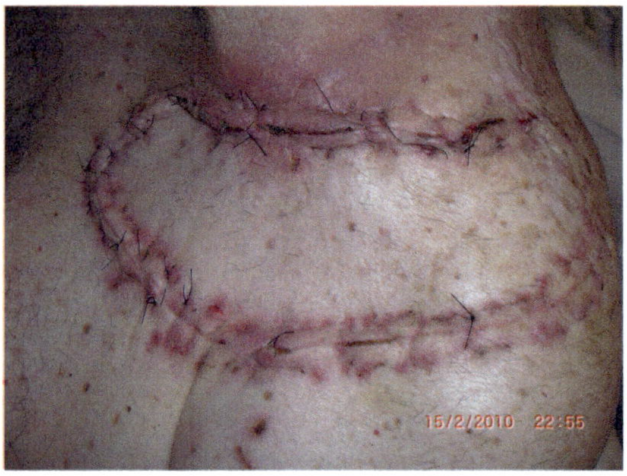

Fig. 2.575 The appearance at 10 days with the staged suture removal technique with the cutting of the continuous nylon and some of the interrupted units is shown. The wound dressing is completed at 3.5 weeks for really tight wound closure

In summary, the PACES charactristics of the Keystone were all exemplified in this island flap repair. Using random perforators along the infraclavicular alignment guarantees that the vascular support will achieve wound closure and successful healing.

2.1.6.2 Case 59—Posterior Clavicular Exposure with an Undermined Keystone

Cause 59 features a level II neck melanoma over the prominence of C7 (Figs. 2.577, 2.578, 2.579, 2.580, 2.581 and 2.582).

In summary, the PACES charactristics of the Keystone were all exemplified in this island flap repair.

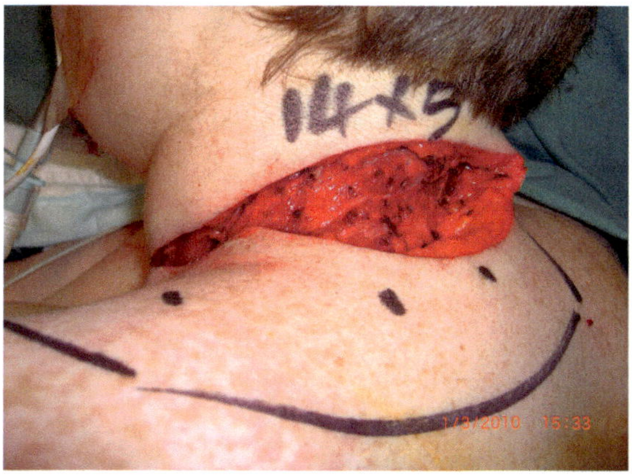

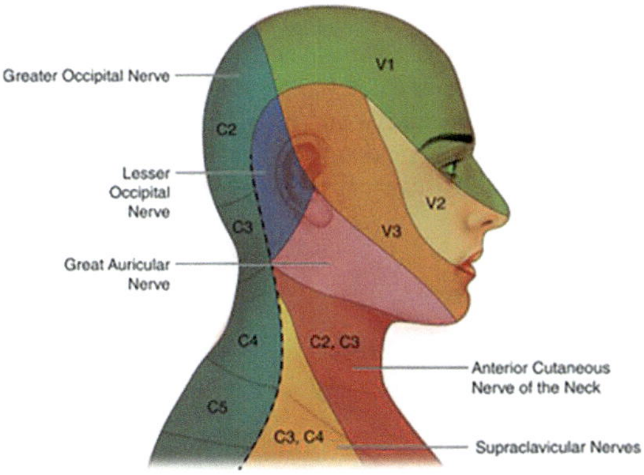

Fig. 2.577 A level II melanoma in the nape of the neck overlying the C7 spinal prominence is shown. The short hair factor may have been an aeteological link in the development of the melanoma. The biopsy confirmed the wide 2 cm clearence margin. The Keystone mark out on the inferior limit of the defect is highlighted, and the dots represent random perforator support in the C5 and C6 dematome, the basis of its vascular support, and these random perforators in the vicinity of the spine of the scapular on either side do not need identification. The dermatomal mark outs become the line of incision of the dermis and epidermis, ensuring that one-third deeply is attached with only partial undermining to facilitate the closure and vascular integrity of the defect. (Reprinted with permission from Atlas, *Reconstructive Technique in Melanoma Management* (p. 19), by Felix Behan, Springer Nature 2023)

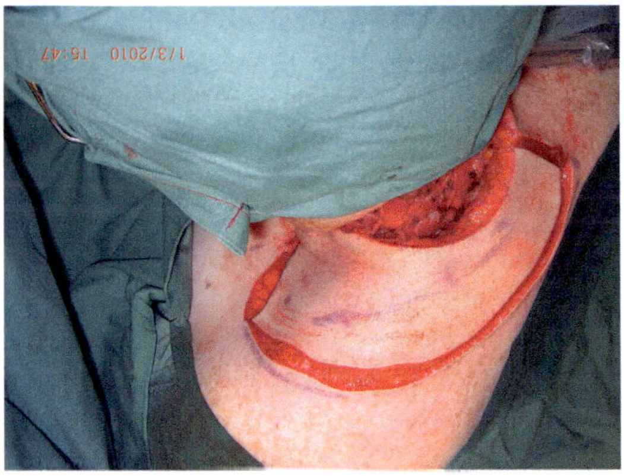

Fig. 2.578 The Keystone mark out of the flap indicates where the medial and lateral parts of the island design are at the epidermal dermal level, and the central part has retained deep attachment

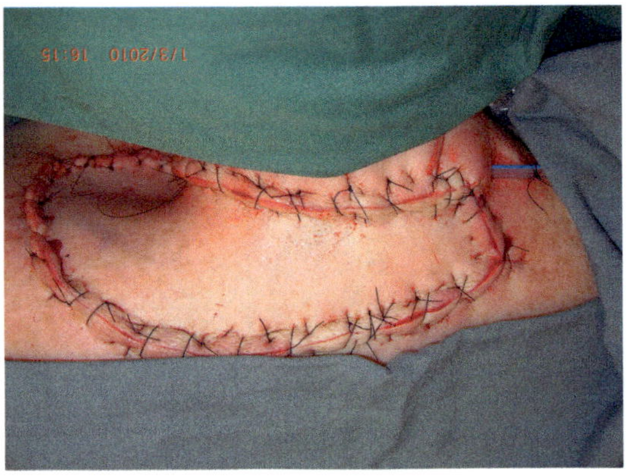

Fig. 2.580 The three-phase single-layer suture technique using locking mattress sutures at the maximum tension points is shown. Ordinary mattress sutures are for wound closure, and a continuous nylon is for an epidermal seal. The wound-dressing technique follows the same 3-week cycle of cutting the loops at 7 days, cutting some of the mattress sutures at 14 days and removing the tension sutures at 21 days or longer if they bleed. If they bleed, leave these in for another week

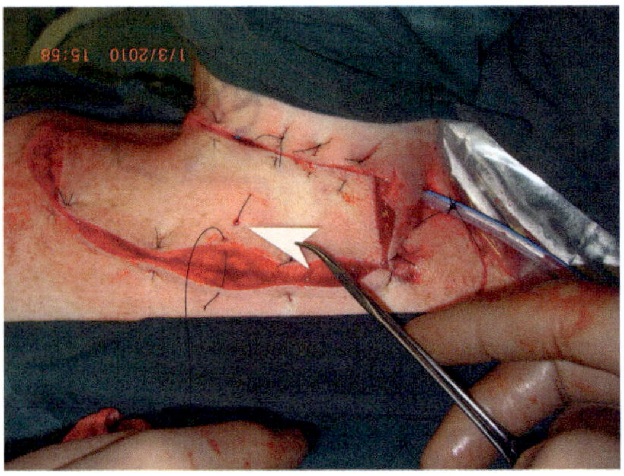

Fig. 2.579 In-transit closure with some extension of the neck, the V-Y points on either extreme close the flap medially and laterally, and the arrow points to the red dot sign, indicating its hyperaemic phase, which ensures sound healing

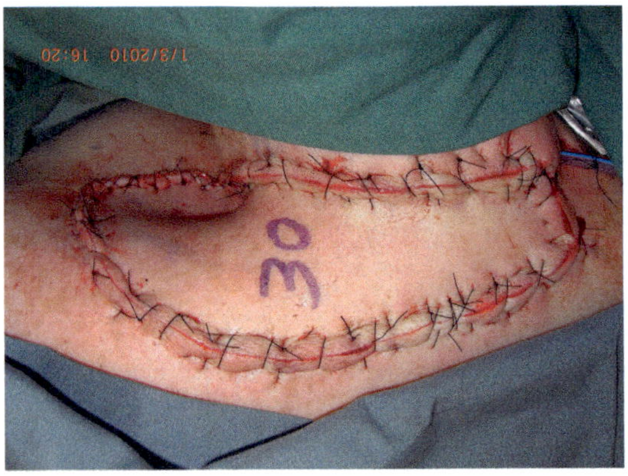

Fig. 2.581 The timeframe for the repair of this defect is 30 min. Note the hyperaemia, indicating the hypervascular phase evident in this Keystone island flap technique, which ensures sound healing

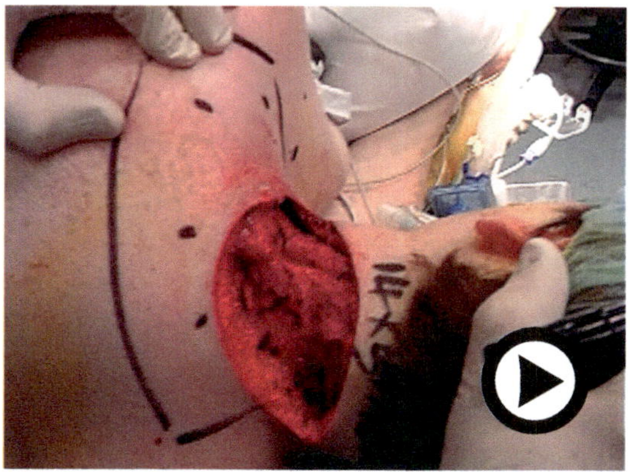

Fig. 2.582 Video 2.81 The planned Keystone along the C7 dermatome alignment (▶ https://doi.org/10.1007/000-k8e)

2.1.6.3 Case 60—L Mastoid Region

Case 60 features a level II melanoma over mastoid and parotid areas in this 78-year-old man with extensive comorbidities. The defect size was 12 × 6 cm (Figs. 2.583, 2.584, 2.585, 2.586, 2.587, 2.588 and 2.589).

In summary, the hyperaemic phase of the Keystone principle has ensured vascular perfusion and therefore healing in this melanotic excisional defect in a 78-year-old patient with extreme comorbidities.

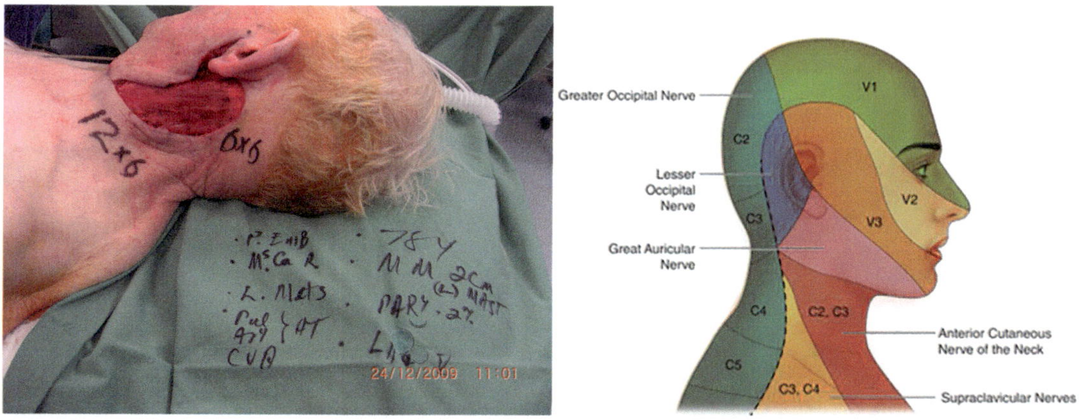

Fig. 2.583 A list of the comorbidities, including vascular abnormalities (see video). The dermatomal mark outs become the line of incision of the dermis and epidermis, ensuring that one-third deeply is attached with only partial undermining to facilitate the closure and vascular integrity of the defect. (Reprinted with permission from Atlas, *Reconstructive Technique in Melanoma Management* (p. 19), by Felix Behan, Springer Nature 2023)

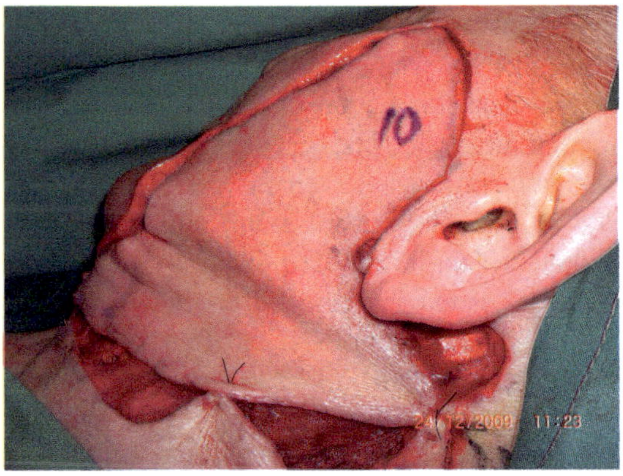

Fig. 2.584 The island Keystone is closed at various tension points, as indicated

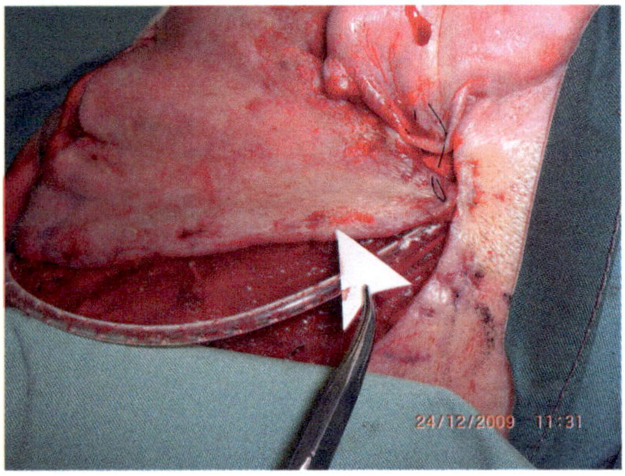

Fig. 2.585 The closure of the neck wound overlying the Redivac drainage system is shown, and the arrow points to the red dot signs on the cervical tissue, which are indicators of the hyperaemia created by the island flap design and an endorsement of potential safe postoperative healing

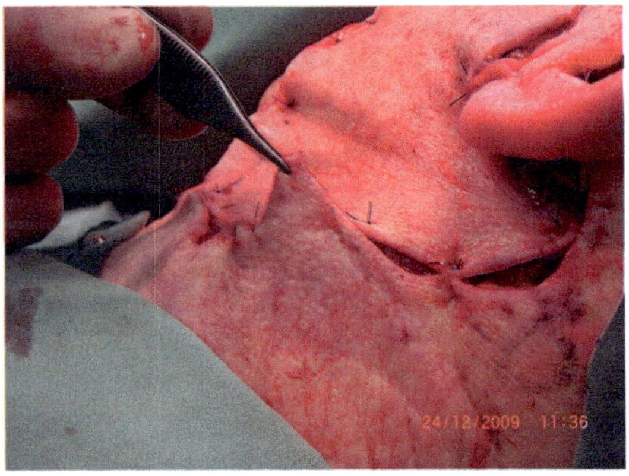

Fig. 2.586 The closure is refined by closing off excess tissue. Note the comparison of the hyperaemic phase of the Keystone used in the wound closure and the somewhat tardy circulatory flow with the neck tissue, where the cyanosis of the attached neck tissue provides remarkable contrast against the undermined island flap

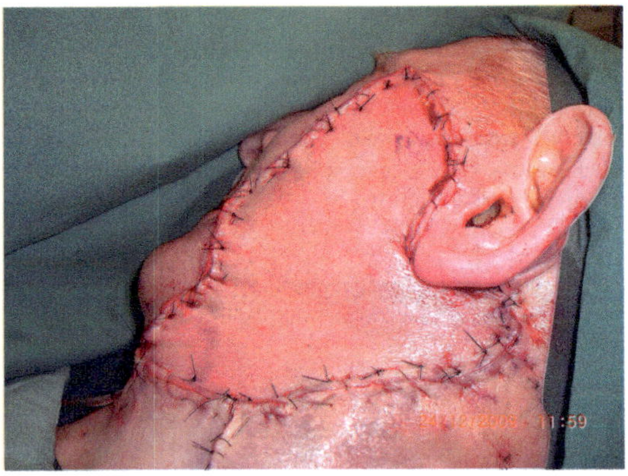

Fig. 2.587 The postoperative appearance at approximately 60 min later is shown, after employing the three-phase single-layer suture technique for closure. The outline of the flap, including neck tissue and cervical extension, becomes hyperaemic, which ensures wound healing

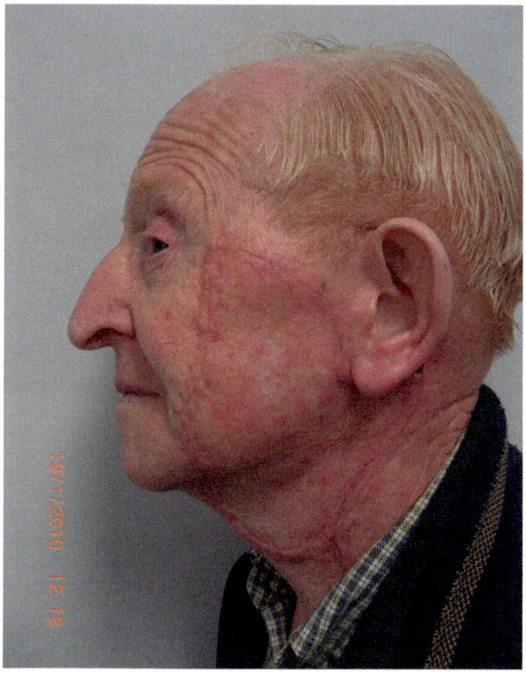

Fig. 2.588 The postoperative appearance at approximately 3 weeks is shown. The PACES characteristics of the Keystone were all exemplified in this elderly man with extensive comorbidities

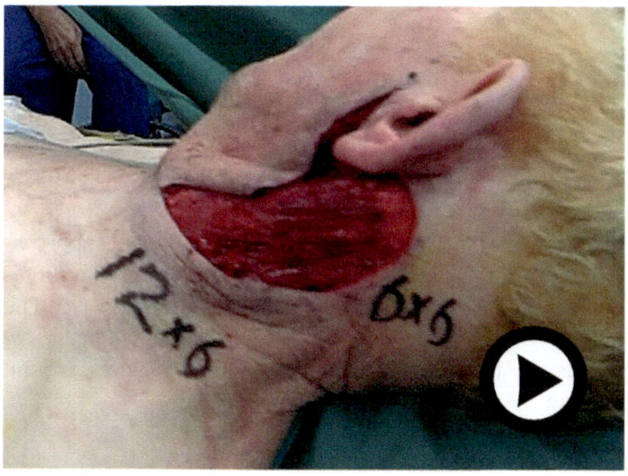

Fig. 2.589 Video 2.82 The planned supraclavicular Keystonereconstruction(▶https://doi.org/10.1007/000-k8f)

2.1.6.4 Case 61—Supraclavicular Melanoma L Neck: Unknown Primary

Case 61 features the salvage procedure of undermined neck dissection flaps C2 and C3 neck dissection. The Keystone principles are created by the island design, as illustrated. This island flap obviates the development of any tissue necrosis in this neck dissection in association with the tumour mass removal. This would otherwise happen with closure under tension at this oncological site in this 66-year-old man, and this case is another example of tissue expansion where the Keystone is expanded to fill the defect, as happens with tailoring (Figs. 2.590, 2.591, 2.592, 2.593, 2.594, 2.595 and 2.596).

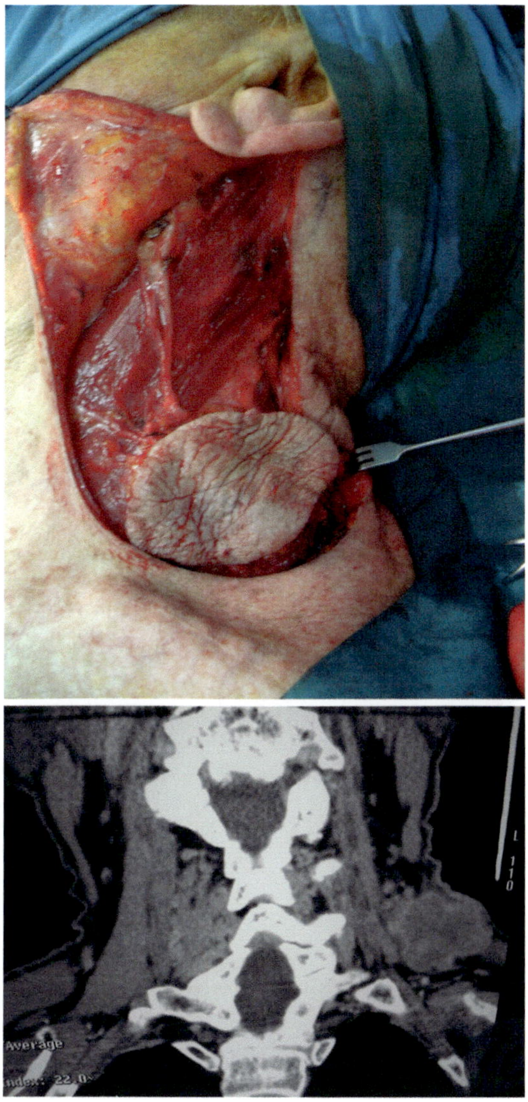

Fig. 2.590 The 9 × 8 cm surgical defect and CT confirmation

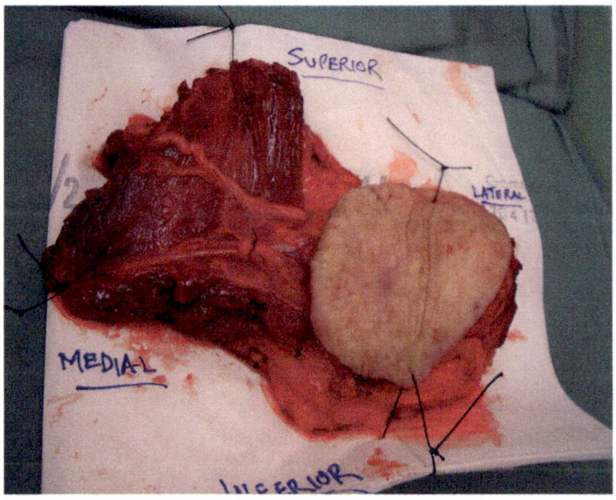

Fig. 2.591 Pathology specimen including nodal clearance from levels II, III and IV

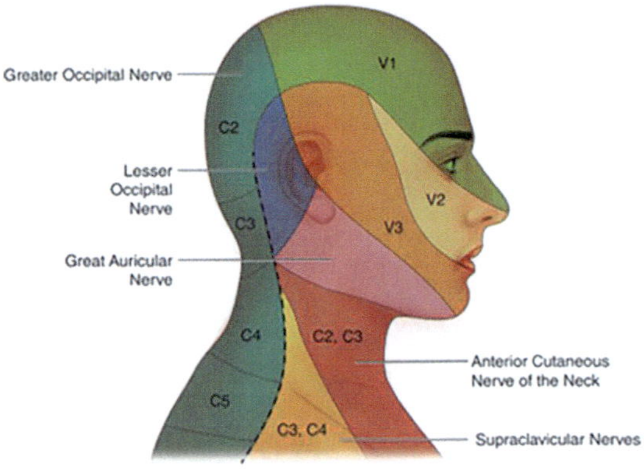

Fig. 2.592 The dermatomal mark outs become the line of incision of the dermis and epidermis, ensuring that one-third deeply is attached with only partial undermining to facilitate the closure and vascular integrity of the defect. (Reprinted with permission from Atlas, *Reconstructive Technique in Melanoma Management* (p. 19), by Felix Behan, Springer Nature 2023)

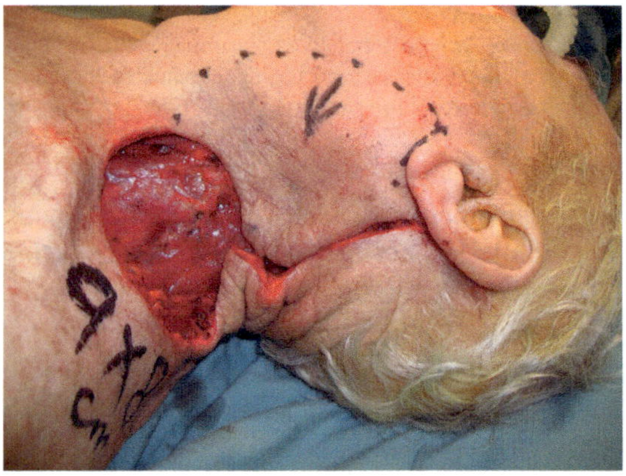

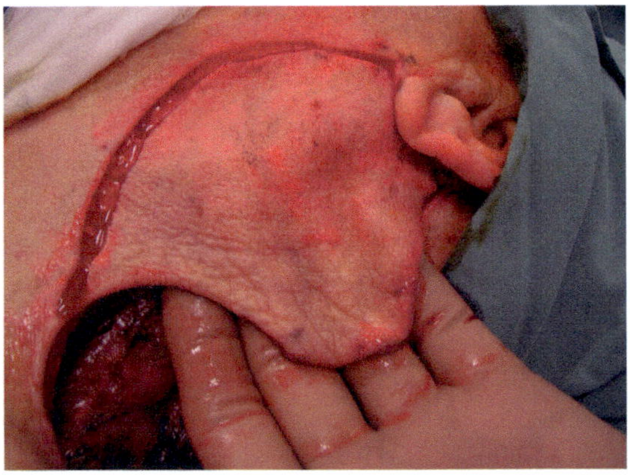

Fig. 2.593 This is the important slide in that the undermined area of the flap is cyanotic and arrowed. To overcome this problem, the cervical neck flap is islanded, leaving one-third of deep attachment, which produces a hypervascularised phase with increased flow, eliminating the cyanotic appearance (a sympathectomy effect). The operator's digits are placed under the undermined flap, essentially leaving one-third deep attachment. The reflex hyperaemia takes 10–15 min to develop this vascular change. This allows closure under tension for the 9 × 8 cm defect, which otherwise would create a risk due to the hypervascularisation. In other words, immediate tissue expansion occurs when the flap is stretched to fill the defect, like an element of tailoring

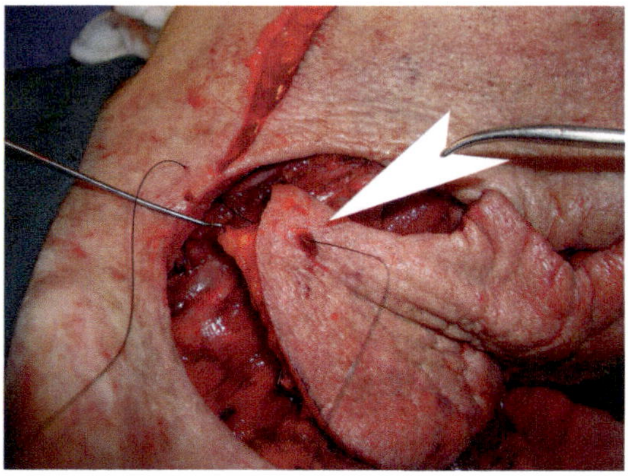

Fig. 2.594 The Keystone characteristic red dot sign indicates the hyperaemia bleeding more on the flap side than on the receiving site. This is an integral part of the excellent healing evidenced in Keystone reconstruction. The closure of the defect with the Keystone exemplifies all its characteristics, whereas the upper preauricular flap has been hypervascularised via delineation around the dermatomal alignment

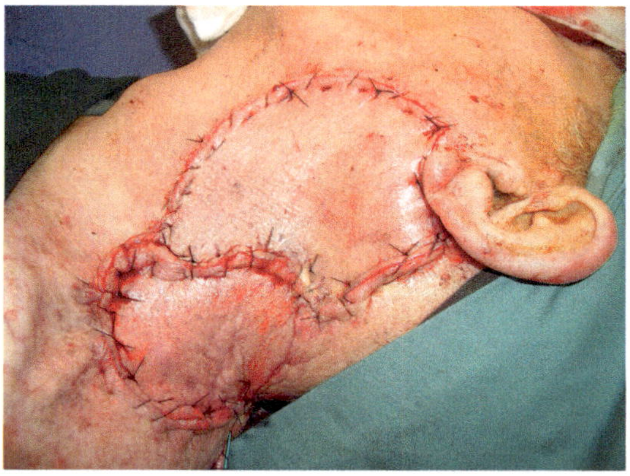

Fig. 2.595 A second Keystone with Redivac drainage from the cervical region (C2, C3) helps to close the defect to eliminate any element of tension. Note the vascular suffusion through both flaps, reflecting the hyperaemic phase, which contrasts with the appearance of the surrounding tissues

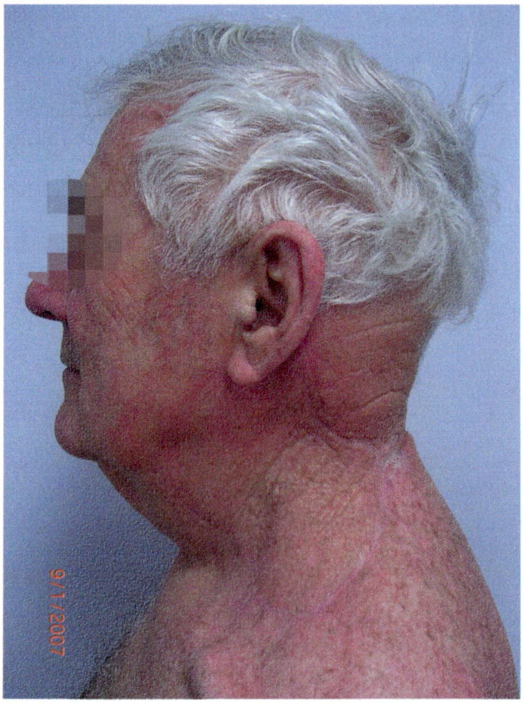

Fig. 2.596 The postoperative appearance shows no indication of flap necrosis, and the appearance of the facial expression mirrors the patients' satisfaction

In summary, islanding tissue while leaving one-third deep attachment of the undermined flap (Fig. 2.588) allows the locoregional flap of the integument to achieve surgical healing in this melanoma of an unknown primary thanks to hyperaemic hypervascularity. All the PACES charactristics are again exemplified.

2.1.7 Scalp

The applications of the Keystone on the scalp are based on neurovascular supply at various sites, but closure under tension is almost the norm. The mismatch of free tissue transfer is an obvious aesthetic disadvantage but often also a necessity because of the nature of the reconstructive challenge and the malignancy [21, 22]. Sometimes skin grafting is a necessary accompaniment to the Keystone because of tensional closure restrictions and restraints over the bony vault. However, the aesthetic advantage of the Keystone is obvious, and it shows all the Keystone's PACES characteristics.

Advancement and rotational flap techniques all apply, often with the delineation of various defined neurovascular structures (superficial temporal neurovascular structures and postauricular and occipital neurovascular structures). Microvascular variants of fascio-cutaneous latissimus dorsi flaps and rectus abdominus flaps have not been part of this reconstructive repertoire [23, 24].

2.1.7.1 Case 62—1.5 cm Scalp Melanoma Level II (Figs. 2.597, 2.598, 2.599, 2.600, 2.601, 2.602 and 2.603)

In summary, the pain-free postoperative phase of and the absence of necrosis in—and the characteristic of increasing hair growth—of the Keystone in the scalp were not compromised by complications. Expeditious execution is the key here—the timestamp confirms the 1 h timeframe with sensory recovery within 3 weeks.

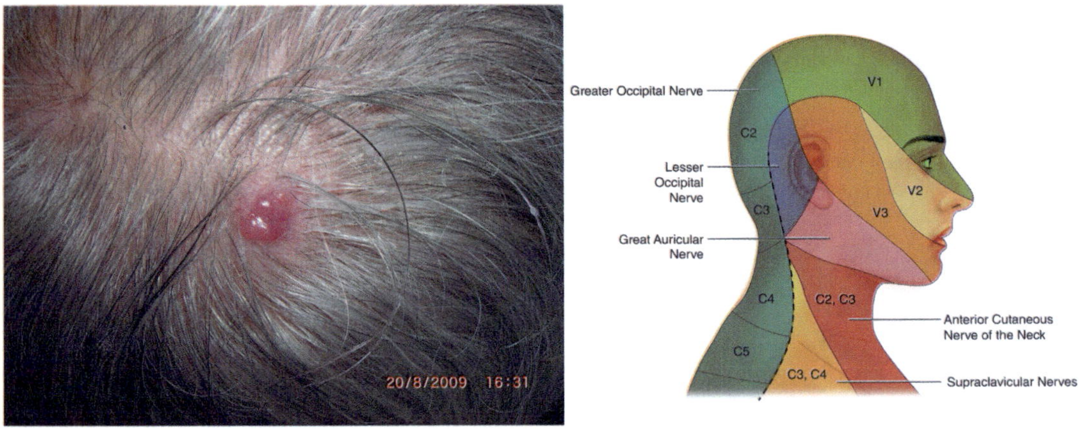

Fig. 2.597 The melanotic lesion is shown. The dermatomal mark outs become the line of incision of the dermis and epidermis, ensuring that one-third deeply is attached with only partial undermining to facilitate the closure and vascular integrity of the defect. (Reprinted with permission from Atlas, *Reconstructive Technique in Melanoma Management* (p. 19), by Felix Behan, Springer Nature 2023)

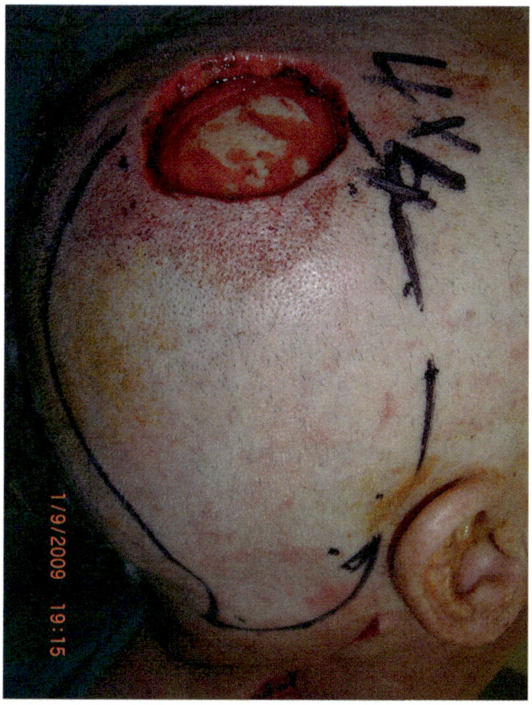

Fig. 2.598 A 4 × 4 cm clearance is shown, including pericranium. The mark out of the island flap design sits in the region of the occipital branch of the postauricular artery in the C2 and C3 origin

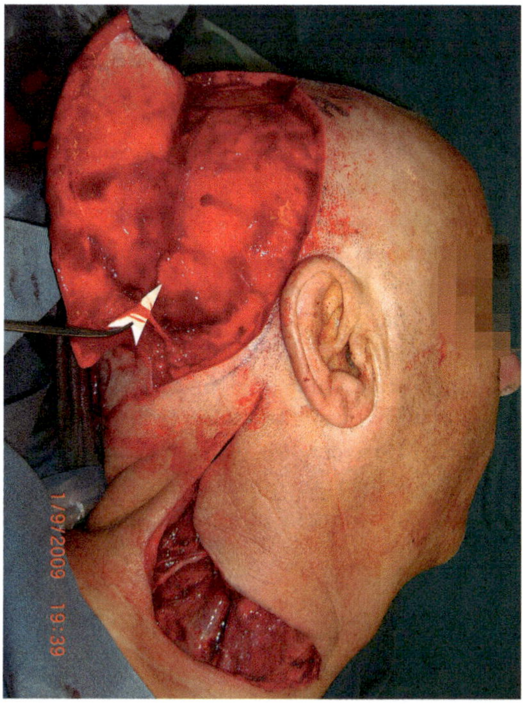

Fig. 2.599 The neurovascular axes supporting the flap are freed from the surrounding tissues, but the structures are not skeletonised, to maintain autonomic, somatic and venous support to the arterial stalk of the occipital branch of the posturicular artery (arrowed)

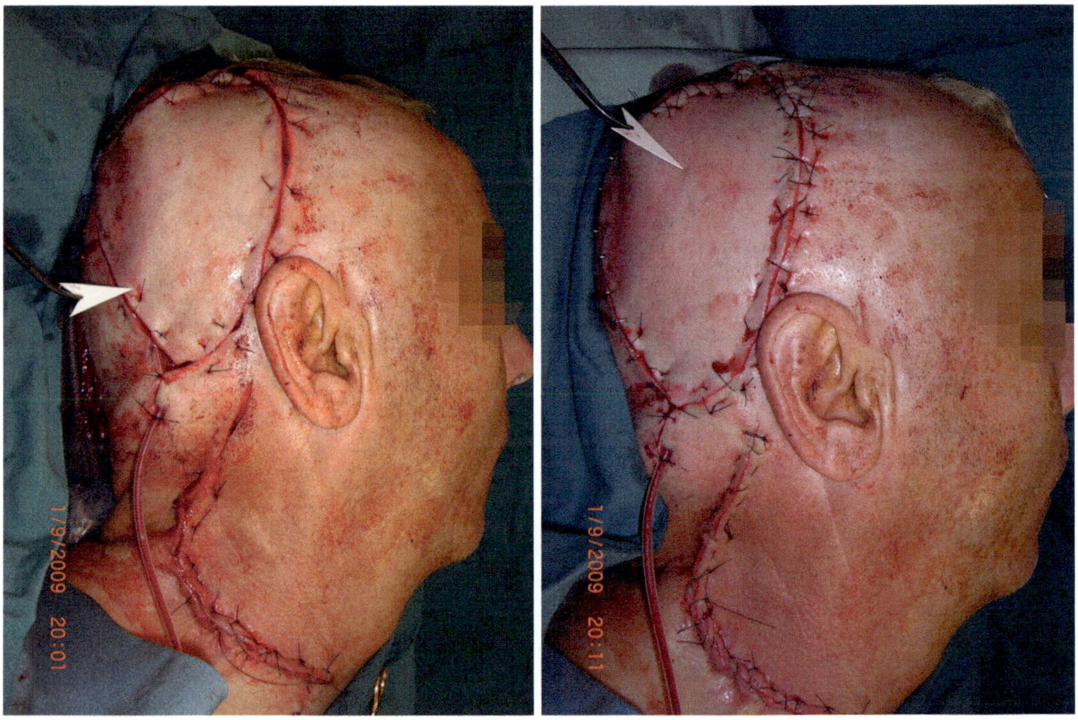

Fig. 2.600 The three-phase suture closure technique, with locking mattress sutures at the points of maximum tension, mattress sutures to close the wound and a continuous nylon around the periphery for epidermal seal, is shown. The lines of tension at the key points are locking mattress sutures. The remaining loose neck in the skin is trimmed accordingly. The hyperaemia, a Keystone characteristic, is evident in the island flap

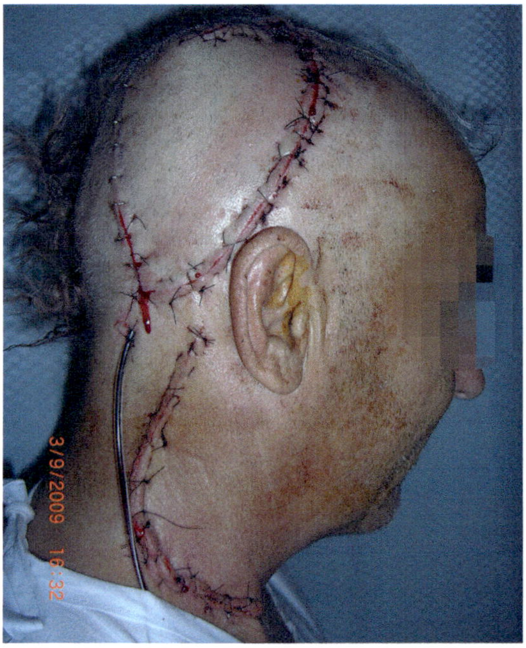

Fig. 2.601 Appearance at 2 days with drain tubes functioning

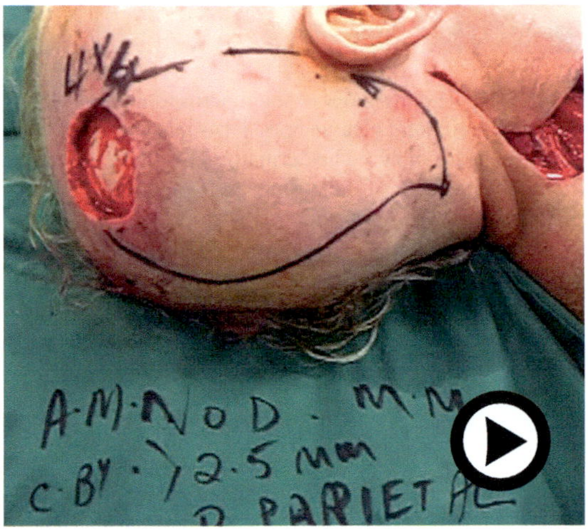

Fig. 2.602 Video 2.83 The Keystone mark out based on theoccipitalcirculation(▶https://doi.org/10.1007/000-k8g)

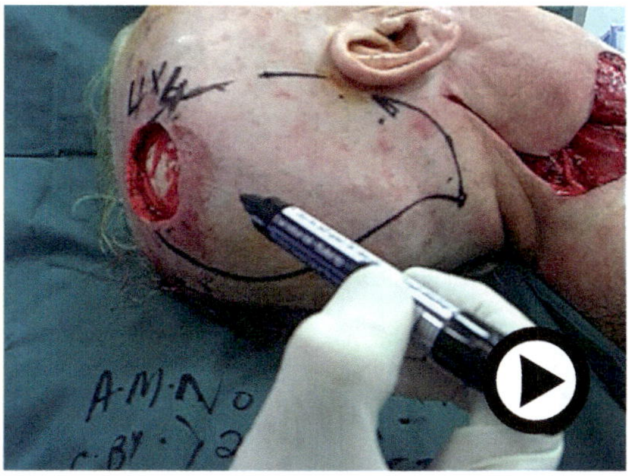

Fig. 2.603 Video 2.84 Planned operative sequence (▶ https://doi.org/10.1007/000-k8h)

2.1.7.2 Case 63—Mitotic Lesion Recurrence Involving the Outer Table of the Skull

The tumour defect on the vertex of the scalp produced an oncological clearance of a defect 8 × 8 cm (Figs. 2.604, 2.605, 2.606, 2.607, 2.608, 2.609, 2.610, 2.611 and 2.612).

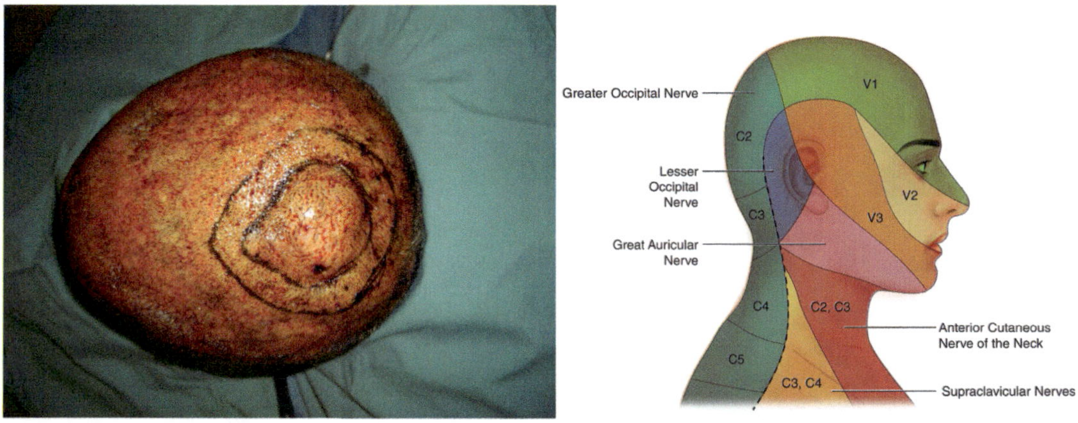

Fig. 2.604 The mark out of the macroscopic tumour and the 2 cm peripheral clearance of 1 cm into the outer table of the scalp are shown. The dermatomal mark outs become the line of incision of the dermis and epidermis, ensuring that one-third deeply is attached with only partial undermining to facilitate the closure and vascular integrity of the defect. (Reprinted with permission from Atlas, *Reconstructive Technique in Melanoma Management* (p. 19), by Felix Behan, Springer Nature 2023)

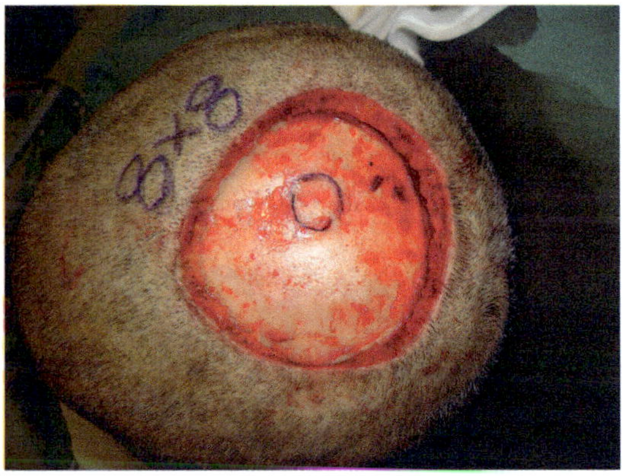

Fig. 2.605 The peripheral clearance before the additional removal of the outer skull table producing an 8 × 8 cm scalp defect

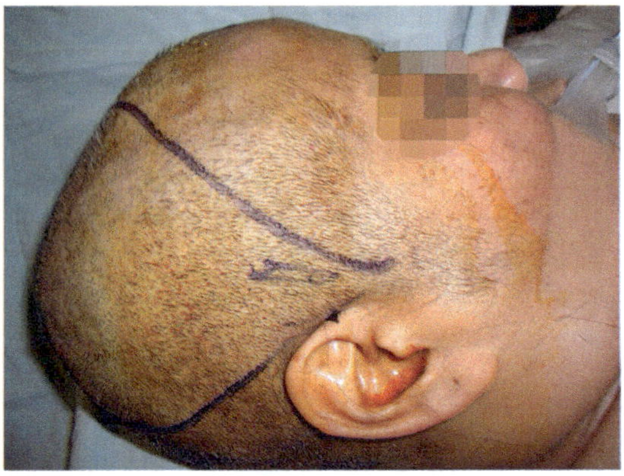

Fig. 2.606 A superficial temporal artery mark out is shown. The flap is raised, retaining and not skeletonising the axial neurovascular structures. This retains periadventitial tissue to ensure autonomic and somatic input

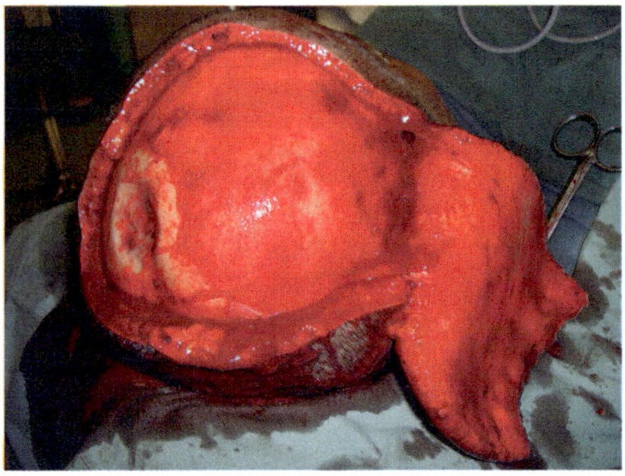

Fig. 2.607 Raising the flap using blunt dissection once the integument has been divided around the periphery

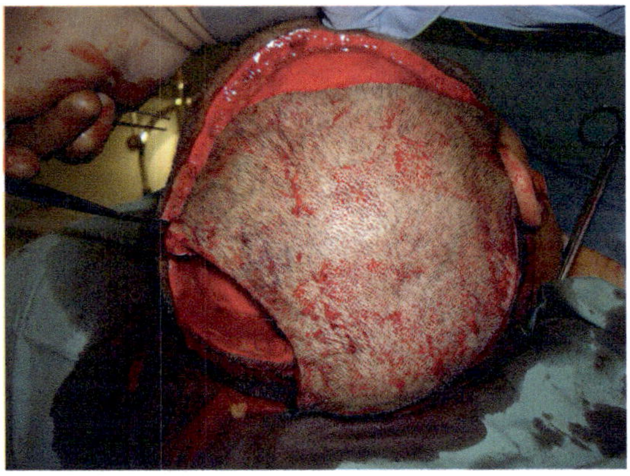

Fig. 2.608 Staged closure sequence

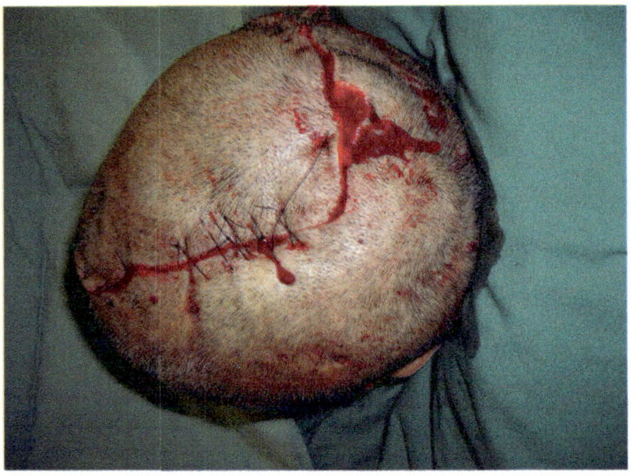

Fig. 2.609 The locking mattress sutures at the points of maximum tension are used to close the defect before ordinary mattress sutures produce wound closure

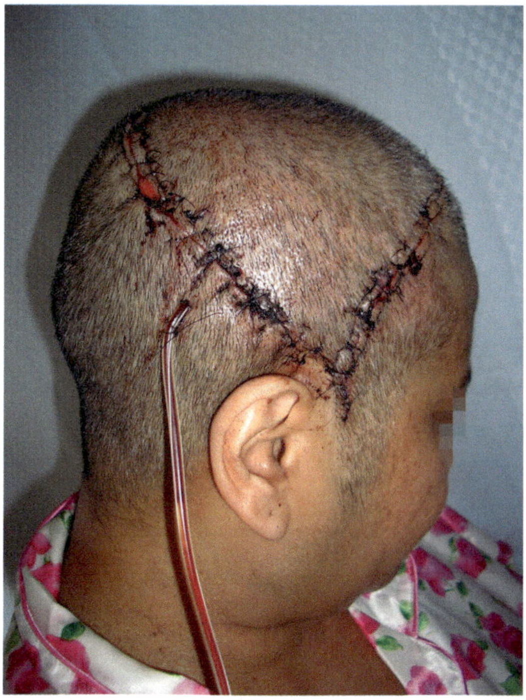

Fig. 2.610 Completion with Redivac drainage is shown. Note the hyperaemic flare in the island flap compared with the image of the surrounding scalp

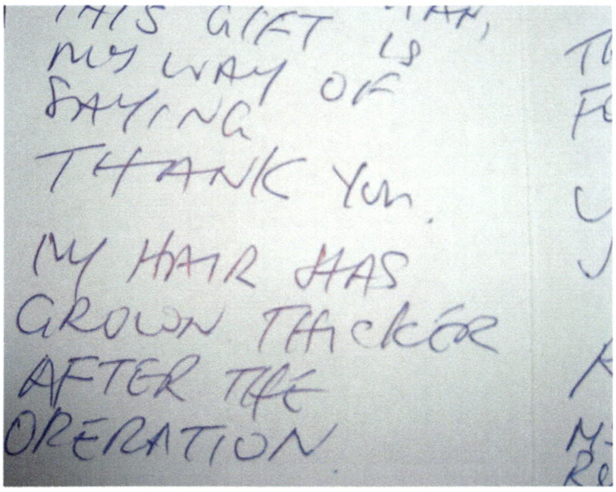

Fig. 2.612 The patient's Christmas card thanking me for the surgical procedure and stating that her hair is now growing thicker as a result of the Keystone reconstruction. This exuberant growth is a reflection of the hypervascularity phase produced with islanding

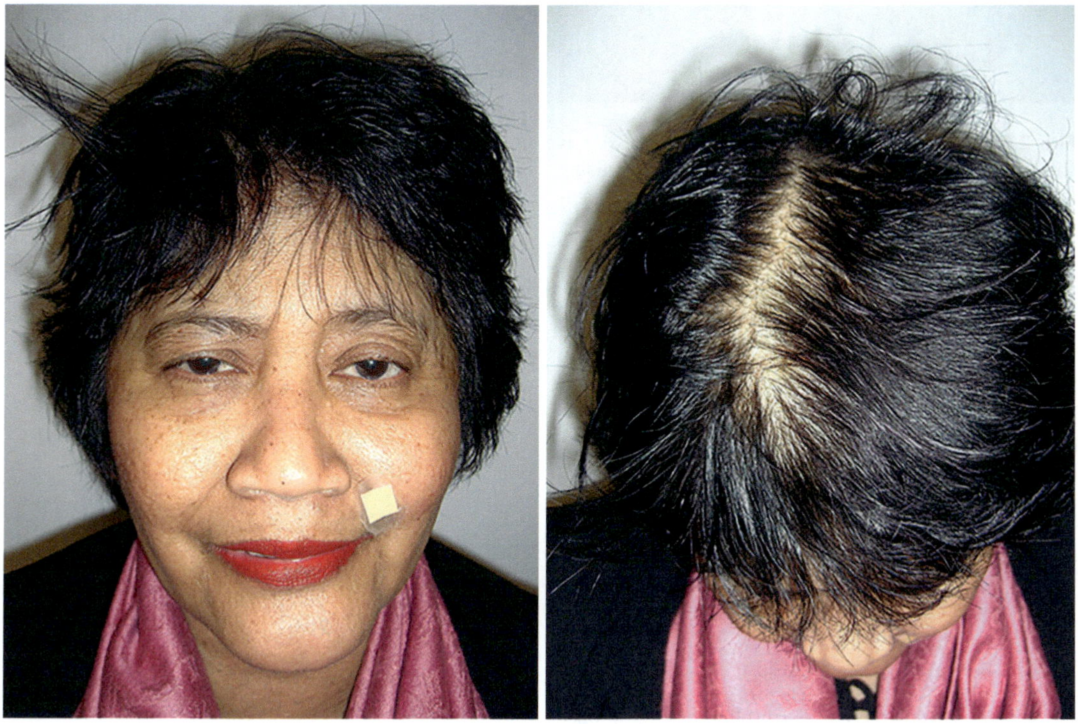

Fig. 2.611 The appearance 6 months later is shown, and note the patient's observation of the increased hair growth and thickness. Again, a clinical outcome of hypervascularity in the scalp is produced. The hair is parted to show the suture line

The PACES characteristics were all exemplified: pain-free, aesthetic, no vascular complications, economical in terms of time and sensory recovery with the resolution of oedema.

2.1.7.3 Case 64—Local Recurrence into the Occipital Glands Following a Melanoma of a Previously Grafted Scalp

Case 64 features a level II melanoma of the scalp in a 62-year-old male golfer, with a secondary melanoma of the R neck (T2N2) and occipital nodes. The tumour-free interval was 15 months (Figs. 2.613, 2.614, 2.615, 2.616 and 2.617).

In summary, islanding in the Keystone manner has hypervascularised the flap, allowing a large oncological defect of secondary melanoma to be successfully closed. All the PACES characteristics were evident throughout the procedure, indicating that the Keystone principles apply in this reconstruction.

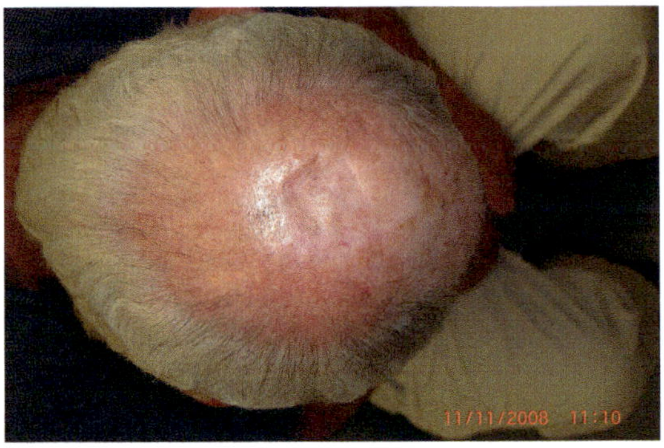

Fig. 2.613 The postoperative melanoma appearance of a graft on the scalp prior to regional dissemination into the R occipital glands

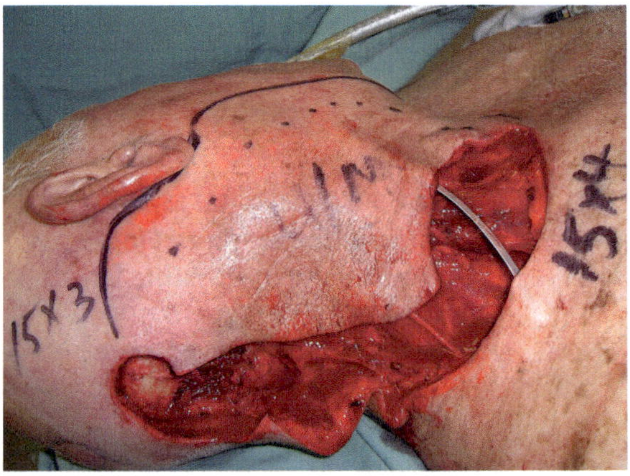

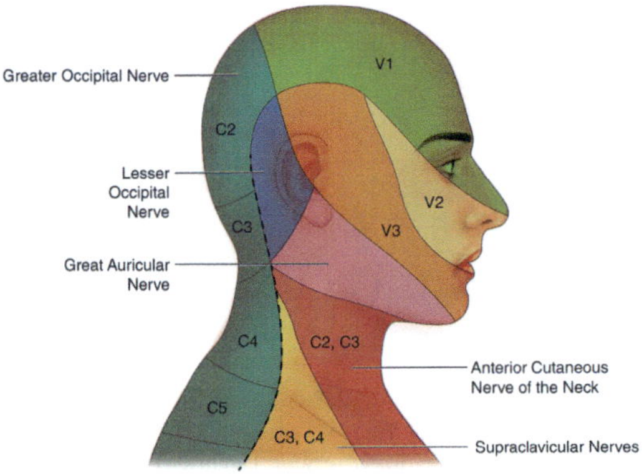

Fig. 2.614 The surgical clearance of the occipital glands and level II, III and IV neck glands is shown. The dissection created a 15 × 3 cm defect over the occiput and a 15 × 4 cm defect in the neck, which was performed by Professor Andrew Sizeland of the Peter MacCallum Cancer Institute. The flap undermining is defined by the suction drainage tubing (arrowed) in situ and the distal incision, where leaving one-third of deep attachment anterially guarantees the flow at the fascial level and the hyperaemic vascular apperance. This leaves 30% of deeper attachment along the chin and anterior neck, supplied by the facial artery and branches but lying within the C3, C4 and C5 neuro-dermatomes. Without using the skin incision to create the island of skin and subcuataneous tissue, the reflex hyperaemia would not occur and flap viability would be questionable. This simple idea of incising the skin and then surgically closing the wound creates this biological phenomenon of hypraemia to ensure the absence of necrosis in flap reconstruction. The dermatomal mark outs become the line of incision of the dermis and epidermis, ensuring that one-third deeply is attached with only partial undermining to facilitate the closure and vascular integrity of the defect. (Reprinted with permission from Atlas, *Reconstructive Technique in Melanoma Management* (p. 19), by Felix Behan, Springer Nature 2023)

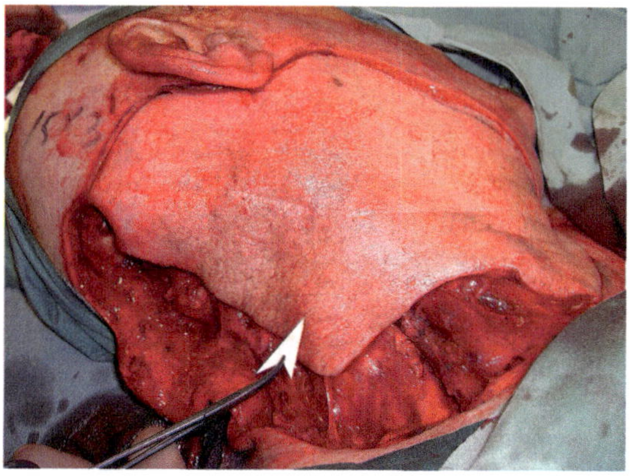

Fig. 2.615 The Keystone principle of using a quadrilateral design in this case is evident. The island design anteriorly penetrates only the dermal-epidermal line into the subcutaneous tissues. Hypervascularisation becomes evident within a 10–15 min timeframe. It is hypothesised, which is a sympathectomy effect at the epidermal level that increases flow. If this island is not created, flap necrosis will occur

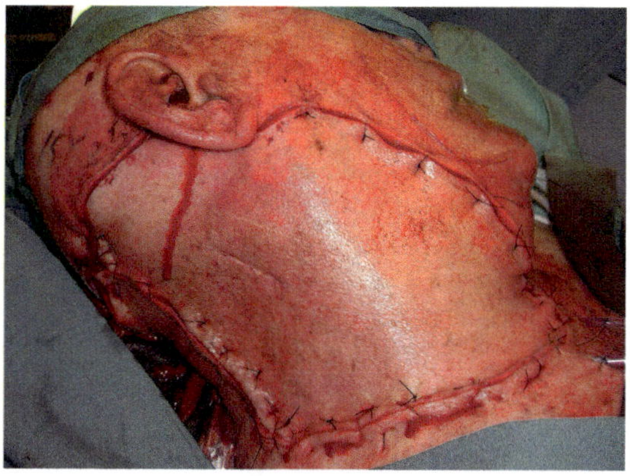

Fig. 2.616 Staged closure using the three-phase suture technique of locking mattress sutures at the points of maximum tension to achieve cover is shown; these sutures stay in for 21 days. The remaining wound is closed by interrupted mattress sutures, which stay in for 14 days. Then a continuous nylon is used to achieve wound seal, which stays in 7–10 days. The vascular hyperaemia is evident

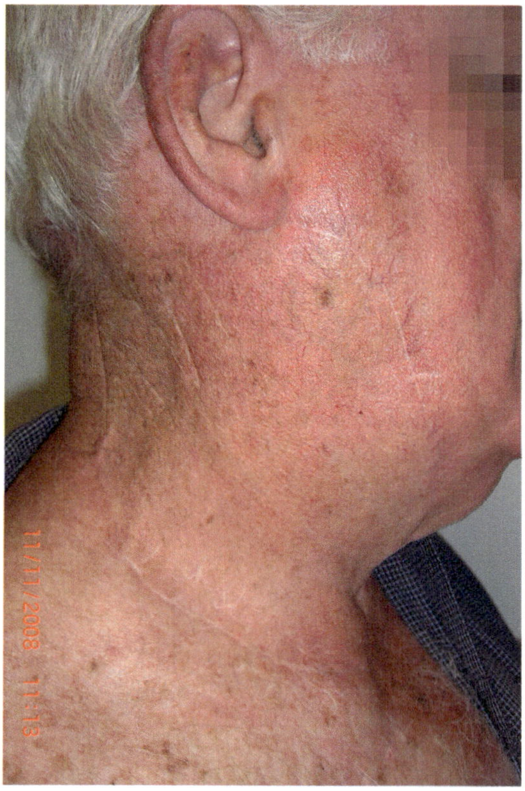

Fig. 2.617 The postoeprative healed wound appearance at 6 months—no evidence of necrosis throughout

2.1.7.4 Case 65—R Occipital Mass Closing a Undermined Flap Under Tension is Possible Using Keystone Mark Outs to Hypervascularise the Tissue

Case 65 features a secondary melanoma dissemination into the posterior neck over the mastoid in a 77-year-old man following a scalp excision of the melanotic region 12 months earlier (Figs. 2.618, 2.619, 2.620, 2.621 and 2.622).

In summary, all the PACES characteristics were evident throughout the procedure. It was done as a duet procedure with Professor Andrew Sizeland at the Peter McCallum Cancer Institute.

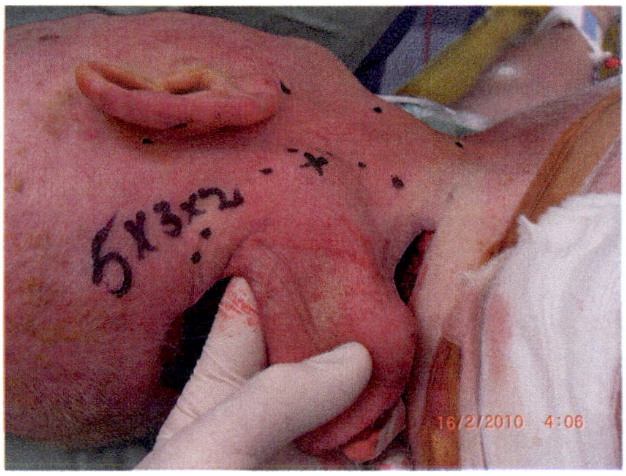

Fig. 2.618 The melanoma mass measured 5 × 3 × 2 cm in the hands of the operator before detachment and neck gland clearance

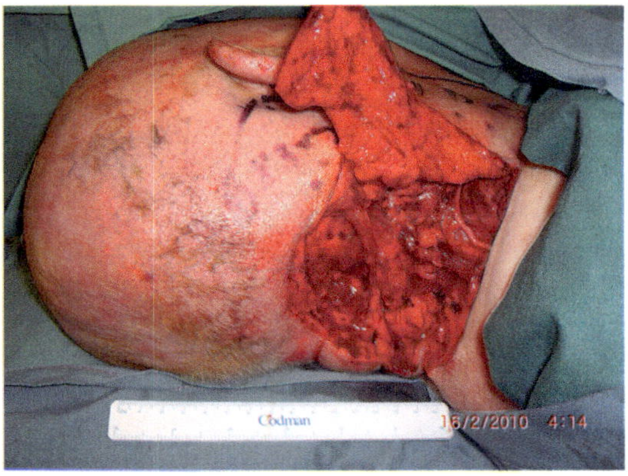

Fig. 2.619 Level 5 cervical nodes in the R posterior triangle were used for clearance. The surgical defect with undermined anterior neck flaps was used for closure, leaving one-third deep attachment. The pyramidal Keystone is goverened by the surgical defect but leaves one-third deep attachment below the R ear

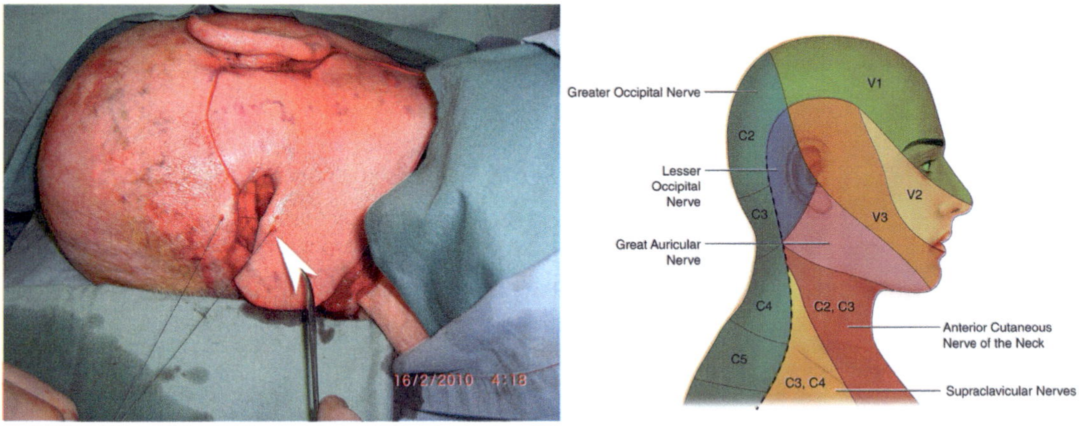

Fig. 2.620 For neck flap closure, the neck flaps are islanded in the region of the sternomastoid at the dermal-epidermal level. This Keystone variant fits into the oncological defect. The white arrow indicates the hyperaemia and the red dot sign—a Keystone characteristic. The dermatomal mark outs become the line of incision of the dermis and epidermis, ensuring that one-third deeply is attached with only partial undermining to facilitate the closure and vascular integrity of the defect. (Reprinted with permission from Atlas, *Reconstructive Technique in Melanoma Management* (p. 19), by Felix Behan, Springer Nature 2023)

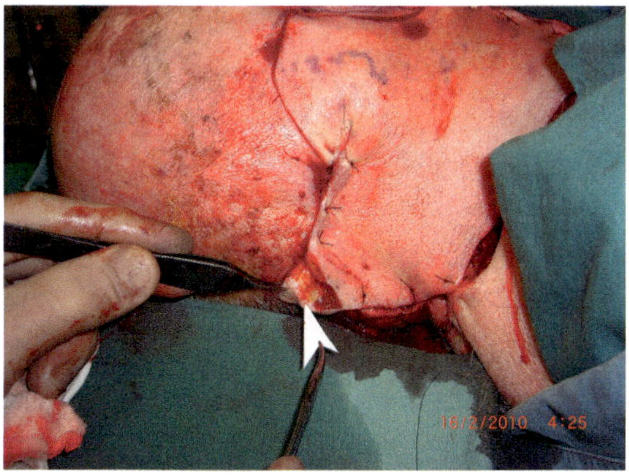

Fig. 2.621 Redundant tissue is being trimmed out, and the arrow indicates the generous subdermal flow that ensures healing without necrosis

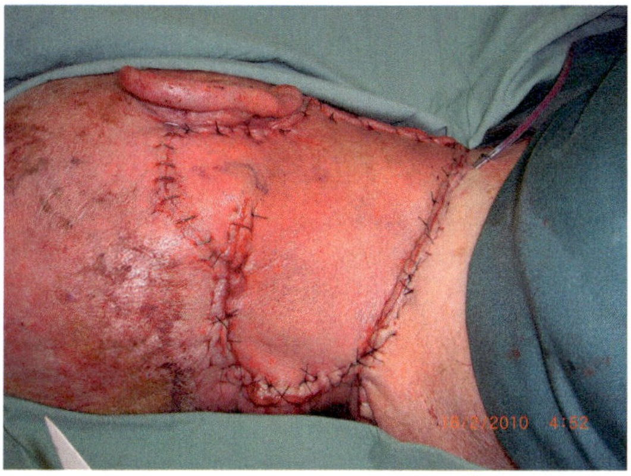

Fig. 2.622 The time taken from the timestamped images is 45 min. The three-phase suture technique of using locking mattress sutures at tension points, ordinary mattress sutures and a continuous nylon for epidermal closure is used here, as is routine. Suction drainage is mandatory

2.1.7.5 Case 66—Melanoma Secondary over the Occiput with a Graft Site Above (Figs. 2.623, 2.624, 2.625, 2.626, 2.627, 2.628, 2.629, 2.630, 2.631, 2.632 and 2.633)

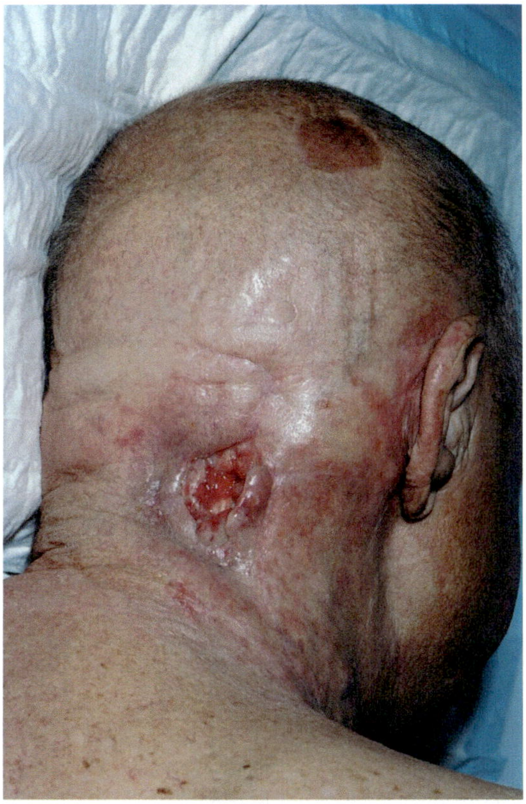

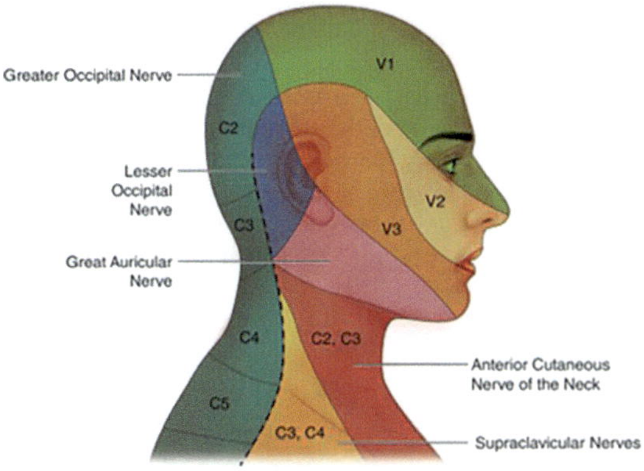

Fig. 2.623 The ulcerated lesion that needs wide excision is shown. The dermatomal mark outs become the line of incision of the dermis and epidermis, ensuring that one-third deeply is attached with only partial undermining to facilitate the closure and vascular integrity of the defect. (Reprinted with permission from Atlas, *Reconstructive Technique in Melanoma Management* (p. 19), by Felix Behan, Springer Nature 2023)

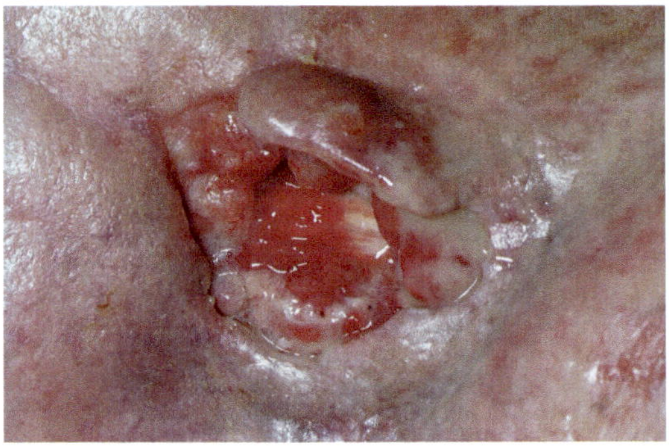

Fig. 2.624 Closeup of the pathology

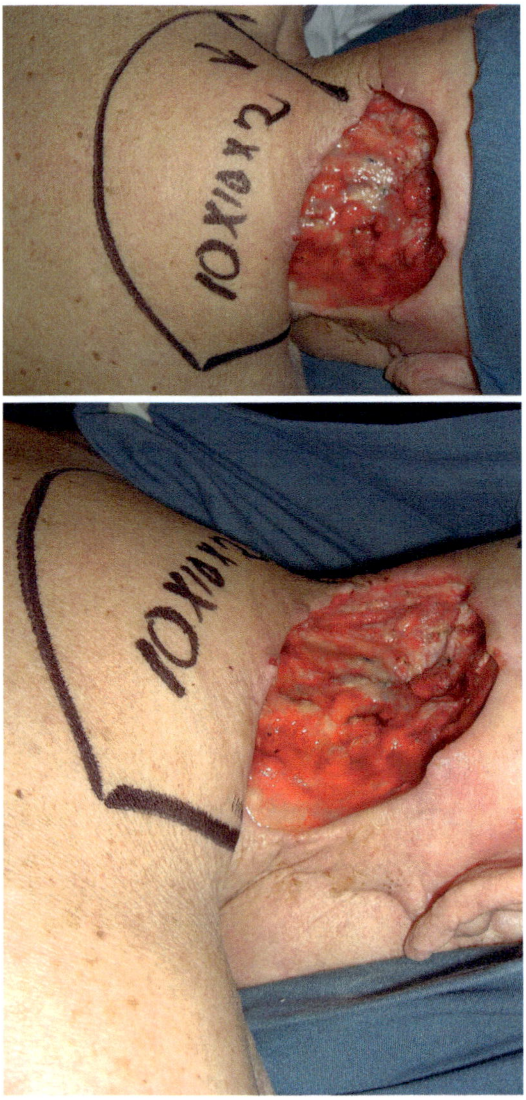

Fig. 2.625 The excisional defect, the 10 × 10 × 5 cm Keystone mark out and the planned Keystone from the area of C7

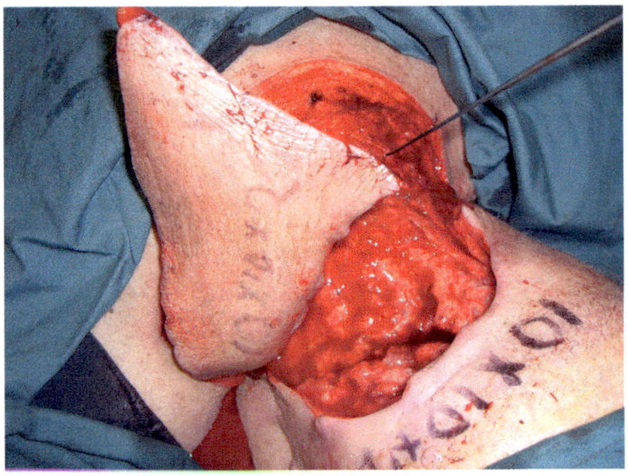

Fig. 2.626 The 10 × 10 × 2 in depth cm defect

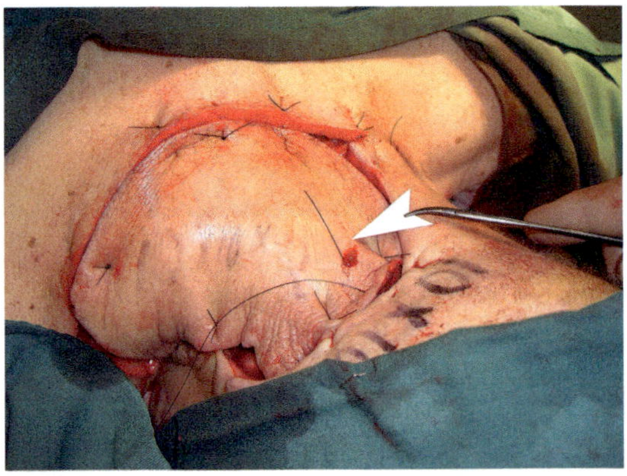

Fig. 2.627 The red dot sign indicating the Keystone's vascular integrity

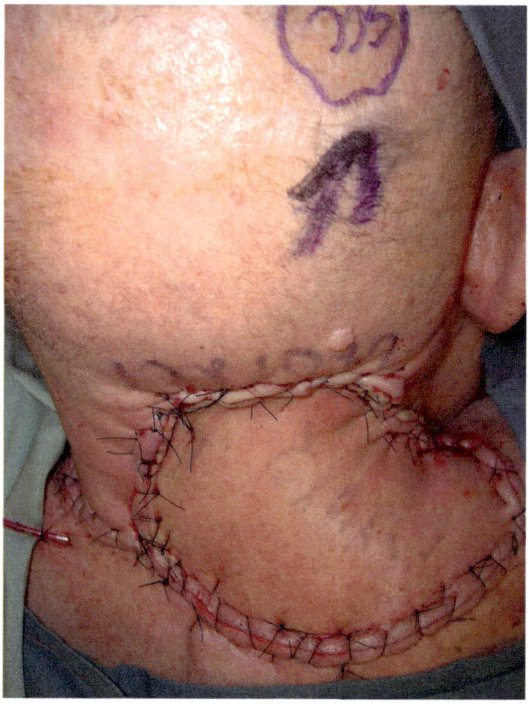

Fig. 2.628 The original SCC lesion that was grafted and the spread of nodes to the region of the cervical spine

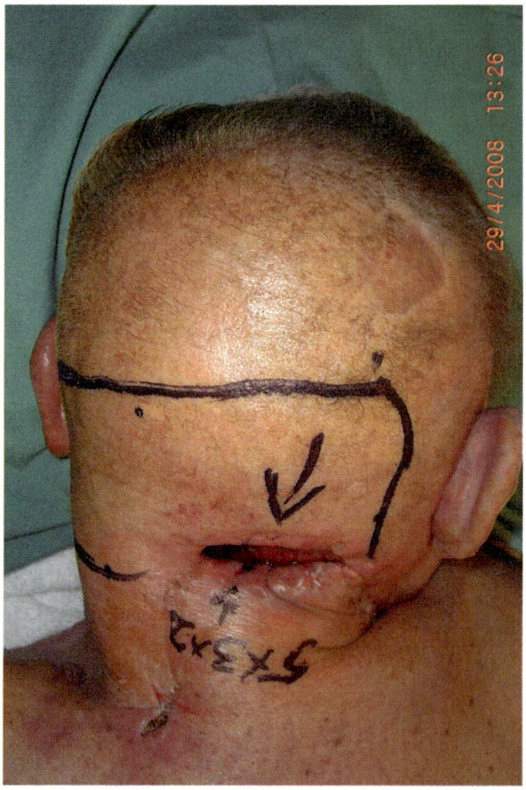

Fig. 2.630 The Keystone mark out

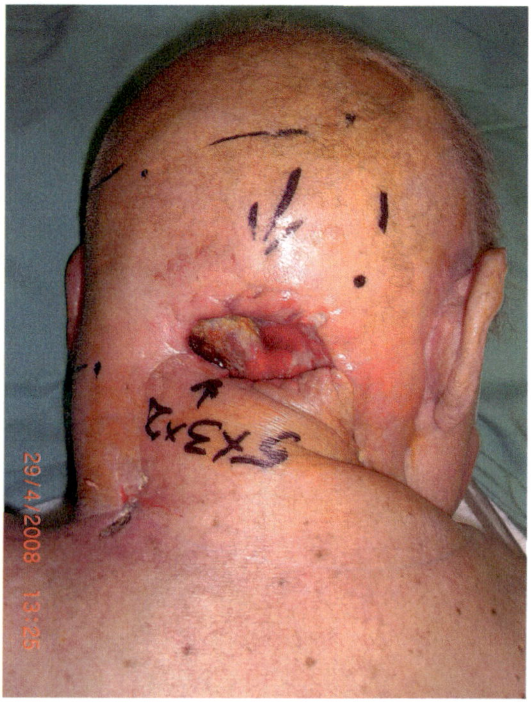

Fig. 2.629 Another lesion in the same patient spread down over the occiput to the region of the cervical spine

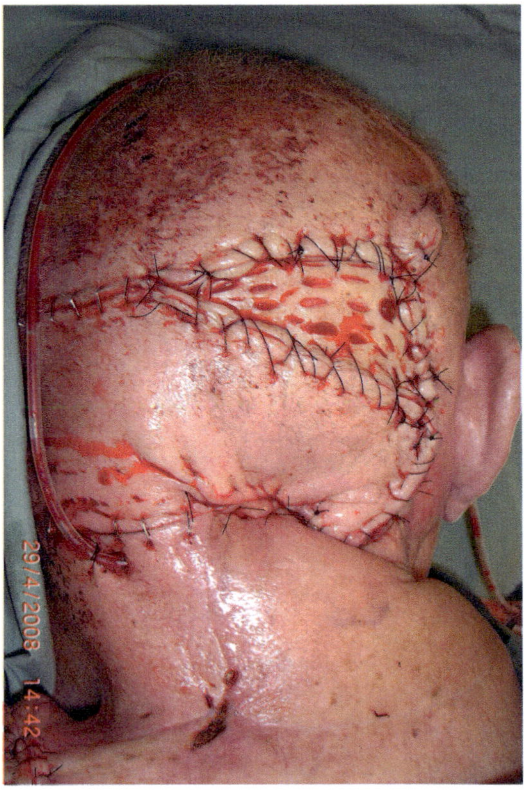

Fig. 2.631 To avoid lines of tension with drainage installed, the Keystone is rotated and the secondary defect is grafted

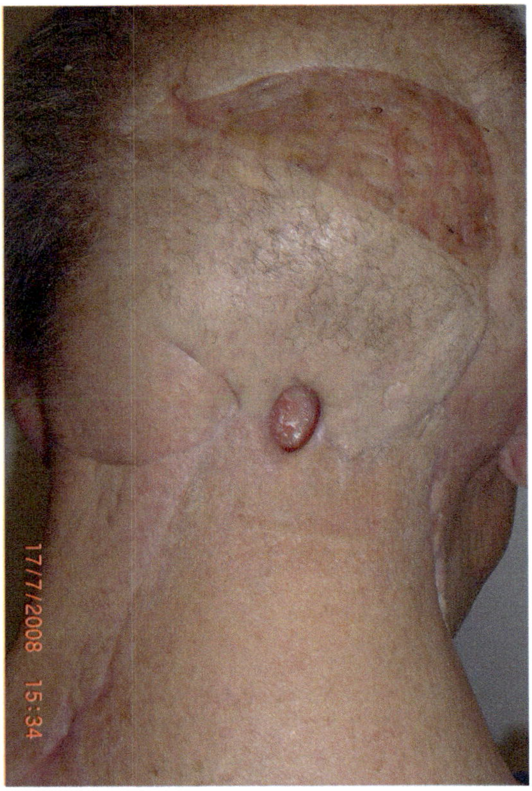

Fig. 2.632 Recurrence after 3 months

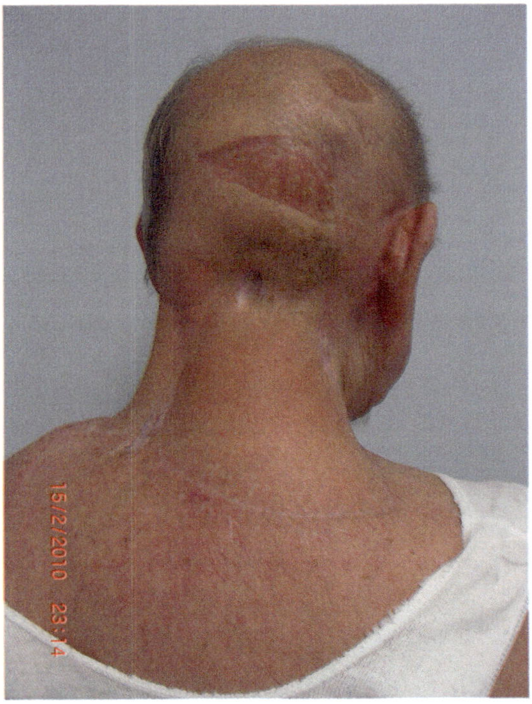

Fig. 2.633 Appearance at 2 years

The PACES characteristics were all exemplified: pain-free, aesthetic, no vascular complications, economical in terms of time and sensory recovery with the resolution of oedema.

2.1.7.6 Case 67—Lesion of the Temple Closed with a Scalp Rotation Flap (Figs. 2.634, 2.635, 2.636, 2.637 and 2.638)

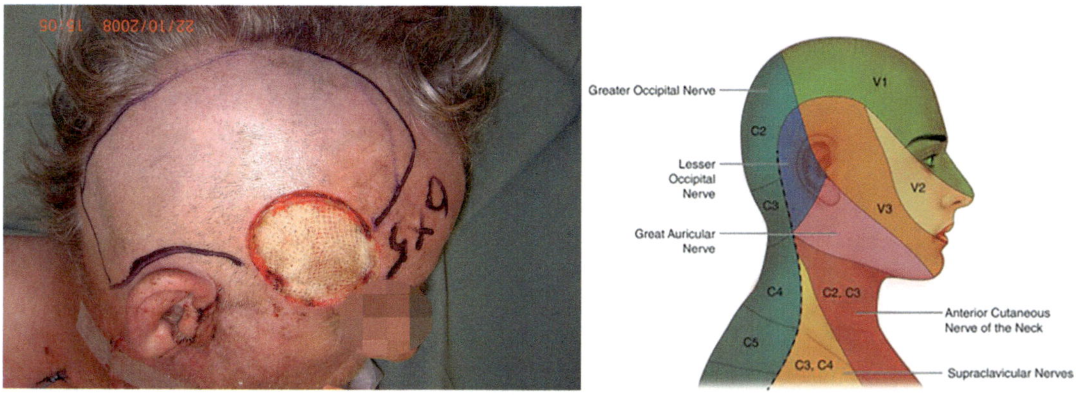

Fig. 2.634 The 6 × 5 cm defect is shown prior to flap rotation before grafting the secondary defect to avoid tension. The dermatomal mark outs become the line of incision of the dermis and epidermis, ensuring that one-third deeply is attached with only partial undermining to facilitate the closure and vascular integrity of the defect. (Reprinted with permission from Atlas, *Reconstructive Technique in Melanoma Management* (p. 19), by Felix Behan, Springer Nature 2023)

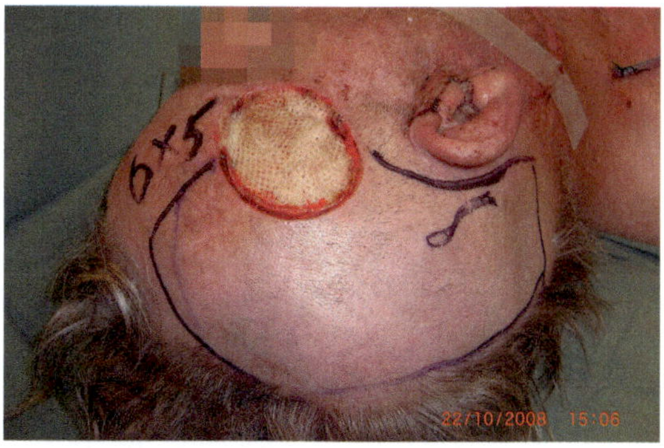

Fig. 2.635 The mark out prior to transfer, which covers the defect

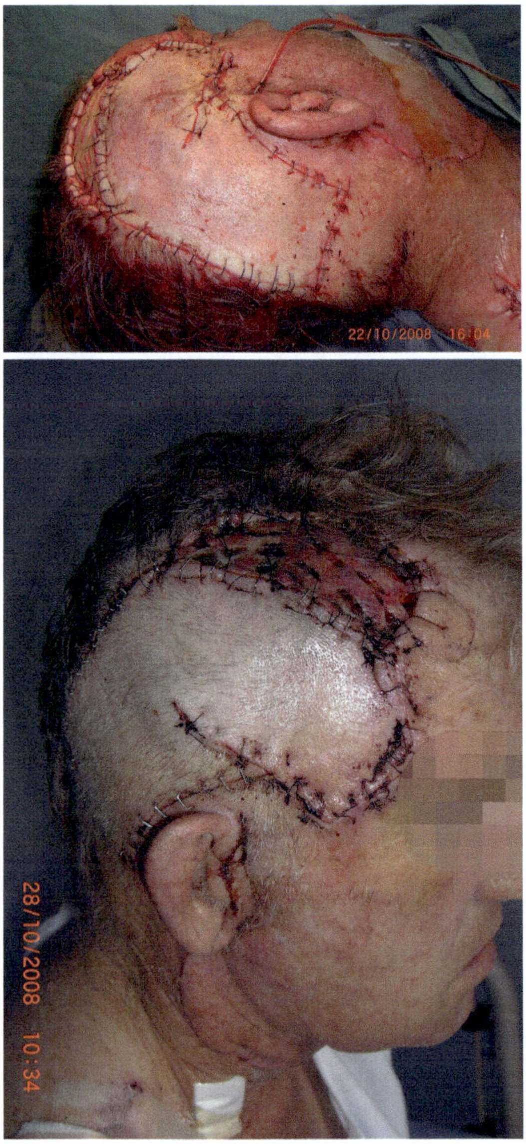

Fig. 2.636 This is the element of poor perfusion over the temple warranting an alternative use of a skin graft. The 6-day appearance with the fenestrated full-thickness graft in situ is shown

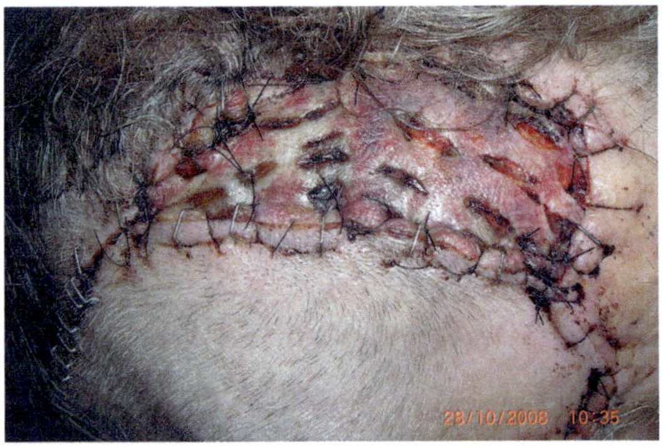

Fig. 2.637 Appearance at 6 days of the fenestrated full-thickness graft

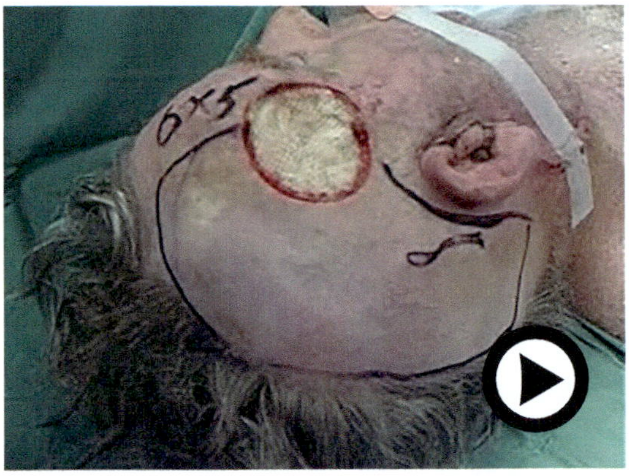

Fig. 2.638 Video 2.85 The mark out of the scalp Keystone flap prior to insertion using Keystone principles (▶ https://doi.org/10.1007/000-k8j)

The PACES characteristics were all exemplified: pain-free, aesthetic, no vascular complications, economical in terms of time and sensory recovery with the resolution of oedema)

2.1.7.7 Case 68—Scalp Keystone Using Extension into the Occipital Region to Facilitate Rotation and Advancement (Figs. 2.639, 2.640, 2.641, 2.642 and 2.643)

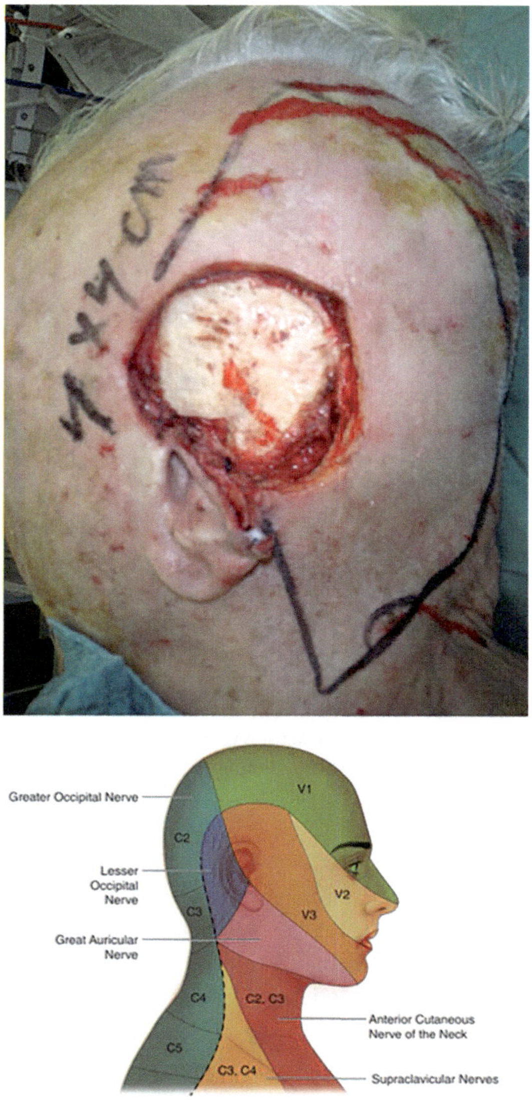

Fig. 2.639 The 7 × 7 cm surgical defect with exposed skull is shown. The dermatomal mark outs become the line of incision of the dermis and epidermis, ensuring that one-third deeply is attached with only partial undermining to facilitate the closure and vascular integrity of the defect. (Reprinted with permission from Atlas, *Reconstructive Technique in Melanoma Management* (p. 19), by Felix Behan, Springer Nature 2023)

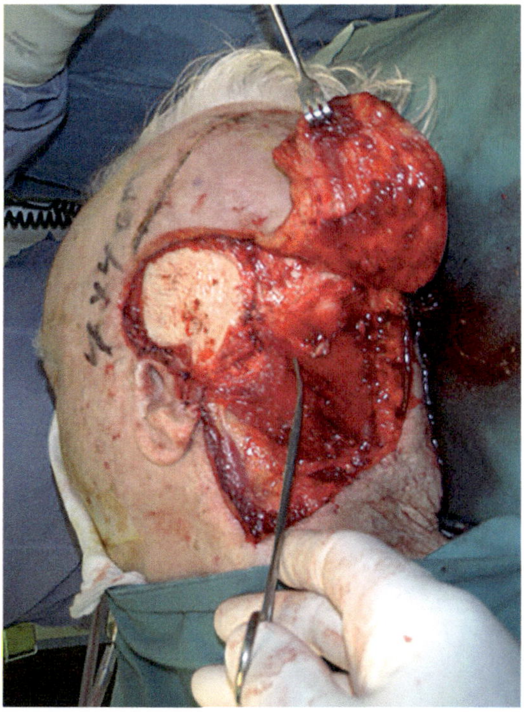

Fig. 2.640 The exposed skull surface must be covered with the flap

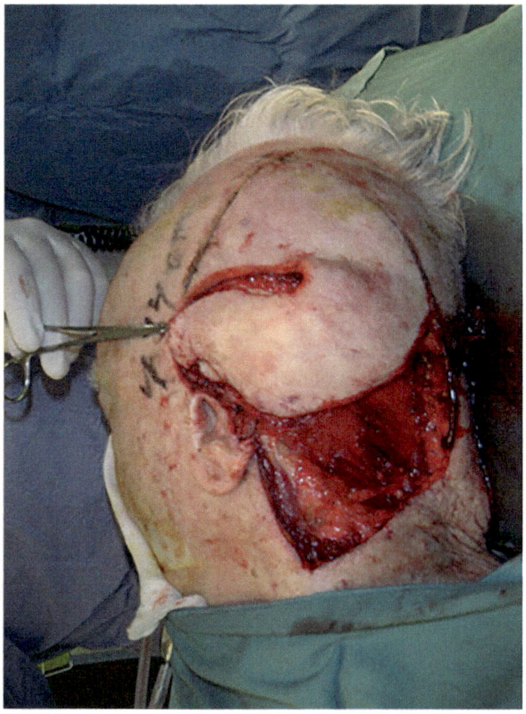

Fig. 2.641 The insertion covers the skull by rotating the Keystone, and the secondary defect is grafted to avoid undue tension

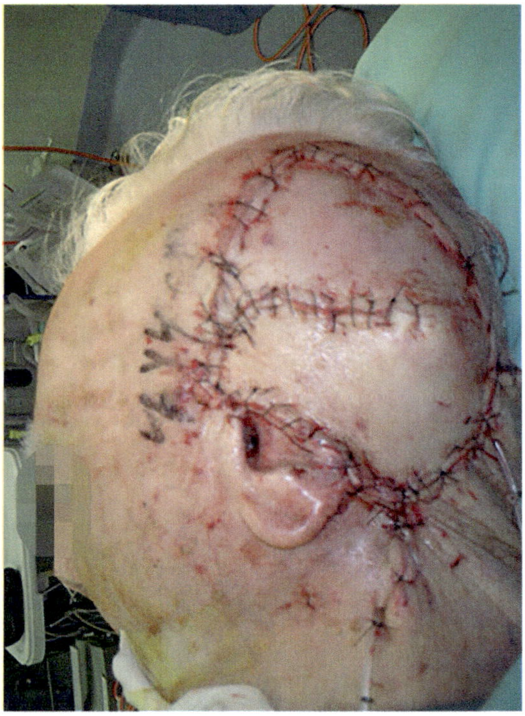

Fig. 2.642 On completion

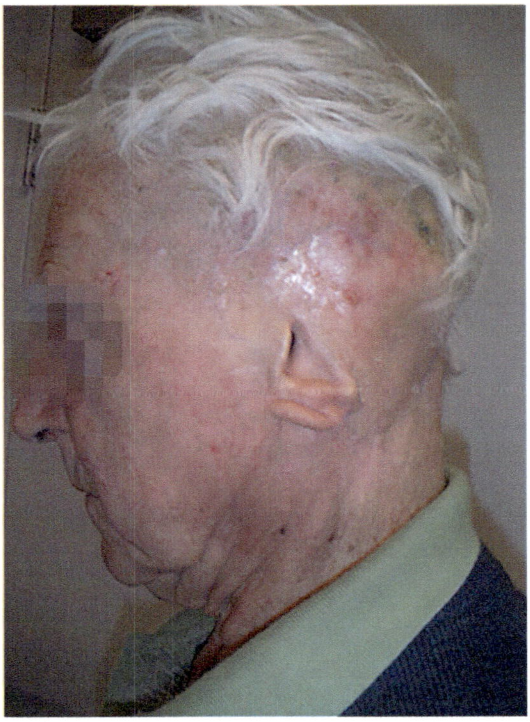

Fig. 2.643 The definitive outcome with a remnant of the patient's L ear for his spectacles

The PACES characteristics were all exemplified: pain-free, aesthetic, no vascular complications, economical in terms of time and sensory recovery with the resolution of oedema.

2.1.7.8 Case 69—A Scalp Rotation and Advancement with a Keystone Design and Grafting the Small Secondary Defect over the Fontanel (Figs. 2.644, 2.645, 2.646 and 2.647)

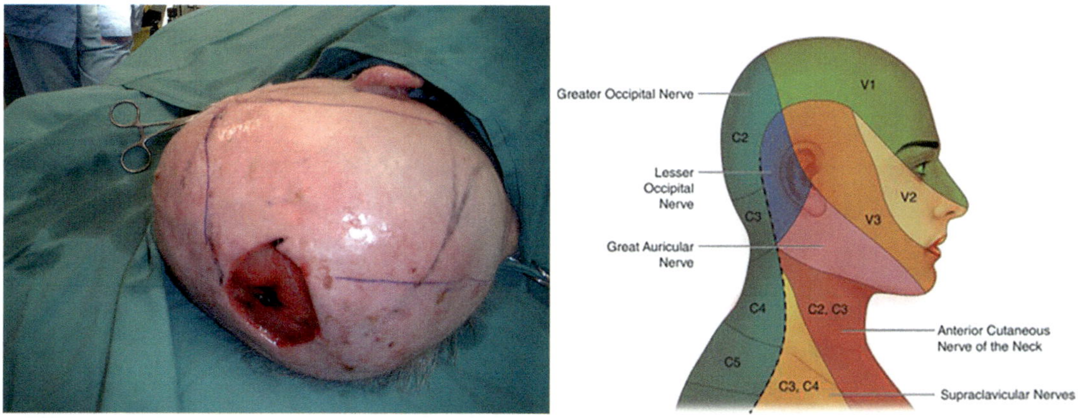

Fig. 2.644 The surgical defect and the mark out of the scalp flap are indicated thanks to occipital perforators. The dermatomal mark outs become the line of incision of the dermis and epidermis, ensuring that one-third deeply is attached with only partial undermining to facilitate the closure and vascular integrity of the defect. (Reprinted with permission from Atlas, *Reconstructive Technique in Melanoma Management* (p. 19), by Felix Behan, Springer Nature 2023)

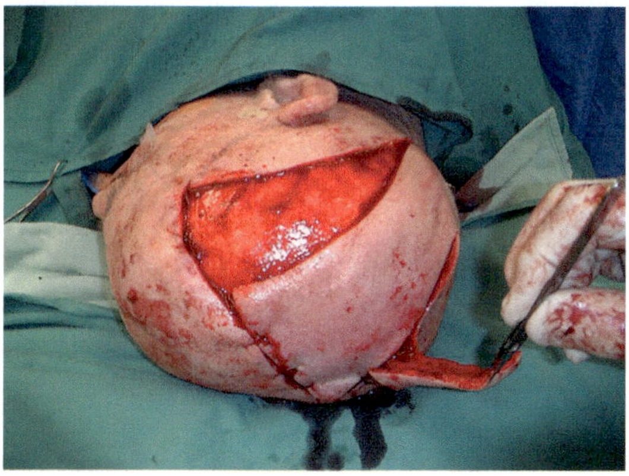

Fig. 2.645 Excising redundant tissue

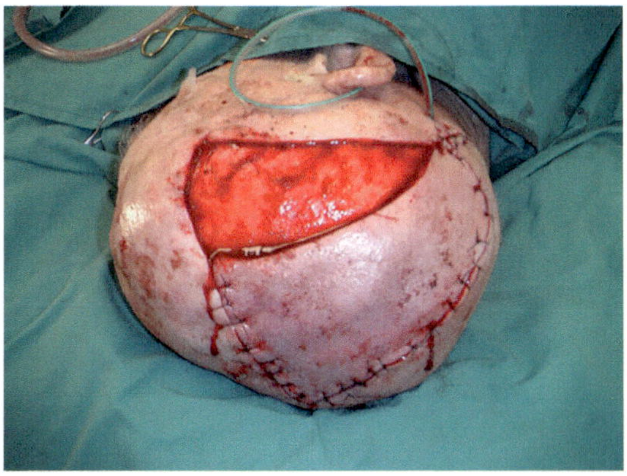

Fig. 2.646 Full dynamic perfusion when based on Keystone principles and the axis of rotation in the vicinity of the occipital vasculature

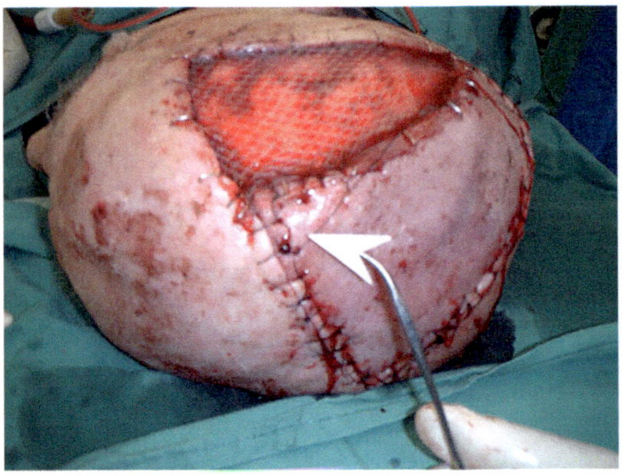

Fig. 2.647 Grafting the secondary defect to avoid tension

The PACES characteristics were all exemplified: pain-free, aesthetic, no vascular complications, economical in terms of time and sensory recovery with the resolution of oedema.

References

1. Haddad-Tame JL, et al. Reconstruction of the aesthetics units of the face with microsurgery: experience in five years. Microsurgery. 2000;20:211–5.
2. Gonzalez-Ulloa M. Restoration of the face covering by means of selected skin in regional aesthetic units. Br J Plast Surg. 1956;9:212–21.
3. Gonzalez-Ulloa M, Stevens E. Reconstruction of the nose and forehead by means of regional aesthetic units. Br J Plast Surg. 1960;13:305–9.
4. Gillies H, Millard D. The principles and art of plastic surgery. London: Butterworth; 1957.
5. Karapandzic M. Reconstruction of lip defects by local rotation arterial flaps. Br J Plast Surg. 1974;27:93–7.
6. Zimany A. The bi-lobed flap. Plast Reconstr Surg. 1953;11(6):424–34.
7. Dufourmentel C. Closure of limited loss of cutaneous substance. So-called 'LLL' diamond-shaped L rotation-flap. Ann Chir Plast. 1962;7:60–6.
8. Belt PJ, Emmett A. Local transposition flap repair of the pectoralis major myocutaneous flap donor site. Plast Reconstr Surg. 2004;114(3):732–7.
9. Barron J, Emmett A. Subcutaneous pedicle flaps. Br J Plast Surg. 1965;18:51–78.
10. Behan F. Atlas of keystone reconstructive technique in the management of melanoma. Springer Nature; 2024.
11. McGregor JC. A critical assessment of the biolbed flap. Br J Plast Surg. 1981;34:197–205.
12. Nordstrom RE, Devine JW. Scalp stretching with a tissue expander for closure of scalp defects. Plast Reconstr Surg. 1985;75:578–81.
13. Behan F, et al. Island flaps including the Bezier type in the treatment of malignant melanoma. Aust N Z J Surg. 1995;65(12):870–80.
14. Dufourmentel C. Stag-beetle flap. Sliding island flap with plasty in VY. Ann Chir Plast. 1970;15(4):344–7.
15. Behan F, et al. Oncologic clearance with preservation of reconstructive options: literature review and the 'delayed reconstruction after pathology evaluation (DRAPE)' technique. ANZ J Surg. 2012;82(11):780–5.
16. Wagh MS, Dixit V. Tissue expansion: concepts, techniques and unfavourable results. Indian J Plast Surg. 2013;46(2):333–48. https://doi.org/10.4103/0970-0358.118612.
17. Balch C. Modification of cross-lip flap. Plast Reconstr Surg. 1978;61(3):457–8.
18. Driscol BP, Baker SR. Reconstruction of nsasal alar defects. Arch Facial Plast Surg. 2001;3:91–9.
19. Burget GC, Menick FJ. Aesthetic reconstruction of the nose. St Louis: Mosby-Year Book; 1994.
20. Behan F. Surgical tips and skills illustrating the keystone principle. Sydney: Elsevier Textbook Churchill Livingstone; 2014.
21. Lee B, Bickel K, Levin S. Microsurgical reconstruction of extensive scalp defects. J Reconstr Microsurg. 1999;15:255–62.
22. Beasley N, et al. Scalp and forehead reconstruction using free revascularized tissue transfer. Arch Facial Plast Surg. 2004;6(1):16–20.
23. Lipa J, Butler C. Enhancing the outcome of free latissimus dorsi muscle flap reconstruction of scalp defects. Head Neck. 2003;26:46–53. https://doi.org/10.1002/hed.10338.
24. TerKonda RP, Sykes JM. Concepts in scalp and forehead reconstruction. Otolaryngol Clin North Am. 1997;30(4):519–39.

3 Complications and Final Insights on Keystone Flap Applications in Head and Neck Reconstruction

Contents

3.1 Clinical Case Studies and Surgical Outcomes in Head and Neck Keystone Flap Reconstruction

3.1.1 Adverse Outcomes Are Rare Complications of Keystone Flap Surgery

3.1.1.1 Hypertrophic Scarring Followed by Scar Revisional Surgery [1]

Hypertrophic scarring is a rare occurrence in Keystone reconstruction and reflects the nature of the physiology of the patient and his ethnic background (Maltese origin). This unusual case of hypertrophic scarring in a Keystone of the L neck along the line of the sternomastoid was the only case in this series featuring a large focus on head and neck reconstruction that experienced any scarring. A patient with this hypertrophic potential develops this complication only if they have this physiological tendency. According to simple observational conclusions on the pull of the sternomastoid, which is directly beneath the hypertrophic outline, this hypertrophy might reflect muscle activity in a person with a hypertrophic diathesis along the dermatomal mark out (Fig. 3.1).

3.1.1.2 Dermal Necrosis in an Island Flap

Often when the integument features mitotic development, which sometimes broaches the periosteum of the underlying tissue, this may have an antiangiogenesis factor in operation and may lead to superficial necrosis in any reconstructive flap, such as in this case, featuring

F. Behan, *Keystone Reconstructive Solutions for Major Surgical Defects*,
https://doi.org/10.1007/978-3-032-21716-5_3

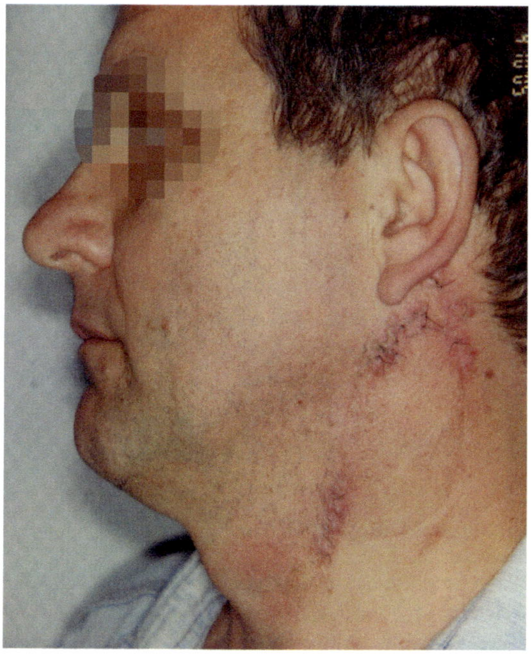

Fig. 3.1 A Keystone L neck level II melanoma is shown. Hypertrophic scarring may occur in a person with this potential. This delineation of a Keystone closure along the lines of the sternomastoid and hypertrophic scarring might reflect closure under tension, and the increase in vascularity and the hyperaemic effect, a characteristic of the Keystone, lead to this final, definitive outcome—a rare event in our Keystone series

an 88-year-old man with a superficial temporal artery island flap covering a desmoplastic melanoma in the midline of the forehead (Figs. 3.2, 3.3, 3.4, 3.5, 3.6 and 3.7).

3.1.2 Complications of Wound Healing

Melanoma of the forehead in a patient with chronic lymphatic leukeamia caused a delay in the angiogenesis factor of wound healing, which ultimately resolved (Figs. 3.8 and 3.9).

3.1.3 A Microsurgical Reconstructive Alternative for Parotid Defects

The unit's (Peter MacCallum Cancer Centre and Western Hospital) experience of the Keystone provides an acceptable alternative to the closure of defects in the vicinity of the parotid for melanoma and other mitotic lesions. The cases illustrated in this book reveal surgical outcomes where the PACES characteristics are quite evident. However, when Keystones are used to close a defect of the parotid and a recurrence occurs, we are obliged to use microsurgical repair because all the lax tissue employed in the initial Keystone units, the laxity of which the Keystone is dependent on, can be substituted only with a free flap microsurgical repair (Figs. 3.10, 3.11 and 3.12).

Free flaps with a microsurgical technique become an option depending on the experience of the operator, and this case illustrates some of those limitations in relation to aesthetic outcomes. The widespread use of free flaps in head and neck reconstruction by plastic surgeons and other surgeons has its place but often at an economic and aesthetic reconstructive cost. This is emphasised when the burden of deformity for patients with poor facial reconstructions is considered (Figs. 3.13, 3.14 and 3.15).

In summary, the psychological disturbance is always something to be considered by any oncological team working on major head and neck reconstructions. This must be part of the preoperative consultation on informed consent.

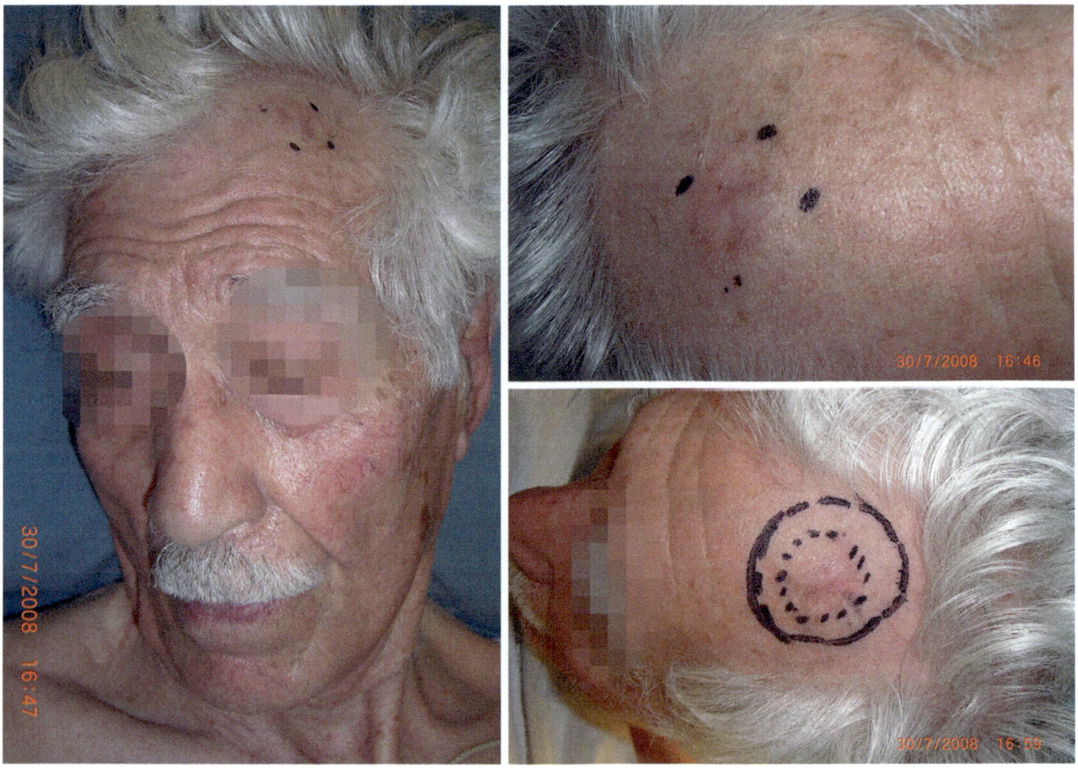

Fig. 3.2 Biopsy excision

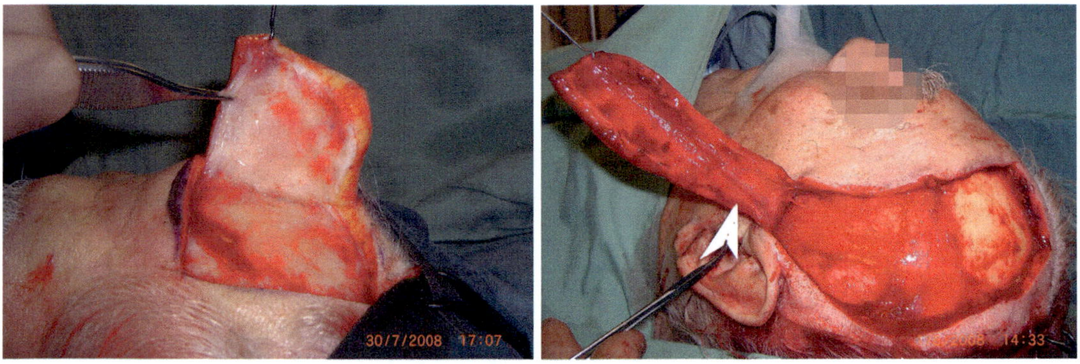

Fig. 3.3 Island flap on the superficial temporal artery (not skeletonised)

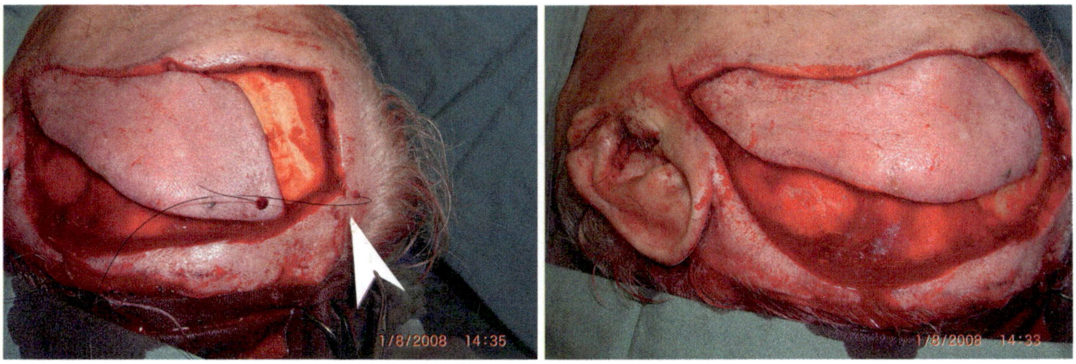

Fig. 3.4 Island flap on the superficial temporal artery (not skeletonised) is shown. Note the hyperaemia in the flap and the red dot sign—Keystone characteristics

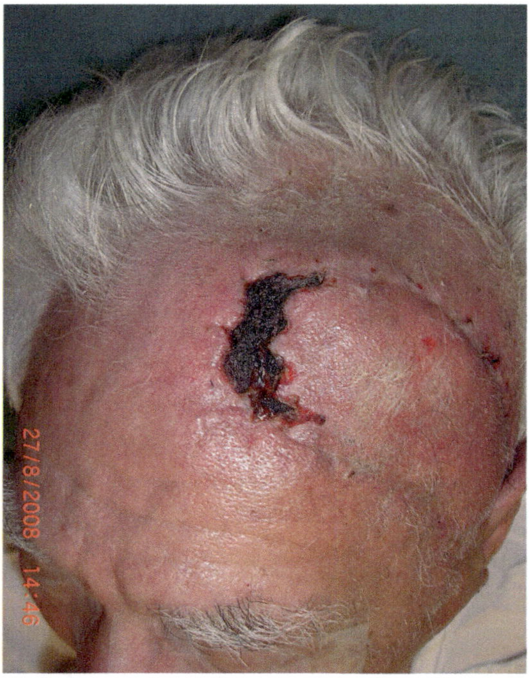

Fig. 3.5 Superficial distal necrosis in a viable flap is a rare finding, and it most likely confirms the manifestation of an underlying mitotic element and impedes angiogenesis and tissue healing as part of the underlying pathology

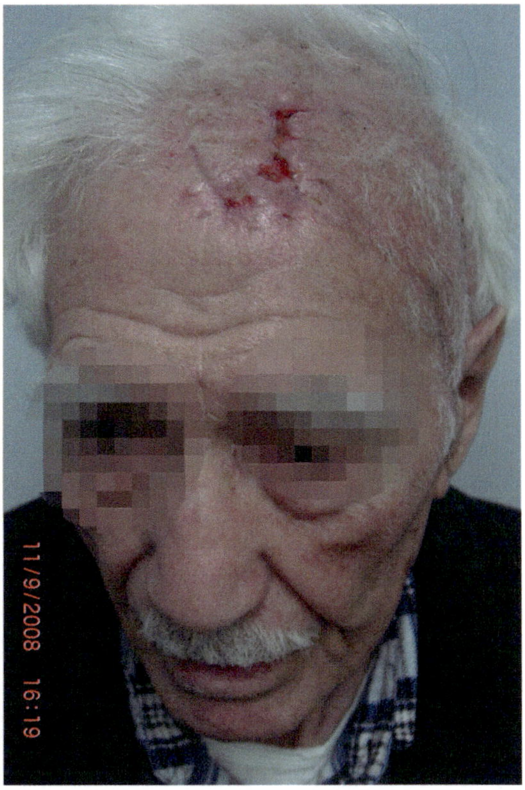

Fig. 3.6 After debridement and wound closure

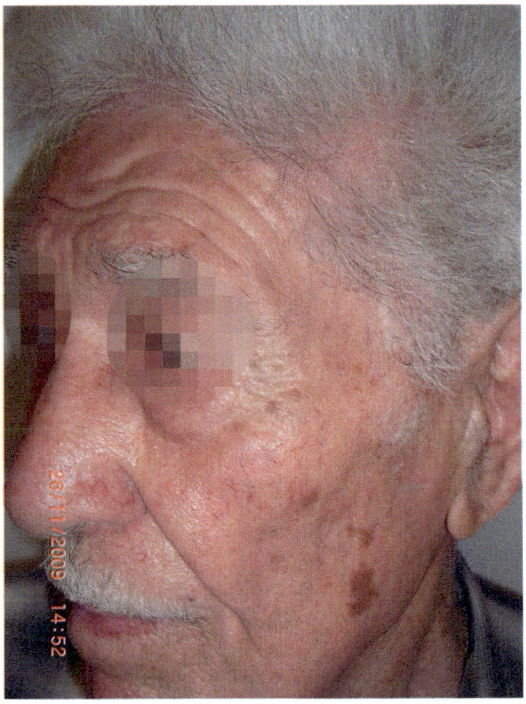

Fig. 3.7 The postoperative appearance—tumour-free interval at 18 months and no sign of integumentary recurrence

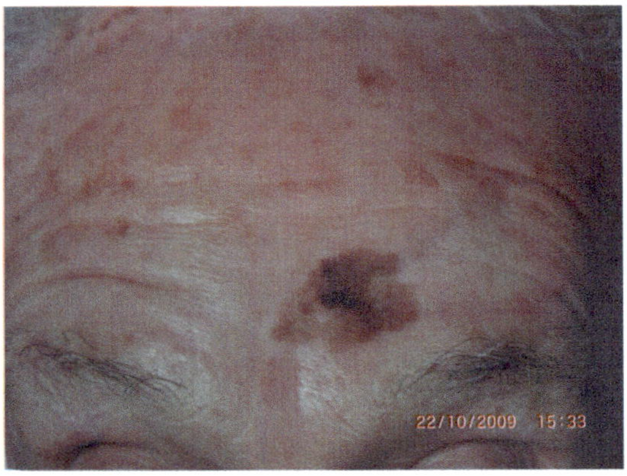

Fig. 3.8 The patient presents with a 3 × 3 cm lesion of the glabella and a Hutchinson melanotic freckle level I melanoma

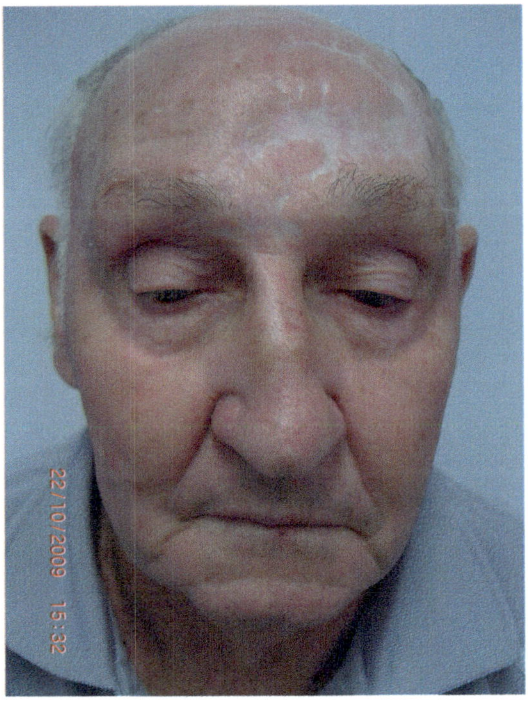

Fig. 3.9 Finally healed after reconstruction

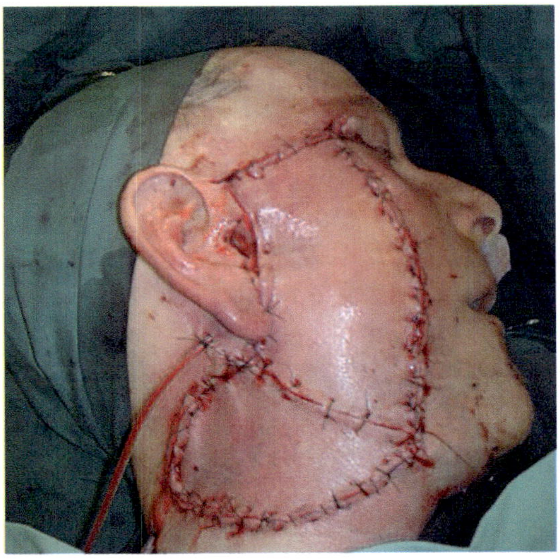

Fig. 3.10 Double Keystone repair for the initial preauricular problem over the parotid and closure

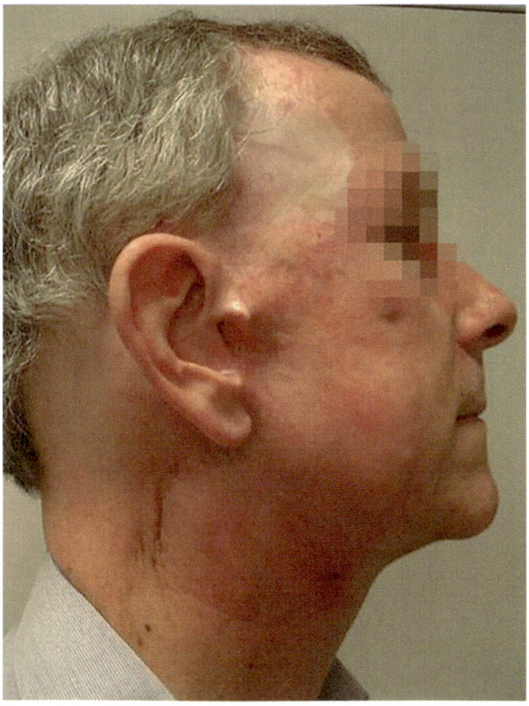

Fig. 3.11 Appearance at 5 months following external radiation therapy (XRT) and a tumour-free interval of 5 years, followed by recurrence needing a free flap reconstruction because the initial Keystone design took the laxity of tissue away, preventing repeat Keystone applications

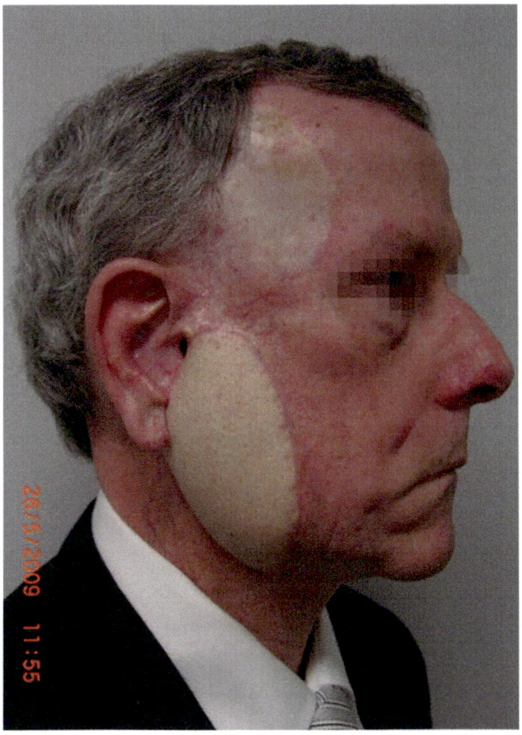

Fig. 3.12 Postoperative appearance with free flap following recurrence—the only reconstructive option available because of tissue tightness, which precludes the reuse of a Keystone

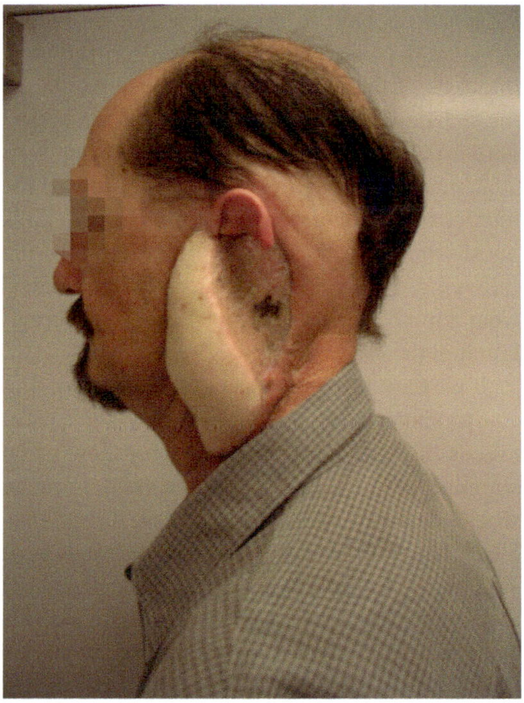

Fig. 3.13 This borrowed case from another unit with a free flap reconstruction helps to emphasise the poor aesthetic outcome for large parotid defects. In the parotid section, it makes valid comparisons with the Keystone closures for large melanoma defects over the parotid with or without subsequent radiation. This aesthetic deformity, lacking refinement, has created a psychological worry for the patient, so much so that he wears head gear to disguise the deformity when he goes out in public for social gatherings, shopping, etc.

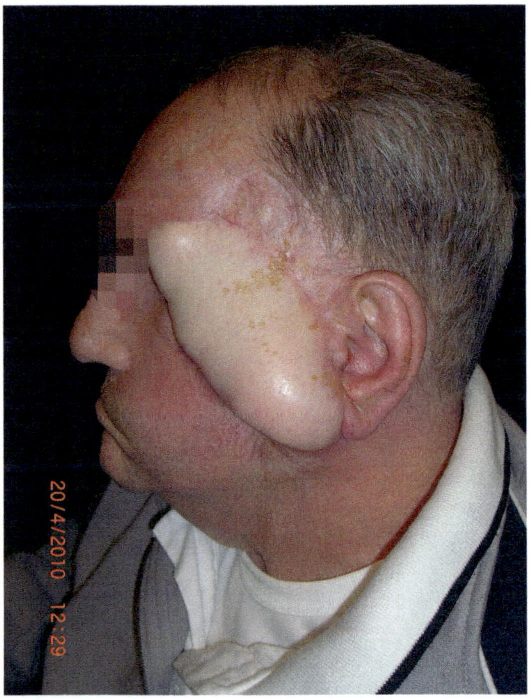

Fig. 3.14 A microsurgical alternative which needs no elaboration when one compares the PACES characteristics of the Keystone concept with this outcome, which is fairly standard

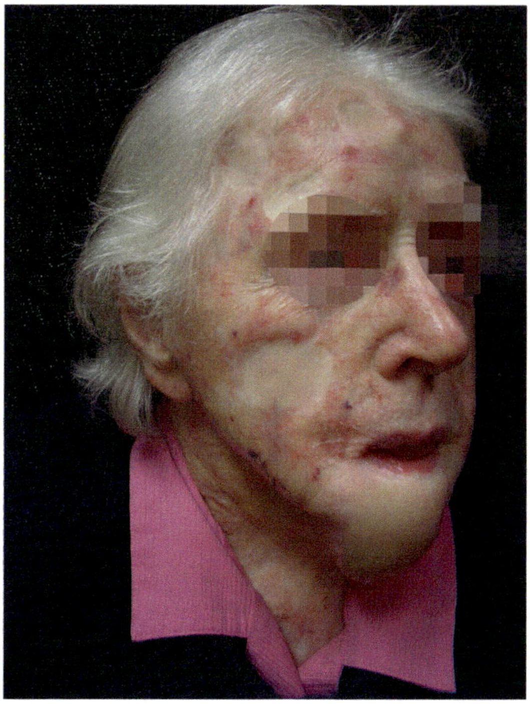

Fig. 3.15 This alternative method of lower lip reconstruction uses a microvascular technique, which makes for an interesting comparison with a similar defect in Case 36 using Keystone concepts. This could precipitate psychological changes when similarly treated patients become social outcasts

3.2 Strategic Insights and Future Perspectives on Keystone Flap Use in Head and Neck Surgery

After a career in reconstructive surgery of being somewhat adventurous, where rules are broken (les règles sont enfreintes) because of clinical necessity and where the closure of wounds under tension has become a necessity, certain clinical findings have emerged. **I would not be publishing such remarks if the complications were clinically adverse, preventing the repetition of the technique and forming a cloud over repeat performances.**

Every Keystone flap features a hypervascularity flare developing as it is designed within the dermatomal precincts, which is an aide-mémoire to the physician in charge or a guide to young surgeons on how to design a Keystone reconstructive flap. The mark out of the dermatome is the basis of the reconstruction, where the flap is incised only at the epidermal level and raised with a fascial support, leaving one-third of deep attachment. We have hypothetically surmised the red dot sign to be a sympathectomy effect that is not dissimilar to the pink foot that develops the following day in old vascular cases that underwent a lumbar sympathectomy to improve circulation in the lower limb.

If we have this sympathectomy effect, nothing else promotes healing like blood flow, and a natural conclusion from increasing blood flow is the stimulus of angiogenesis—a stepping stone in wound healing promoted under these restrictions. I have cases on hand of some Keystone reconstructions which have suffered complications, and only after some years did a retrospective analysis yield some inkling of why the Keystone failed.

I refer you to a referral case from Professor Michael Henderson in Volume II of cancer of the breast requiring a reconstructive closure which was simply organised by using the redundant tissue of the contralateral breast after the lumpectomy to close the wound. The vascular necrosis, a rare complication for Keystones, did eventuate, resulting in a second Keystone design to close the wound. Again, this second procedure suffered a similar outcome, and I said the following to my consultant associate who referred the reconstruction: "This does not happen with Keystones. Is there another explanation?" Next, 3 years later, when the explanation surfaced, the postradiation necrosis of the chest wall was revealed to have been the focal point for the development of the sarcoma, and it, belatedly, led me to the conclusion that the undiagnosed sarcoma may have been the hindrance or restriction preventing normal angiogenesis and Keystone healing. This patient subsequently had an omentum repair and a split skin graft to cover the wound and close the defect.

In other words, as William Osler said when he was a professor of medicine at Oxford University, observation is the basis of ongoing teaching. His other famous quote is that the patient always gets the diagnosis right. Thus, here, I have achieved a successful clinical outcome on the basis of observational findings, the basis of the vascular changes in the Keystone.

A recent publication has just been published, [2] titled 'Late Spontaneous Head and Neck Free Flap Failure'. It features a case of late spontaneous free flap failure and describes the clinical background of this concept with a literature review, where the complex interplay of radiotherapy, immunotherapy and chemotherapy are all discussed. This could be a sign of things to come.

Professor Andrew Sizeland's concluding remarks elaborate on the characteristics of the Keystone's PACES characteristics—pain-free, aesthetically matching, complications are rare, economical in terms of time and efficiency and sensory recovery in the integumentary flap with the resolution of oedema: The Keystone reconstruction in the head and neck is the most efficient available technique to repair large soft-tissue defects. Compared with alternatives, it takes less time (and therefore less anaesthetic time for the patient), results in less postoperative pain, avoids donor site morbidities and has a much shorter postoperative recovery period (and therefore a shorter hospital stay). It enables close collaboration between the surgeon undertaking the resection and the reconstructive surgeon, which maximises the chances of curing the disease and achieving the best cosmetic and functional outcome for the patient. The use of tissue adjacent to the defect results in a vastly superior cosmetic result, and function returns quickly (sensation recovers, and the tissues are supple and mobile). Complications are rare, and if they occur, they occur early. The Keystone has been successfully used to repair heavily irradiated tissue. It has had no late complications. Given our extensive experience of the Keystone flap repairing parotid defects, scalp defects, the loss of the entire lip and given the outstanding functional and cosmetic results, it has been our repair technique of first choice for several years for thousands of cases.

References

1. Amadeu T, et al. Vascularization pattern in hypertrophic scars and keloids: a stereological analysis. Pathol Res Pract. 2003;199(7):469–73.
2. Ferdinands T, et al. Late spontaneous head and neck free flap failure: a case report. Australas J Plast Surg. 2025;8(2):132352.

GPSR Compliance

The European Union's (EU) General Product Safety Regulation (GPSR) is a set of rules that requires consumer products to be safe and our obligations to ensure this.

If you have any concerns about our products, you can contact us on ProductSafety@springernature.com

In case Publisher is established outside the EU, the EU authorized representative is:

Springer Nature Customer Service Center GmbH
Europaplatz 3
69115 Heidelberg, Germany

Batch number: 10731385

Printed by Printforce, the Netherlands